ALZHEIMER'S DISEASE: ABSTRACTS OF THE PSYCHOLOGICAL AND BEHAVIORAL LITERATURE

Paul T. Costa, Jr.
James R. Whitfield
Donna Stewart
Editors

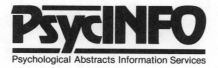

Psychological Abstracts Information Services

Bibliographies in Psychology No. 4

American Psychological Association

Library of Congress Cataloging-in-Publication Data

Alzheimer's disease: abstracts of the psychological and behavioral
        literature / Paul T. Costa, Jr., James R. Whitfield, Donna Stewart, editors.

p. cm--(Bibliographies in psychology; no. 4)
        Includes bibliographies and index.
        1. Alzheimer's disease--Abstracts
I. Costa, Paul T. II. Whitfield, James R. III. Stewart, Donna IV. Series.
[DNLM: 1. Alzheimer's Disease--abstracts.   ZWM 220 A47
RC523.A375 1989   616.8'3--dc19   89-360
ISBN: 1-55798-049-7

Published by the
American Psychological Association
1200 Seventeenth Street, N.W.
Washington, DC 20036

Copies may be ordered from:
Order Department
P.O. Box 2710
Hyattsville, MD 20784
Item No. 4900040

Printed in the United States of America

Acknowledgments

We gratefully acknowledge the assistance of the following persons: Alain Dessaint for guiding its publication, Maurine Jackson for attending to modifications of the programming and photocomposition specifications, Karen Monroe for modifying computer programs to structure the output of the data, Jody Kerby for the classification and proofreading of the records, Barbara McLean for assistance in the development of the ad hoc classification scheme and editorial processes, and Brenda Evans for desktop publishing parts of this book.

TABLE OF CONTENTS

An Overview of Recent Relevant Psychological and Behavioral Research on
Alzheimer's Disease: A Foreword

Originally described over 80 years ago by the German physician Alois Alzheimer, senile dementia of the Alzheimer's type (SDAT) or Alzheimer's disease (AD) is a progressive degenerative disorder, characterized by memory loss and a variety of cognitive disabilities. AD is one of more than 75 disorders within the syndrome of dementia.

Age is one of the few reliable risk factors for AD. While AD can occur at ages from 40 upwards, advancing age brings increased incidence. AD has its highest rates in the 85 and over age group, the population group that is also the fastest growing sub-group of the population.

As a syndrome of a group of clinical syndromes, dementia involves intellectual declines and impairments in memory, other cognitive abilities, and adaptive behavior. Dementia can be caused by numerous pathological processes that affect the brain. Dementia states may be classified as reversible and irreversible. Clinical states of dementia that are produced, for example by intoxications, infection, metabolic and nutritional disorders, vascular conditions, space-occupying lesions, or affective disorders are potentially arrestable or reversible causes of dementia. By comparison, Alzheimer's dementia, classified as a primary degenerative dementia, is considered to be an irreversible disease primary to the brain.

Even though AD is viewed as irreversible, it is not thought to be a fundamental part of normal human aging. The separation of disease processes that are age-associated from the universal processes of aging is one of the most important challenges in this area. Cognitive aging involves different patterns and rates of change that depend upon the type of mental ability under consideration. The declines that occur with normal aging after the sixth or seventh decade of life are, for the most part, modest and gradual.

Only about 10% of the elderly population show clinically significant cognitive deficits. The prevalence estimates for AD are even smaller: Only about 5-6% of the population over 65 is estimated to be affected by this neurological disease. Nevertheless, this means that between 2.5 and 3 million people have AD in some stages. AD is the most prevalent cause of cognitive disorder in later life.

Estimated costs for AD alone, including nursing home care, is currently about $38 billion per year. More than 50% of nursing home residents are thought to have some form of mental impairment, and a significant number of these have AD.

Observations on AD-Related Behavioral Research

Partly in response to these urgent concerns, APA's PsycINFO has assembled this bibliography on AD from the psychological and behavioral literature. These 1334 articles were drawn from over 1300 journals covered in the PsycINFO databases.

The bibliography classifies abstracts into four domains: (1) Etiology and Neuropathological Aspects; (2) Epidemiology and Diagnosis, including clinical, cognitive, and neuropsychological/behavioral and physiological aspects; (3) General Issues and Research; and (4) Treatment and Counseling.

The number and dates of abstracts published reveals that there has been a veritable explosion of research publication in the last 6 years. Fewer than 100 abstracts were found in the period from 1974 to 1982. By contrast, more than 1200 abstracts were found from 1983 to the present.

As Section One (403 abstracts) of this bibliography shows, there is considerable interest in genetic factors and hereditary contributions to AD, particularly in its association with Down's syndrome. Although few reliable risk factors have been identified, proposed risks have included exposure to aluminum, slow virus, thyroid disease, and head trauma.

Research on the etiology and neuropathology of this dementing disorder covers a broad range of topics in the neurobiology of aging, including basic neuronal changes in circuits, intracellular systems, proteins, and genes. In addition to the hallmark pathological lesions of AD (neuritic plaques and neurofibrillary tangles), research interest has also centered on cyclic AMP, viruses, somatostatin deficits, changes in neurotransmitters and receptors (particularly the cholinergic system), and neurotropic factors and modulators.

The Second Section (Epidemiology and Diagnosis) includes 492 abstracts. This underscores the importance attached to improving screening and differential diagnosis. Estimates are that 10% to 20% of persons 65 and older, identified as having intellectual impairment (which, as noted earlier, is a little over 10% of the elderly population), may have reversible brain disorders that are amenable to treatment. What makes diagnosis so difficult is that cognitive deterioration in the early stages of AD consists mainly of an exaggeration of the cognitive declines associated with normal aging. Repeated testing and evaluation are critical for accurate detection and diagnosis.

As might be expected, a relatively large number of studies are found that deal with the investigation of intellectual and cognitive performance characterizing AD patients. Subjects of investigation have included memory deficits in both short and long term memory, and in prose, non-verbal, spatial, and tactile memory. There are also many useful articles reported here that examine other cognitive and psychological processes, including language and communicative behavior, memory loss, sleep deprivation, and coping. Surprisingly, there are as yet only a few studies examining the relationship between personality and AD.

In future bibliographies or updates of the present one, we anticipate increased research emphases on behavioral, clinical, and psychometric descriptions of the clinical phases and stages of AD. Specifically, more studies on neuropsychological screening for AD, biological and chemical markers of AD, and neuroimaging tests such as PET and NMR are suggested by current research cited in this bibliography.

Section Three (General Issues and Research) contains 35 articles on the history, diagnostic nosology, and legal aspects of the disorder as well as other topics of broad interest.

Section Four covers treatment and counseling, and it includes 258 abstracts. A preponderance of abstracts involve drug studies. Interestingly, there are more reviews in this section than in any of the others. Lecithin, physostigmine and other cholinergic drugs have been popular agents under study, but the abstracts reveal a wide variety of other agents that have been studied, including opiate antagonists, neuroleptics, muscarinic and dopaminergic drugs and MAO inhibitors.

Also documented in this section is the growing recognition and importance of the role of caregivers and family processes in AD. AD not only affects its primary victims, but it also has widespread impact on family members. The burdens and stress of caregivers form a separate stream of research. Issues of social support, both formal and informal, along with social policy in the arena of long-term care, are important topics for future research.

The last part of the bibliography includes 146 citations to the most recent journal literature received by PsycINFO through December 1988. As it is not yet fully abstracted and indexed, it is not formally in the publicly available PsycINFO system. Nonetheless, we are able to include the basic citations here.

Keeping Informed: Updating This Bibliography

Keeping up with the literature on AD is a matter of concern to psychologists, behavioral scientists, and medical professionals. A major, but sometimes overlooked, tool for staying abreast of developments and research is *Psychological Abstracts* and its electronic counterparts, PsycINFO online and PsycLIT on CD-ROM Disc.

The search strategy employed to retrieve references for this bibliography is described in the Appendix. The search strategy can be repeated again by readers who wish to update this bibliography with the very latest references on PsycALERT (which makes available citations and indexing within weeks of an article's publication) or PsycINFO (when complete abstracting and indexing are desired). The strategy can also serve as a model for conducting bibliographic research on other topics.

Paul T. Costa, Jr., Ph.D.
    Chief, Laboratory of Personality and Cognition, Gerontology
        Research Center, National Institute on Aging, Francis Scott Key Medical Center, Baltimore, MD
Gary R. VandenBos, Ph.D.
    Executive Director, Office of Publications and Communications, APA
Lois W. Granick
    Director, PsycINFO, APA

Section I. Selected References to Journal Articles and Dissertations on Alzheimer's Disease

This section contains a selective bibliography of annotated references from the journal literature and citations of the dissertation literature on Alzheimer's disease. Entries are organized alphabetically by author within 9 categories.

ETIOLOGY & NEUROPATHOLOGICAL/ NEUROCHEMICAL ASPECTS

1. Adolfsson, Rolf; Gottfries, C. G.; Roos, B. E. & Winblad, Bengt. (1979). **Changes in the brain catecholamines in patients with dementia of Alzheimer type.** *British Journal of Psychiatry,* 135, 216–223.
Brain monoamine concentrations were determined postmortem in 19 patients with dementia of Alzheimer type. Samples were taken from 10 parts of the brain and compared with an age-matched control group. There were lower mean concentrations of dopamine in the demented group of patients in 7 regions of the brain, and 2 of these were at a significant level. There were also significantly lower concentrations of homovanillic acid in the nucleus caudatus and in the putamen. The means of the concentrations of noradrenaline were also lower, and in the putamen and the cortex gyrus frontalis significant differences were observed. The 5-hydroxytryptamine concentrations were slightly lower in the demented group, but the differences did not reach significance. The degree of intellectual deterioration was negatively correlated with the noradrenaline concentrations in the hypothalamus and the cortex gyrus cinguli. (54 ref).

2. Ahlberg, J.; Blomstrand, C.; Ronquist, G. & Wikkelsö, Carsten. (1985). **Dementia—and adenylate kinase activity in cerebrospinal fluid.** *Acta Neurologica Scandinavica,* 72(5), 525–527.
When 22–82 yr old patients admitted for dementia and/or normal pressure hydrocephalus (NPH) were evaluated for adenylate kinase activity in cerebrospinal fluid (CSF), no differences could be found between the 16 Ss diagnosed as having NPH, the 15 Ss suffering from multi-infarct dementia, and the 11 Ss with dementia of the Alzheimer type. (13 ref).

3. Alfrey, Allen C. (1986). **Systemic toxicity of aluminum in man.** Special Issue: Controversial topics on Alzheimer's disease: Intersecting crossroads. *Neurobiology of Aging,* 7(6), 543–545.
Responds to D. R. Crapper McLachlan (1986), by asserting that although systematic aluminum (AL) has clearly been shown to be toxic in humans, the evidence for a role in the pathogenesis of Alzheimer's disease (AD) is lacking. Given the relatively small concentrations of AL found in AD brains, and the clinical and anatomical dissimilarities between AD patients and other maladies with an established AL relationship, it seems unlikely that AL plays an important role in the pathogenesis of AD. More likely, the increased AL reported in AD brains is a result of damage associated with the disease and not a cause.

4. Allsop, David; Kidd, Michael; Landon, Michael & Tomlinson, Annette. (1986). **Isolated senile plaque cores in Alzheimer's disease and Down's syndrome show differences in morphology.** *Journal of Neurology, Neurosurgery & Psychiatry,* 49(8), 886–892.
Frontal and temporal cortical tissue from the brains of elderly cases of Down's syndrome was used to make preparations of neuronal cell bodies containing senile plaque cores. Polarization microscopy revealed normal classical plaque cores and also a high proportion of unusual amorphous plaque cores not seen in Alzheimer's disease. The 2 forms were easily distinguished by electron microscopy. It is suggested that late Down's syndrome may not be an exact model for Alzheimer's disease.

5. Anderton, B. A. (1986). **The origin of the structural proteins found in plaques and tangles.** Special Issue: Controversial topics on Alzheimer's disease: Intersecting crossroads. *Neurobiology of Aging,* 7(6), 443–444.
Responds to D. J. Selkoe's (1986) article by emphasizing that careful biochemical analysis is still required to establish the complete chemical composition of tangles and amyloid typical of Alzheimer's disease pathology. It is argued that although evidence implicates the cytoskeleton in paired helical filaments composition, the precise cytoskeletal components that are involved are still far from being defined.

6. Anderton, Brian H. (1987). **Progress in molecular pathology.** *Nature,* 325(6106), 658–659.
Discusses the relationship between the A4 component of the core of extracellular plaque and the paired helical filament proteins found in neurofibrillary tangles, both of which are found in patients with senile dementia of the Alzheimer type. It is suggested that the posttranslational changes that produce A4 from its precursor are similar to those that affect the cytoskeleton of paired helical filaments.

7. Anderton, Brian H. et al. (1982). **Monoclonal antibodies show that neurofibrillary tangles and neurofilaments share antigenic determinants.** *Nature,* 298(5869), 84–86.
Neurofibrillary tangles are a prominent feature in the pyramidal cells of the hippocampus and in neurons of the cerebral cortex of senile dementia patients with Alzheimer's disease. Similar neuronal changes also occur in elderly Down's syndrome patients and to a lesser degree in intellectually normal people. Postmortem samples were collected from 1 normal and 1 Down's syndrome S and from 3 cases of senile dementia. Monoclonal antibodies demonstrated that neurofilament antigens are present in neurofibrillary tangles. (22 ref).

8. Anderton, Brian & Miller, Chris. (1986). **Proteins in a twist: Are neurofibrillary tangles and amyloid in Alzheimer's disease composed of the same protein?** *Trends in Neurosciences,* 9(8), 337–338.
Discusses research findings with regard to the pathogenesis of neurodegeneration and theories concerning the pathogenesis of tangles and plaques. The possibility of a candidate for a protein component of Alzheimer amyloid is discussed.

9. Ansari, Khurshed A. (1986). **Olfactory mucosa, aluminosilicates and Alzheimer's disease.** Special Issue: Controversial topics on Alzheimer's disease: Intersecting crossroads. *Neurobiology of Aging,* 7(6), 575–576.
Comments on the hypothesis by E. Roberts (1986), by noting that age-related degenerative changes in mucosal epithelium may result in decreased barrier function. This change may predispose the adjacent brain areas to invasion by organisms and toxins leading to regional tissue damage as seen in Alzheimer's disease (AD). Age-related decrease in nasal mucosal barrier function, however, would explain some but not all the pathologic changes associated with AD.

1

10. Appel, Stanley H. & McManaman, James L. (1986). **Is a breakdown of the blood-brain barrier cause or effect?** Special Issue: Controversial topics on Alzheimer's disease: Intersecting crossroads. *Neurobiology of Aging,* 7(6), 512–514.
Proposes several alternative explanations for the pathogenesis of Alzheimer's disease (AD) proposed by J. A. Hardy et al (1986). The present authors question the explanation concerning the amyloid deposition and alterations in the blood brain barrier in AD. They suggest instead a process involving formation of neuritic plaques that increasingly engulf presynaptic and postsynaptic neuronal constituents as well as surrounding glia. Such a process could then result in degeneration of the projecting cells and impairment of cognitive function characteristic of AD.

11. Arai, Heii; Moroji, Takashi; Kosaka, Kenji & Iizuka, Reiji. (1986). **Extrahypophyseal distribution of α-melanocyte stimulating hormone (α-MSH)-like immunoreactivity in postmortem brains from normal subjects and Alzheimer-type dementia patients.** *Brain Research,* 377(2), 305–310.
Using a sensitive double-antibody, solid-phase enzyme immunoassay method, alpha-MSH-like immunoreactivity (AMSHLI) was measured in 21 regions of postmortem brains from 8 normal Ss and 5 patients with Alzheimer-type dementia. In the brains from the normal Ss, the highest concentration of AMSHLI was found in the hypothalamus. In the Alzheimer brains, although the temporal cortex and hippocampus had normal concentrations of AMSHLI, the cingulate cortex, caudate, and substantia nigra showed significantly lower concentrations of AMSHLI than those of the control brains.

12. Arai, Heii et al. (1984). **A preliminary study of free amino acids in the postmortem temporal cortex from Alzheimer-type dementia patients.** *Neurobiology of Aging,* 5(4), 319–321.
Measured concentrations of free amino acids in the temporal cortex of postmortem brains from 4 histologically verified cases (aged 45–84 yrs at death) with Alzheimer-type dementia (ATD) and 8 age-matched histologically normal controls. The concentrations of taurine, glutamate, and GABA, which are all neurotransmitter candidates, were significantly lower in the ATD brains than in the controls. Findings suggest that the involvement of amino acid neurons in ATD cannot be ruled out. (17 ref).

13. Arai, Heii et al. (1985). **Free amino acids in postmortem cerebral cortices from patients with Alzheimer-type dementia.** *Neuroscience Research,* 2(6), 486–490.
Investigated concentrations of free amino acids in the cerebral cortices of postmortem brains from 5 histologically verified cases (mean age at death 61.6 yrs) of Alzheimer-type dementia (ATD) and 8 histologically normal controls (mean age at death 69.6 yrs). Concentration of glutamate in the ATD brains was significantly lower in the superior frontal, orbital, and cingulate and in the inferior temporal cortices when compared with the control brains. Concentrations of taurine and gamma-aminobutyric acid (GABA) in the ATD brains were significantly lower in the inferior temporal cortex. Findings suggest that amino acid neurons could be involved in ATD. (21 ref).

14. Baker, H. & Margolis, F. L. (1986). **Deafferentation-induced alterations in olfactory bulb as a model for the etiology of Alzheimers disease.** Special Issue: Controversial topics on Alzheimer's disease: Intersecting crossroads. *Neurobiology of Aging,* 7(6), 568–569.
In response to E. Roberts's (1986) hypothesis, the present author notes that the ability of exogenous agents to enter the brain by way of the olfactory nerve coupled with the early anatomical and behavioral pathology observed in patients has led to the hypothesis that Alzheimer's disease may be of environmental etiology. Studies of the influence of peripheral olfactory deafferentation on the expression of olfactory bulb neuron phenotype suggest that this approach may be a useful model in which to explore the validity of the hypothesis.

15. Ball, M. J. (1987). **Pathological similarities between Alzheimer's disease and Down's syndrome: Is there a genetic link?** *Integrative Psychiatry,* 5(3), 159–163.
Discusses 3 aspects of the similarity in the brains of patients with Alzheimer's disease and Down's syndrome. The aspects of the relationship discussed include the histological parallels between the central nervous system (CNS) lesions found in the 2 diseases; the apparent lack of concordance between the existence of dementia in some cases of Down's syndrome and the near categorical presence of Alzheimer-type lesions in Down's syndrome cases aged 40+ yrs; and clinical evidence that certain families may share a genetic propensity for the 2 disorders. It is suggested that research efforts such as gene linkage analyses and chromosome mapping in appropriate pedigrees may shed light on the functioning of Chromosome 21 and the pathogenesis of both diseases.

16. Ball, Melvyn J. (1986). **Herpesvirus in the hippocampus as a cause of Alzheimer's disease.** *Archives of Neurology,* 43(4), 313.
Discusses recent findings with regard to the storage of memories by the hippocampal formation and contends that repeated reactivation of herpes virus from the trigeminal ganglia may represent an etiological infrastructure for the clinical syndrome of Alzheimer's dementia.

17. Barbaccia, Maria L.; Costa, Erminio; Ferrero, Patrizia; Guidotti, Alessandro et al. (1986). **Diazepam-binding inhibitor: A brain neuropeptide present in human spinal fluid: Studies in depression, schizophrenia, and Alzheimer's disease.** *Archives of General Psychiatry,* 43(12), 1143–1147.
Investigated differences in the cerebrospinal fluid (CSF) content of diazepam-binding inhibitor (DBI) immunoreactivity in patients with neuropsychiatric disorders. Study 1 involved 21 depressed Ss (mean age 37.4 yrs) and 28 controls (mean age 28.9 yrs); Study 2 involved 6 Ss with Alzheimer's disease (mean age 60.2 yrs), 8 depressed Ss (mean age 62.1 yrs), and 7 controls (mean age 65 yrs); Study 3 involved 15 schizophrenics (mean age 29.6 yrs) and 27 controls (mean age 29.2 yrs). Results show that Ss with major depression had significantly higher concentrations of DBI immunoreactivity in the CSF than did the controls. Findings suggest a functional disinhibition of GABAergic neurotransmission associated with depression. (21 ref).

18. Barclay, Laurie L. (1986). **Genetics in Alzheimer's disease: Methodological problems, research strategies, and practical applications.** Special Issue: Controversial topics on Alzheimer's disease: Intersecting crossroads. *Neurobiology of Aging,* 7(6), 479–480.
Refers to P. Davies's (1986) article and suggests that pedigree analysis in Alzheimer's disease (AD) requires well-defined diagnostic criteria and verification of family history. Before generalizations concerning genetic transmission in AD can be extrapolated from early onset, autosomal dominant cases to all subgroups, clinical, pathological, and neurochemical comparisons between groups must be completed. Differences in presentation may reflect genetic heterogeneity or interaction of genetic and environmental factors. Genetic markers may identify Ss at risk for AD which would facilitate counseling, therapy, or even prophylaxis.

19. Barclay, Laurie L.; Zemcov, Alexander; Blass, John P. & McDowell, Fletcher H. (1984). **Rates of decrease of cerebral blood flow in progressive dementias.** *Neurology,* 34(12), 155–1560.
Studied ^{133}Xe washout at 2 or 3 different times in 23 demented patients (aged 56–83 yrs) to determine whether cere-

bral blood flow (CBF) progressively decreases as dementia progresses. All 15 Ss with Alzheimer's and 5 of 8 Ss with vascular dementias had more rapid declines of CBF than did 30 nondemented age-matched controls. Mean rate of change in Alzheimer's disease was -.60 per month, compared with +.29 per month in 4 controls tested twice. Regression analysis of CBF with age in 30 controls tested once showed a decline of CBF with aging at a rate of -.013 per month. The rates of CBF decline in dementia were significantly correlated with rates of change of behavioral score measuring functional impairment. It is concluded that the accelerated decrease of CBF in patients with progressive dementia may be a more sensitive indicator of abnormality than single measurements of CBF. CBF should corroborate the diagnosis of organic dementia when there is doubt about organic and functional elements. (14 ref).

20. Barnes, Deborah M. (1987). **Defect of Alzheimer's is on chromosome 21.** *Science,* 235(4791), 846–847.
Presents data suggesting that one or more genes causing familial Alzheimer's dementia (AD) are located on the same region of chromosome 21; one of the genes in this region produces the beta amyloid protein that forms the core of neuritic plaques in AD and aged Down's syndrome brains.

21. Bartus, Raymond T.; Dean, Reginald L.; Pontecorvo, Michael J. & Flicker, Charles. (1985). **The cholinergic hypothesis: A historical overview, current perspective, and future directions.** *Annals of the New York Academy of Sciences,* 444, 332–358.
The authors discuss the cholinergic hypothesis of geriatric memory dysfunction, which proposes the following: (1) Significant, functional disturbances in cholinergic activity occur in the brains of aged and especially demented patients; (2) these disturbances play an important role in memory loss and related cognitive problems associated with old age and dementia; and (3) proper enhancement or restoration of cholinergic function may significantly reduce the severity of the cognitive loss. The initial empirical foundation for the cholinergic hypothesis can be traced to at least 4 distinct areas of study: biochemical determinations of human brain tissue, particularly from Alzheimer's patients; animal psychopharmacological studies; clinical pharmacological observations; and basic neuroscience research. The current status of treatment approaches with cholinomimetic agents is that there is hope for future drug development, but there is no immediate promise of effective therapeutic intervention. Future directions for research include the development of characteristic-specific cholinergic agents and reliable animal models of primary symptoms. (177 ref).

22. Bauer, Anne M. & Shea, Thomas M. (1986). **Alzheimer's disease and Down syndrome: A review and implications for adult services.** *Education & Training of the Mentally Retarded,* 21(2), 144–150.
Reviews the literature on Alzheimer's disease (AD) and Down's syndrome (DS), noting that neurological changes associated with AD have been consistently documented in individuals with DS 35 yrs of age or older. A genetic relationship has been suggested between DS and AD. The diagnosis of AD and its progressive behavioral impact on persons with DS are discussed. Implications and suggestions for care and service provision for adults with DS are presented, including maintaining skills as long as possible, adjusting communication to the individual's needs, and responding to the behaviors indigenous to AD in practical ways. (32 ref).

23. Beal, M. Flint et al. (1985). **Reduced numbers of somatostatin receptors in the cerebral cortex in Alzheimer's disease.** *Science,* 229(4710), 289–291.

Measured somatostatin receptor concentrations (SRCs) in 12 Alzheimer's disease patients (aged 72–90 yrs) and in 13 controls (aged 36–86 yrs). Results indicate that, in the frontal cortex (Brodmann areas 6, 9, and 10) and temporal cortex (Brodmann area 21), the Alzheimer SRCs were reduced to approximately 50% of control values, and a 40% reduction was seen in the hippocampus. Somatostatinlike immunoreactivity was significantly reduced in both the frontal and temporal cortex and was linearly related to somatostatin-receptor binding in the cortices of Alzheimer's patients.

24. Beal, M. Flint; Benoit, Robert; Mazurek, Michael F.; Bird, Edward D. et al. (1986). **Somatostatin-28$_{1-12}$-like immunoreactivity is reduced in Alzheimer's disease cerebral cortex.** *Brain Research,* 368(2), 380–383.
Measured concentrations of somatostatin-28$_{1-12}$-like immunoreactivity in 8 cortical regions from 12 patients (aged 62–90 yrs) with Alzheimer's disease (AD) and 13 controls (aged 36–86 yrs). Significant reductions were found in all cortical regions examined, with the largest decrease in temporal lobe, and they were significantly correlated with decreases in somatostatin-14-like immunoreactivity in the same regions. The similar reductions of 2 prosomatostatin-derived peptides in AD cerebral cortex supports the contention that decreased somatostatin immunoreactivity in AD is caused by a degeneration of somatostatin cortical neurons and terminals.

25. Beal, M. Flint; Growdon, John H.; Mazurek, Michael F. & Martin, Joseph B. (1986). **CSF somatostatin-like immunoreactivity in dementia.** *Neurology,* 36(2), 294–297.
Examined cerebrospinal fluid (CSF) concentrations of somatostatinlike immunoreactivity (SLI) in 40 55–78 yr old patients with Alzheimer's disease (AD), 5 patients with multiinfarct dementia, 12 Ss with normal pressure hydrocephalus, 6 patients with Parkinson's disease, and 12 patients with Huntington's disease. Results show that SLI concentrations were reduced in AD and multi-infarct dementia, suggesting that reduced SLI content in AD cerebral cortex is reflected in CSF. However, changes in CSF SLI had no diagnostic specificity. (28 ref).

26. Beal, M. Flint & Growdon, John H. (1986). **CSF neurotransmitter markers in Alzheimer's disease.** *Progress in Neuro-Psychopharmacology & Biological Psychiatry,* 10(3–5), 259–270.
A review of the literature indicates that cerebrospinal fluid (CSF) neurotransmitter markers may reflect neurochemical alterations in Alzheimer's disease (AD). Studies concerning CSF acetylcholine markers, monoamines, amino acids, neuropeptides, somatostatin, and vasopressin in AD are reviewed. It is concluded that although no individual CSF neurochemical markers are specific for AD, it may be possible to develop a profile of several neurochemical markers that will have enhanced specificity.

27. Beal, M. Flint; Mazurek, Michael F. & Martin, Joseph B. (1986). **Somatostatin immunoreactivity is reduced in Parkinson's disease dementia with Alzheimer's changes.** *Brain Research,* 397(2), 386–388.
Somatostatinlike immunoreactivity (SLI) was measured in postmortem brain tissue from 15 control patients, 7 nondemented parkinsonian (NDP) patients and 7 demented parkinsonian (DP) patients who had Alzheimer-type cortical pathology (all Ss aged 23–88 yrs). The NDP Ss had normal concentrations of SLI in various areas (e.g., the cerebral cortex). DP Ss had significantly reduced (approximately 40%) levels of SLI in both the frontal and temporal cortex.

28. Beck, Charles H. (1980). **Normal aging of the human brain potentiates the neuropathologies of Parkinson's disease, depression, and Alzheimer's disease: Behavioural implications.** *Canadian Counsellor,* 14(2), 110–120.

Notes that the normal aging process of the human brain involves neuropathological changes that potentiate the progress of Parkinson's disease, depression, and Alzheimer's disease. Thus the old person is not just a younger person afflicted with an especially stressful array of environmental contingencies. The professional should be prepared for the insidious development of milder forms of the symptoms of these diseases in normal aging persons. As a corollary, parkinsonism, depression, and Alzheimer's disease may be viewed as accelerations of normal aging. (French abstract) (4½ p ref).

29. Bird, Thomas D. (1986). **Problems and limitations in studying a genetic component of Alzheimer's disease.** Special Issue: Controversial topics on Alzheimer's disease: Intersecting crossroads. *Neurobiology of Aging,* 7(6), 477–478.
Emphasizes 4 issues raised by P. Davies (1986) concerning Alzheimer's disease (AD) and argues that difficulties with conclusively diagnosing Alzheimer's patients and the apparent multifactorial, genetic/environmental interactions of AD continue to complicate attempts to study and understand AD. Although families with an apparent autosomal dominant trait are potentially quite valuable in studying a possible genetic etiology, small numbers of such families, small numbers of living members within such families, and possible genetic heterogeneity will make their evaluation a complex task.

30. Bisso, G. M.; Masullo, C.; Michalek, H.; Silveri, Maria C. et al. (1986). **Molecular forms of cholinesterases in CSF of Alzheimer's disease/senile dementia of Alzheimer type patients and matched neurological controls.** *Life Sciences,* 38(6), 561–567.
Acetylcholinesterase (AChE), pseudocholinesterase, and their molecular forms were measured in the cerebrospinal fluid (CSF) of 6 56–78 yr old patients affected by Alzheimer's disease and 5 63–80 yr old matched neurological controls. Three different molecular forms of ChE were found in the CSF of both groups of patients, but only 2 of them belonged to "true" AChE. No differences were found between Alzheimer's Ss and controls in all the examined parameters.

31. Bondareff, William. (1984). **Neurobiology of Alzheimer's disease.** *Psychiatric Annals,* 14(3), 179–185.
Alzheimer's disease is an age-related disorder of neurotransmission involving noncortical neurons from which major ascending cholinergic and monoaminergic pathways originate. Local pathology and functional decline of postsynaptic neurons in the higher brain centers are associated with the clinical signs and symptoms of the disorder, which then appear to reflect impaired transmission in cholinergic and noradrenergic systems associated with memory, learning, and a variety of higher cortical functions. (68 ref).

32. Bondareff, William; Mountjoy, Christopher Q.; Roth, Martin; Rossor, Martin N. et al. (1987). **Age and histopathologic heterogeneity in Alzheimer's disease: Evidence for subtypes.** *Archives of General Psychiatry,* 44(5), 412–417.
Followed up 46 elderly persons (mean age at death 77.73 yrs) satisfying Diagnostic and Statistical Manual of Mental Disorders (DSM-III) criteria for dementia during the course of their disease in a geriatric or psychogeriatric ward in 1 of 4 British hospitals. Sequential longitudinal study during the course of their illness had indicated that each S met DSM-III criteria for primary degenerative dementia and strongly suggested a diagnosis of Alzheimer's disease (AD). Postmortem histopathological examination of the brains was conducted. A control group comprised 44 brain specimens selected from Ss (mean age at death 80.84 yrs) not known to have been demented during life. Postmortem counts of the total number of nucleus locus ceruleus (nLC) neurons confirmed that AD exists in 2 subtypes differentiated by the number of nLC neurons and the age at death.

33. Bondareff, William & Mountjoy, Christopher Q. (1986). **Number of neurons in nucleus locus ceruleus in demented and non-demented patients: Rapid estimation and correlated parameters.** *Neurobiology of Aging,* 7(4), 297–300.
Counted the total number of neurons in nucleus locus ceruleus (nLC) in 20 patients (age at death 63–91 yrs) with dementia (19 with dementia of the Alzheimer type) and 10 nondemented patients (age at death 71–93 yrs) with the assistance of an image analyzer. The average number of neurons in a single representative section of nLC through the site maximal neuronal density was then determined in each case. Both the mean total neuronal count and the average number of neurons in single sections correlated significantly with age, severity of dementia, and length of nLC. The mean total number of neurons for demented and nondemented Ss differed significantly.

34. Bouras, Constantin; de St Hilaire-Kafi, Sarah & Constantinidis, Jean. (1986). **Neuropeptides in Alzheimer's disease: A review and morphological results.** *Progress in Neuro-Psychopharmacology & Biological Psychiatry,* 10(3–5), 271–286.
Reviews the anatomic distribution of classical neurotransmitters in the postmortem autopsied brains of Alzheimer's disease (AD) patients. It is concluded that the reviews give evidence for the change of a large number of neuropeptides in AD on the basis of immunohistochemical criteria. Somatostatin changes in postmortem brain material of 3 cases of AD and 2 controls (aged 63–87 yrs) were observed by means of immunohistochemical methods. In animal studies, an interaction between somatostatin and acetylcholine turnover in the substantia innominata has been reported.

35. Bowen, D. M. & Davison, A. N. (1980). **Biochemical changes in the cholinergic system of the ageing brain and in senile dementia.** *Psychological Medicine,* 10(2), 315–319.
Maintains that one-third of nerve cell components are lost from the temporal lobe of patients with senile dementia of Alzheimer's type as compared to age-matched controls. It is suggested that the alteration, marked by the loss of choline acetyltransferase activity (especially in the hippocampus), is parallel to the intensity of neuropathological damage and relates to prior mental impairment. (29 ref).

36. Bracha, Haim S. & Kleinman, Joel E. (1984). **Postmortem studies in psychiatry.** *Psychiatric Clinics of North America,* 7(3), 473–485.
Contends that postmortem neurochemical studies have led to positive findings in schizophrenia, depression and suicide, and Alzheimer disease and Huntington's chorea. In schizophrenia, many positive findings have not been replicated, and the confounding treatment effects of neuroleptics may account for many, if not all, of these findings. Nevertheless, support has been found for the hypotheses that involve catecholamines and peptides in schizophrenic symptomatology. Most of the evidence in affective disorders and suicide may favor some disorder of the serotonin system, probably at the receptor level. In Alzheimer disease, the dementia and decreased cholinergic activity appear related to the loss of cholinergic neurons from the nucleus basalis of Meynert. There is a marked paucity or total lack of neurochemical studies in some affective illnesses (e.g., delusional depression, bipolar disorder, and major depression). The findings in victims of suicide suggest that borderline personality disorders may be a worthwhile group to examine. It is suggested that studies of eating disorders and panic disorders may also warrant examination. (28 ref).

37. Brandenburg, Nancy A. (1986). **The familial aggregation of Down's syndrome, senile dementia of the Alzheimer type, and other clinical disorders.** *Dissertation Abstracts International,* 46(11-B), 3709.

38. Breitner, John C. (1986). **On methodology and appropriate inference regarding possible genetic factors in typical, late-onset AD.** Special Issue: Controversial topics on Alzheimer's disease: Intersecting crossroads. *Neurobiology of Aging,* 7(6), 476–477.
Endorses points raised by P. Davies (1986), suggesting that diagnosis of Alzheimer's disease (AD) in both probands and relatives, and its typically late onset, pose difficulties for the interpretation of its apparent familial aggregation—a possible indicator of genetic causes. Recent methodologic improvements have ameliorated these difficulties somewhat, and new studies incorporating these improvements suggest much greater familial risk in AD than has been previously reported. Actual risk to aged relatives remains a topic of controversy, and the true role of genetic factors in the etiology of AD will probably require the application of the classical genetic methods of twin and linkage studies.

39. Breitner, John C.; Folstein, Marshal F. & Murphy, Edmond A. (1986). **Familial aggregation in Alzheimer Dementia: I. A model for the age-dependent expression of an autosomal dominant gene.** *Journal of Psychiatric Research,* 20(1), 31–43.
To evaluate the possible genetic transmission of Alzheimer's disease (AD) from its familial aggregation, a provisional biomathematical genetic model was developed from the empirical age-specific incidence of AD in 3 familial data sets collected by T. Larsson et al (1963), L. L. Heston et al (1981), and the 1st 2 authors (1984). Based on the premise of an autosomal dominant AD gene in proband families, the modeling technique provides estimates of the proportion of genetic index cases and the parameters of age-dependent gene expression. With appropriate parameters, the model accurately reflects the age-specific familial risk of AD, suggesting the appropriateness of its underlying assumptions. The estimated proportions of genetic index cases indicate that heritable disease constitutes a majority of AD. In cases ascertained by the presence of aphasia or apraxia, the estimated proportion of genetic cases was 100%.

40. Breitner, John C.; Murphy, Edmond A. & Folstein, Marshal F. (1986). **Familial aggregation in Alzheimer Dementia: II. Clinical genetic implications of age-dependent onset.** *Journal of Psychiatric Research,* 20(1), 45–55.
Applied a biomathematical genetic model proposed by the present authors (1986) for the age-specific risk of Alzheimer's disease (AD) to 2 problems in the clinical genetics of this disorder. In a test of the ability of a clinical marker specifically to identify genetic AD, cases grouped by the phenotype of amnesia with aphasia or apraxia were shown to have familial risk that suggested a pure genetic illness, and differed significantly from cases without this phenotype. The model was also used to assess the probability that individual cases had hereditary disease, given their family history. Even with no affected relatives, there is a substantial likelihood that many AD cases may have a genetic illness, suggesting that one cannot reliably classify individual cases as "familial" or "sporadic" from family history alone. Findings show that the clinical phenotype may better indicate genetic AD than does the observed familial aggregation in single index cases.

41. Briley, Mike; Chopin, Philippe & Moret, Chantal. (1986). **New concepts in Alzheimer's disease.** *Neurobiology of Aging,* 7(1), 57–62.
Describes some presentations that were offered at a 3-day symposium on "New Concepts in Alzheimer's Disease" held in France in October 1985. Topics included neuropharmacology of central cholinergic and other neurotransmitter systems, biochemical and immunological markers of cholinergic neurons, the differentiation of cholinergic neurons in culture, genetic studies, and neuron grafting.

42. Brion, S.; Plas, J. & Massé, G. (1986). **Maladie d'Alzheimer et noyau basal de Meynert: Point de vue anatomo-clinique. / Alzheimer's disease and nucleus basalis of Meynert: An anatomo-clinical point of view.** *Encéphale,* 12(3), 111–114.
Studied the histologic quality and significance of lesions in the nucleus basalis of Meynert (NBM) in 10 56–68 yr olds with Alzheimer's disease and 6 73–88 yr olds with senile dementia. A cellular count and histologic observation of the NBM were done on slides imbedded in paraffin. The cortex was studied in the classical way. The occurrence and importance of neurofibrillary tangles in the NBM and neuron loss were compared in the 2 groups of Ss. (English abstract).

43. Brun, A. & Gustafson, L. (1976). **Distribution of cerebral degeneration in Alzheimer's disease.** *Archiv fur Psychiatrie und Nervenkrankheiten,* 223(1), 15–33.
In 7 cases (3 males and 4 females) of Alzheimer's disease, cerebral degeneration was regularly found to be most pronounced in certain areas. Maximal cortical degeneration occurred in the medial temporal (limbic) area and, in the lateral hemisphere, consistently within a field expanding from the posterior inferior temporal areas to the adjoining portions of the parieto-occipital lobes. In addition, the posterior cingulate gyrus was severely involved. Certain areas were notably and consistently spared or less involved, mainly the anterior cingulate gyrus and the calcarine and central sensory motor areas (primary projection areas). The frontal lobes occupied an intermediate position, being less severely involved than is usually reported. The clinical symptoms correlated well with this pattern of degeneration. Groups of symptoms, such as memory dysfunction, emotional and personality alterations, and some symptoms of the Kluver-Bucy syndrome, were referable to the limbic lesions. The pattern described may be related to ontogenetic features, and the tendency to focalization to the age of disease onset. The role of genetic factors and of other diseases in the development of the disease is discussed. (German summary) (75 ref).

44. Brun, A. & Gustafson, L. (1978). **Limbic lobe involvement in presenile dementia.** *Archiv für Psychiatrie und Nervenkrankheiten,* 226(2), 79–93.
Limbic lobe involvement in presenile dementia was studied from neuropathological and neuropsychiatric viewpoints. The material consisted of 7 cases of Alzheimer's disease, 4 cases of Pick's disease, and 4 cases of Jacob-Creutzfeldt's disease. The Alzheimer group had a mainly temporoparieto-occipital and posterior cingulate gyrus involvement. The Pick group generally showed an inverse distribution with frontotemporal and anterior cingulate gyrus accentuation of the damage. Basal temporal limbic areas were involved in both groups. The Jacob-Creutzfeldt group had a less schematic lesion pattern, without involvement of limbic areas. From a neuropsychiatric aspect, these differences were reflected in symptoms that could be referred both to areas spared and those more pronouncedly destroyed by the degenerative process. Thus the Alzheimer group retained emotional qualities that were lost early in the Pick group. The possible relationship between neurotransmitters and regional accentuation of the degeneration is discussed. (64 ref).

45. Butler, Robert N. (1984). **"Is Alzheimer's Disease inherited? A methodologic review": Commentary.** *Integrative Psychiatry,* 2(5), 173.
Comments on the hypothesis of M. F. Folstein and D. Powell (1984) that most Alzheimer's disease is transmitted as an autosomal-dominant age-dependent disorder. It is suggested that (1) with increasing survival, there will be greater opportunity for pedigree studies; (2) senile dementia of the Alzheimer type may be more than one disease; (3) it is unlikely that deficiency of 1 neurotransmitter system (e.g., the cholinergic system) would be the evolutionary thread; and (4) Alzheimer's disease is a uniquely human disease.

5

46. Carlisle, Edith M. (1986). **A silicon aluminum relationship in aged brain.** Special Issue: Controversial topics on Alzheimer's disease: Intersecting crossroads. *Neurobiology of Aging,* 7(6), 545–546.
Suggests that the review by D. R. Crapper McLachlan (1986) is an informative summary of the research on aluminum (AL) and Alzheimer's disease (AD) and supports the point that to establish a cause and effect relation of AL as a potential factor in the pathogenesis of AD demands a greater understanding of how AL acts at the molecular level in the brain and also the entire body. It is suggested that the effect of silicon should be considered as animal studies indicate a protective action of silicon against AL neurotoxicity in certain tissues.

47. Chase, Gary A. (1986). **Genetic counseling in Alzheimer's disease.** Special Issue: Controversial topics on Alzheimer's disease: Intersecting crossroads. *Neurobiology of Aging,* 7(6), 483–484.
In commenting on the article by P. Davies (1986), the present author contends that it is important to recognize the incomplete state of knowledge concerning the causes of Alzheimer's disease (AD). Along with the phenomenon of delayed onset, which reduces the portion of risk actually experienced by relatives in most instances, genetic heterogeneity must be considered. Differences in published findings may result from methodology, diagnostic techniques, or most likely the presence of several genetic and nongenetic entities within the rubric of AD. Genetic counselors should therefore be cautious in assessment of risks to relatives.

48. Chase, Thomas N.; Burrows, G. Howard & Mohr, Erich. (1987). **Cortical glucose utilization patterns in primary degenerative dementias of the anterior and posterior type.** Eric K. Fernström Foundation Symposium: Frontal lobe degeneration of non-Alzheimer type (1986, Lund, Sweden). *Archives of Gerontology & Geriatrics,* 6(3), 289–297.
Evaluated regional cortical function in 13 patients with primary degenerative dementia and 6 age-matched, neurologically normal controls. Five Ss were selected on the basis of preponderant signs of posterior dementia, 5 mainly had signs of anterior dementia, and the remaining 3 evidenced mixed anterior-posterior cognitive deficits. Positron emission tomographic scans revealed a characteristic pattern of abnormalities in each group. Results indicate that the primary degenerative dementias may reflect a selective abnormality of the frontal and parietal association cortices.

49. Chu, Dorothy C.; Penney, John B. & Young, Anne B. (1987). **Cortical GABA$_B$ and GABA$_A$ receptors in Alzheimer's disease: A quantitative autoradiographic study.** *Neurology,* 37(9), 1454–1459.
Evaluated gamma-aminobutyric acid (GABA)$_B$ and GABA$_A$ binding sites by quantitative autoradiography of ^{3}H-GABA binding in superior frontal gyrus of 4 Ss (mean age 67 yrs) who died with dementia of the Alzheimer's type (DAT) and of 4 age-matched normal controls. Scatchard analysis and competition studies disclosed 48–68% and 25% decrements in receptor density for GABA$_B$ and GABA$_A$ receptors, respectively, in layers II, III, and V of DAT frontal cortex as compared with controls.

50. Chui, Helena C.; Mortimer, James A.; Slager, Ursula; Zarow, Chris et al. (1986). **Pathologic correlates of dementia in Parkinson's disease.** *Archives of Neurology,* 43(10), 991–995.
Examined, through postmortem histopathologic studies, the cerebral cortex, hippocampus, and 3 subcortical nuclei in 4 patients who had had idiopathic Parkinson's disease (PD) and whose mental status had been characterized by neuropsychologic testing and in 5 Alzheimer's disease patients and 5 nondemented elderly patients. Ss' age at the time of death was 57–87 yrs. Results, in part, show that the PD Ss

had significant impairment in intellectual functioning compared with other PD patients; 1 PD S had developed a severe dementia of which a marked language impairment was a principal feature; and in 1 S surviving neurons contained neurofibrillary tangles rather than Lewy bodies.

51. Cohen, Donna; Eisdorfer, Carl & Leverenz, James. (1982). **Alzheimer's disease and maternal age.** *Journal of the American Geriatrics Society,* 30(10), 656–659.
Since previous research has supported an association between Alzheimer's disease (AD) and Down's syndrome (DS), it was hypothesized that similar risk factors may be involved in the pathogenesis of these disorders. An examination of the birth records of 80 AD Ss (mean age 73.2 yrs) showed that the median age of the Ss'. mothers at the time of their birth was 35.5 yrs, compared to 27 yrs in 590 randomly selected birth records. Results support the possibility that an aberration in the mother's aging process may place offspring at heightened risk for dementia. It is possible that a defect in the microtubular structure of the cell, which causes neurofibrillary tangles and chromosomal nondisjunction, may underlie both DS and AD. (35 ref).

52. Colgan, John. (1985). **Regional density and survival in senile dementia: An interim report on a prospective computed tomographic study.** *British Journal of Psychiatry,* 147, 63–66.
Performed computed cranial tomography (CT) on 48 patients with senile dementia of the Alzheimer type (SDAT) who have since been followed up in a continuing prospective study. Ss were administered a geriatric mental state schedule and tests of memory and orientation. At 6-mo follow-up, 10 Ss (mean age 77 yrs) had died; these did not differ significantly from the survivors (mean age 78 yrs) either in mean age or duration of dementia. Despite having shorter histories, the deceased had performed worse on initial testing with several cognitive measures, and this was significant for the mental test score; this suggests that some Ss may have a more rapidly progressive form of SDAT. In a comparison between the CT scan of the deceased and survivors, the deceased were found to have significantly lower mean attentuation densities in the parietal, occipital, and left thalamic regions. The hypothesis that low attentuation density in the parietal regions of the CT scan in SDAT is associated with a more rapid demise is supported for the present period of follow-up. (11 ref).

53. Comfort, Alex. (1984). **Alzheimer's disease or "Alzheimerism"?** *Psychiatric Annals,* 14(2), 130–132.
Discusses symptoms associated with senility not as a normal part of the aging process but as pathologically progressive syndrome, characterized by structural and immunologic changes, genetic association, selective effects on brain areas and neurochemical transmitters, and a resemblance to certain slow-virus conditions. The symptom complex known as "Alzheimerism" is characterized by progressive dementia focusing on associative and recall processes and cortical atrophy due to massive loss of neurons. (20 ref).

54. Corwin, June; Serby, Michael & Rotrosen, John. (1986). **Olfactory deficits in AD: What we know about the nose.** Special Issue: Controversial topics on Alzheimer's disease: Intersecting crossroads. *Neurobiology of Aging,* 7(6), 580–582.
Notes that E. Roberts's (1986) zeolite hypothesis of Alzheimer's disease (AD) rests in part on evidence of olfactory deficits in this disorder. The present authors review this evidence and select evidence for deficits in related disorders and normal aging, stressing gaps in knowledge and problems in assessment. It is concluded that olfactory identification is most likely impaired in AD but that other olfactory functions are poorly characterized at present.

55. Coyle, Joseph T.; Price, Donald L. & DeLong, Mahlon R. (1983). **Alzheimer's disease: A disorder of cortical cholinergic innervation.** *Science,* 219(4589), 1184–1190.
Great emphasis in current research is placed on identification of neurotransmitter systems involved in the symptomatic manifestations of neurological and psychiatric disorders. In the case of Alzheimer's disease, which now seems to be one of the most common causes of mental deterioration in the elderly, evidence has been developed that acetylcholine-releasing neurons, whose cell bodies lie in the basal forebrain, selectively degenerate. These cholinergic neurons provide widespread innervation of the cerebral cortex and related structures and appear to play an important role in cognitive functions, especially memory. These advances reflect a close interaction between experimental and clinical neuroscientists, in which information derived from basic neurobiology is rapidly utilized to analyze disorders of the human brain.

56. Crapper, D. R. & DeBoni, U. (1978). **Brain aging and Alzheimer's disease.** *Canadian Psychiatric Association Journal,* 23(4), 229–233.
The most common cause of senile dementia appears to be a pathological process indistinguishable from that found in presenile dementia of the Alzheimer type. Consideration of the neuropathological changes suggests that this disease may involve the interaction of at least 3 processes: a viral-like infection, a disorder in the immune system, and the neurotoxic effect of an environmental agent. Evidence in support of this hypothesis is reviewed. (French summary) (21 ref).

57. Crapper McLachlan, D. R. (1986). **"Aluminum and Alzheimer's disease": Author's response to commentaries.** Special Issue: Controversial topics on Alzheimer's disease: Intersecting crossroads. *Neurobiology of Aging,* 7(6), 556–557.
The author (1986) responds to comments in a series of papers by H. M. Wisniewski et al, B. Ghetti and O. Bugiani, Z. S. Khachaturian, J. W. Pettegrew, R. S. Jope, G. H. Mayor, A. C. Alfrey, E. M. Carlisle, J. K. Marquis, P. Gambetti, D. P. Perl, L. Liss and D. J. Thornton, and D. C. Gajdusek (1986) concerning his review of the relationship between aluminum neurotoxicity and Alzheimer's disease.

58. Crapper McLachlan, D. R. (1986). **Aluminum and Alzheimer's disease.** Special Issue: Controversial topics on Alzheimer's disease: Intersecting crossroads. *Neurobiology of Aging,* 7(6), 525–532.
A review of the literature suggests that there is now substantial evidence indicating that an accumulation of aluminum (AL) occurs in grey matter in diseases associated with Alzheimer neurofibrillary degeneration. Four principal sites of AL accumulation have been identified in Alzheimer's disease (AD): (1) DNA containing structures of the nucleus, (2) the protein moieties of neurofibrillary tangles, (3) the amyloid cores of senile plaques, and (4) cerebral ferritin. The literature on the toxic effects of AL in these 4 loci strengthens the hypothesis that AL could be important in the pathogenesis of this neurodegenerative process. The evidence, however, does not support an etiological role for AL in AD. The primary pathogenic events responsible for AD are presumed to have affected the genetically determined barriers to AL resulting in increased amounts of this toxic element to vulnerable target sites.

59. Cronin-Golomb, Alice. (1987). **International study group on the pharmacology of memory disorders associated with aging.** *Neurobiology of Aging,* 8(3), 277–282.
Summarizes reports that represent much of the current state of scientific knowledge in regard to Alzheimer's disease (AD). Presentations are summarized under the following headings: neurobiology, phospholipid membranes, clinical advances in AD, and prospects for treatment.

60. Cross, A. J.; Crow, T. J.; Ferrier, I. N. & Johnson, J. A. (1986). **The selectivity of the reduction of serotonin S2 receptors in Alzheimer-type dementia.** *Neurobiology of Aging,* 7(1), 3–7.
Studied the high-affinity binding of ligands to putative neurotransmitter receptors in temporal cortex of 13 control (mean age 78 yrs) and 13 Alzheimer-type dementia (ATD [mean age 78 yrs]) patients whose brains were obtained at autopsy. A selective reduction of serotonin S2 receptors was observed in the ATD patients, with no change in S1 receptors; of the other ligand binding sites only ^{3}H-flunitrazepam binding was significantly reduced. Ligand binding sites that were unchanged in ATD temporal cortex included those labeled by adrenergic, adenosine, histamine, opiate, gamma-aminobutyric acid (GABA), benzodiazepine, and cholinergic ligands. (43 ref).

61. Crow, Timothy J. et al. (1984). **Neurotransmitter receptors and monoamine metabolites in the brains of patients with Alzheimer-type dementia and depression, and suicides.** Spring Meeting of the British Pharmacological Society: 5-HT, peripheral and central receptors, and function (1984, Birmingham, England). *Neuropharmacology,* 23(12-B), 1561–1569.
Compared monoamine turnover and binding to monoamine and other receptors among 32 patients (aged 56–95 yrs) with Alzheimer-type dementia, 9 depressed inpatients (aged 73–84 yrs), 35 normal controls (aged 61–94 yrs), and 17 adult Ss who had committed suicide. Findings indicate a degeneration of the noradrenergic and serotonergic innervation of the cerebral cortices of Ss with dementia. There were no consistent changes in monoamine metabolism in the inpatient and suicidal Ss. Noradrenergic, serotonergic, and other neurotransmitters were unchanged; however, 6 suicidal Ss evidenced a moderate decrease in imipramine binding. (52 ref).

62. Cutler, Neal R. (1986). **Cerebral metabolism as measured with positron emission tomography (PET) and [^{18}F] 2-deoxy-d-glucose: Healthy aging, Alzheimer's disease and Down syndrome.** *Progress in Neuro-Psychopharmacology & Biological Psychiatry,* 10(3–5), 309–321.
Examined the relationship between functional changes and alterations in brain metabolism in aging in studies with 40 healthy men (21–83 yrs old), 12 patients with Alzheimer's disease (AD) and controls (49–81 yrs old), and 14 patients with Down's syndrome and matched controls (19–64 yrs old). Measurements with PET and [^{18}F]fluoro-2-deoxyglucose showed that brain metabolic function was age invariant in healthy Ss. It was significantly reduced throughout the brain in the late-severe form of AD. Marked elevations in metabolism were found in younger Down's syndrome Ss, while age-related declines were found in the older Ss.

63. Cutler, Neal R.; Kay, Arthur D.; Marangos, Paul J. & Burg, Cheryl. (1986). **Cerebrospinal fluid neuron-specific enolase is reduced in Alzheimer's disease.** *Archives of Neurology,* 43(2), 153–154.
Measured neuron-specific enolase (NSE)—a glycolytic enzyme enolase found in the brain—in cerebrospinal fluid (CSF) and serum of 30 patients with presumptive Alzheimer's disease (AD) and 13 healthy control Ss. NSE levels were evaluated as a measure of neuronal functional activity associated with AD. The CSF NSE levels of AD Ss were significantly reduced, and serum NSE levels were significantly increased relative to controls. The increased NSE in serum of the AD Ss may be rather nonspecific and reflect pathology in the spinal cord or differences in platelets or the neuroendocrine system. CSF NSE levels may be indicative of central nervous system (CNS) cell loss or a decrease in neuronal functional activity associated with AD.

7

64. Davies, Peter. (1986). **The genetics of Alzheimer's disease: A review and a discussion of the implications.** Special Issue: Controversial topics on Alzheimer's disease: Intersecting crossroads. *Neurobiology of Aging,* 7(6), 459–466.
Examines the evidence for a genetic etiology of Alzheimer's disease (AD). Three groups of cases are identified—the first being those with a consistently early age of onset, in which autosomal dominant inheritance can be established. There are early onset cases without a strong genetic component, and later onset cases generally show only weak evidence of hereditary disease. Studies of associations between AD and Down's syndrome suggest a role for genes on chromosome 21 in the genesis of the pathologic features. Attempts to link the development of AD to the presence of specific inherited markers have been unsuccessful to date, but there are some promising findings. Progress in understanding the molecular basis of other inherited diseases is reviewed in relation to attempts to understand the molecular basis of AD.

65. Davies, Peter. (1986). **"The genetics of Alzheimer's disease: A review and a discussion of the implications": Author's response to commentaries.** Special Issue: Controversial topics on Alzheimer's disease: Intersecting crossroads. *Neurobiology of Aging,* 7(6), 484–485.
The author (1986) responds to comments in a series of papers by A. D. Roses, W. Henderson, J. F. Gusella, L. J. Whalley, J. C. Breitner, T. D. Bird, L. Barclay, C. A. Marotta, M. Folstein, and G. A. Chase (1986) concerning his review of the genetic hypothesis for the etiology of Alzheimer's disease.

66. Davies, Peter & Wolozin, Benjamin L. (1987). **Recent advances in the neurochemistry of Alzheimer's disease.** *Journal of Clinical Psychiatry,* 48(5, Suppl), 23–30.
Reviews recent progress in research in the genesis of neurochemical changes in the brains of Alzheimer's disease (AD) patients. Research has been conducted primarily in 2 areas: the cellular proteins associated with the pathologic structures and the neurotransmitter changes. Clinical findings in AD, epidemiological and clinical genetic studies, anatomic and biochemical neuropathologies in AD, and recently proposed markers for AD are also examined. Research and clinical implications of recent studies and of works in progress are discussed.

67. Davis, Bonnie M. et al. (1985). **Clinical studies of the cholinergic deficit in Alzheimer's disease: I. Neurochemical and neuroendocrine studies.** *Journal of the American Geriatrics Society,* 33(11), 741–748.
Autopsy studies indicating that cholinergic neurons are selectively lost in patients with Alzheimer's disease (AD) and senile dementia of the Alzheimer type (SDAT) suggest that peripheral markers for central cholinergic activity would be useful in diagnosis. The present studies found that cerebrospinal fluid (CSF) concentrations of acetylcholine (ACh) correlated with the degree of cognitive impairment in 26 49–80 yr olds with AD/SDAT, but metabolites of other neurotransmitters were not related to cognitive state. This suggests that CSF ACh may be a valid measure of cholinergic degeneration. Cortisol and growth hormone were measured in plasma samples drawn from 25 AD/SDAT patients (mean age 66.6 yrs) and 10 normal controls (mean age 59.1 yrs) every 30 min from 9 PM to 11 AM the next day. Mean plasma cortisol concentrations were higher in Ss with AD/SDAT than in controls and correlated inversely with CSF methoxy-hydroxyphenylglycol (MHPG) and positively with degree of cognitive impairment. Because anticholinergic drugs suppress cortisol, this finding indicates that cortisol dysregulation may be a marker for abnormalities in other neurotransmitter systems, particularly the noradrenergic system. Growth hormone secretion was not different in patients and controls but was positively correlated with CSF MHPG. (63 ref).

68. de Estable-Puig, Rosita F.; Estable-Puig, Juan F.; ven Murthy, M. R.; Radouco-Thomas, Simone et al. (1986). **On the pathogenesis and therapy of dementia of the Alzheimer type: Some neuropathological, biochemical, genetic and pharmacotherapeutic considerations.** *Progress in Neuro-Psychopharmacology & Biological Psychiatry,* 10(3–5), 355–390.
Suggests that the extensive literature on dementia of Alzheimer type (DAT) testifies to the enormous progress achieved in the clinical and biochemical delineation of this disease. An overview is presented of major DAT morphological changes, etiopathogenic hypotheses of DAT, recombinant DNA methods for gene analysis, and the pharmacotherapeutic armamentarium used in DAT and senile dementia.

69. Defossez, A.; Persuy, P.; Tramu, G. & Delacourte, A. (1986). **Étude immunohistochimique des lésions élémentaires de la maladie d'Alzheimer. / Immunohistochemical study of Alzheimer's disease lesions.** *Encéphale,* 12(4), 161–168.
Describes the isolation of neurofibrillary tangles (NFTs) and senile (neuritic) plaques (SPs) from an Alzheimer brain and raised antibodies against paired helical filaments (PHFs). The advantages of the immunohistochemical method compared with stainings of NFTs and SPs by the anti-PHF or the classical Bodian silver staining technique are discussed. (English abstract).

70. DeKosky, Steven T. & Bass, Norman H. (1982). **Aging, senile dementia, and the intralaminar microchemistry of cerebral cortex.** *Neurology,* 32(11), 1227–1232.
Compared the microchemical architecture of the right frontal isocortex in the brains of 5 persons (mean age 74 yrs) with senile dementia of the Alzheimer type, 5 age-matched Ss without evidence of intellectual or neurological disability, and 5 younger Ss (mean age 46 yrs) without neurological disease. Results suggest that selective vulnerability of axodendritic arborization of neurons in lower lamina may be correlated with the impaired cognitive functions of senile dementia. (44 ref).

71. de Ruiter, J. P. & Uylings, H. B. (1987). **Morphometric and dendritic analysis of fascia dentata granule cells in human aging and senile dementia.** *Brain Research,* 402(2), 217–229.
Compared cellular morphology (postmortem) in the human fascia dentata of 4 Alzheimer's disease and 1 multi-infarct dementia patients (aged 79–97 yrs) with 5 very old (postmortem) controls (aged 65–94 yrs). In the demented group, there was a significant reduction in thickness of the molecular layer, density of dendritic spines in the middle 3rd of the molecular layer, and total dendritic length, primarily in the inner 3rd of the molecular layer in which the commissural and associational fibers terminate. Results suggest that dendritic degeneration is a predominant process in dementia.

72. de Souza, Errol B. et al. (1986). **Reciprocal changes in corticotropin-releasing factor (CRF)-like immunoreactivity and CRF receptors in cerebral cortex of Alzheimer's disease.** *Nature,* 319(6054), 593–595.
In 11 neurologically normal controls and 14 Ss with Alzheimer's disease (AD), postmortem examinations studied brain pre- and postsynaptic markers of corticotropin-releasing factor (CRF), a hypothalamic peptide regulating pituitary-adrenocortical secretion that also seems to act as a neurotransmitter in the central nervous system (CNS). It was found that in AD Ss, the concentrations of CRF-like immunoreactivity (CRF-IR) were reduced and that there were reciprocal increases in CRF receptor binding in affected cortical areas. These changes were significantly correlated with decrements in choline acetyltransferase activity. Results support a neurotransmitter role for CRF in the brain and demonstrate a modulation of CNS–CRF receptors associated with altered CRF content. Findings suggest a possible role for CRF in the

pathophysiology of the dementia and indicate that therapies directed at increasing CRF levels in brain may prove useful for treatment. (40 ref).

73. Deutsch, Georg. (1986). **Cerebral blood flow indices of structural and functional deficits in dementing pathologies.** *Dissertation Abstracts International,* 46(8-B), 2858.

74. Deutsch, Georg & Tweedy, James R. (1987). **Cerebral blood flow in severity-matched Alzheimer and multi-infarct patients.** *Neurology,* 37(3), 431–438.
Studied cerebral blood flow in 30 patients (mean age 72.7 yrs) meeting research criteria for either Alzheimer's disease or multi-infarct dementia and matched for age and severity of dementia. Results show that in both groups, mean flow was less than in age-matched normal controls, but the Alzheimer Ss also had significantly lower mean flow than the multi-infarct group. It is suggested that this finding helps to resolve discrepancies found in studies with inadequate control for severity. Either global flow or regional left parietal flow can be used to discriminate between these dementia categories with 87% accuracy.

75. Deutsch, Stephen I. et al. (1983). **Acetylcholinesterase activity in CSF in schizophrenia, depression, Alzheimer's disease, and normals.** *Biological Psychiatry,* 18(12), 1363–1373.
Measured acetylcholinesterase (AChE) activity and protein in the CSF of 7 patients with Alzheimer's disease (mean age 59.9 yrs), 11 depressed Ss (mean age 44.2 yrs), 9 schizophrenics with tardive dyskinesia (TD; mean age 48.1 yrs), 10 schizophrenics without TD (mean age 33.6 yrs), and 6 normal controls (mean age 30.5 yrs). No differences between diagnostic groups were found on either measure of AChE when the extraneous factors of age and CSF protein concentrations were controlled, nor were any differences found between groups for CSF protein when age was controlled. (23 ref).

76. Ditter, Susan M. & Mirra, Suzanne S. (1987). **Neuropathologic and clinical features of Parkinson's disease in Alzheimer's disease patients.** *Neurology,* 37(5), 754–760.
Investigated neuropathologic and clinical features of Parkinson's disease (PD) in 20 neuropathologically confirmed Alzheimer's disease (AD) autopsy brains. Findings show that 11 cases (55%) showed PD changes (e.g., Lewy body formation, neuronal loss, gliosis of pigmented nuclei), with no significant difference in age or symptom duration between those cases with and without PD pathology. A history of rigidity in the absence of neuroleptic medication was noted in 80% of those with PD pathology but only 14% of those without PD pathology. Tremor was not observed in either group, suggesting that extrapyramidal signs (e.g., rigidity) noted in many AD patients are related to coexistent PD pathology.

77. Dowson, J. H. (1982). **Neuronal lipofuscin accumulation in ageing and Alzheimer dementia: A pathogenic mechanism?** *British Journal of Psychiatry,* 140, 142–148.
Measured the intraneuronal lipofuscin in the parietal cortex and the inferior olivary nucleus in postmortem tissue affected by Alzheimer dementia from 10 individuals and in specimens from 13 nondemented individuals. Results indicate that there was a linear relationship between the accumulation of cell body lipofuscin and advancing age, both in neuronal populations of the nondemented group and in the olivary neurons of the demented group. The estimated amount of lipofuscin in the olivary neurons in the demented group was significantly higher than in the nondemented, when age was taken into account. Two studies in which centrophenoxine was administered in order to change the neuronal lipofuscin content led to a significant improvement in a new learning task in elderly individuals. (36 ref).

78. Drachman, David A. (1986). **Plaques and tangles in Alzheimer's disease: Cause, consequence or epiphenomenon?** Special Issue: Controversial topics on Alzheimer's disease: Intersecting crossroads. *Neurobiology of Aging,* 7(6), 450–451.
Comments on the article by D. J. Selkoe (1986) on Alzheimer's disease (AD), by arguing that a study of the composition and origin of the plaques, tangles, and amyloid proteins characteristic of AD will be of value in determining the etiology and pathogenesis of AD if they are causally related to the neural damage, but such a study will be of uncertain usefulness if they are merely secondary epiphenomena.

79. Dusheiko, S. D. (1972). **Senile plaques and Alzheimer changes of the neurofibrils in older deceased mental patients.** *Zhurnal Neuropatologii i Psikhiatrii,* 72(7), 1029–1033.
Studied the frequency of senile plaques and Alzheimer changes in brain intracellular neurofibrils in 300 patients wih senile dementia, vascular (atherosclerotic) psychoses, schizophrenia, and manic-depressive and other psychoses. The age of the S at death, irrespective of the diagnosis, had the greatest significance for the studied changes.

80. Elble, Roger; Giacobini, Ezio & Scarsella, Gian F. (1987). **Cholinesterases in cerebrospinal fluid: A longitudinal study in Alzheimer disease.** *Archives of Neurology,* 44(4), 403–407.
Obtained cerebrospinal fluid (CSF) specimens from 39 patients (aged 50–84 yrs) with dementia of Alzheimer type (DAT) and 21 normal controls (aged 52–80 yrs) and compared the levels of acetylcholinesterase (AChE) and butyrylcholinesterase (BuChE) activities at 6-mo intervals for 12 mo. There was no significant change in CSF AChE and BuChE activities and no significant difference between DAT Ss and controls; therefore, it is concluded that these cannot be used to diagnose DAT.

81. Emson, P. C. et al. (1985). **Neurotensin in human brain: Regional distribution and effects of neurological illness.** *Brain Research,* 347(2), 239–244.
Investigated the regional distribution of neurotensin-like immunoreactivity in 76 normal human brains and in 55 brains of patients who had died with neurological illness. In Huntington's disease, neurotensin was increased in the pallidum, but in Parkinson's disease no changes in neurotensin were observed. No changes were found in the telencephalic neurotensin content in senile dementia of the Alzheimer type. High levels of neurotensin-like immunoreactivity, indistinguishable from synthetic neurotensin, were detected in lumbar cerebrospinal fluid. (43 ref).

82. English, Dallas & Cohen, Donna. (1985). **A case-control study of maternal age in Alzheimer's disease.** *Journal of the American Geriatrics Society,* 33(3), 167–169.
In a case-control study of maternal age (less than 25 yrs vs over 40 yrs) as a risk factor for Alzheimer's disease, clinically diagnosed cases of Alzheimer's disease were identified from an outpatient clinic and an organization of relatives of patients with Alzheimer's disease. Controls were spouses of the Alzheimer's disease cases and spouses of patients with Parkinson's disease. Mail questionnaire responses were received for 90 cases and 96 controls. Among the 69 cases and 94 controls whose mothers' ages were known, there was no evidence that the mothers of cases were significantly older than the mothers of controls. (9 ref).

83. Epelbaum, Jacques et al. (1983). **Somatostatin and dementia in Parkinson's disease.** *Brain Research,* 278(1–2), 376–379.
Assessed concentrations of somatostatin in the cortex, hippocampus, and caudate nucleus of 20 68–78 yr old Ss with Parkinson's disease by radioimmunoassay. Somatostatin levels in the frontal cortex were significantly reduced in parkin-

sonian Ss who were slightly or severely demented compared to 15 controls and to nondemented parkinsonians. Significant reductions were also observed in the hippocampus and entorhinal cortex of severely demented Ss. (24 ref).

84. Esiri, Margaret M.; Pearson, R. C. & Powell, T. P. (1986). **The cortex of the primary auditory area in Alzheimer's disease.** *Brain Research,* 366(1–2), 385–387.
Examined the cortex of the superior temporal gyrus in 2 brains with Alzheimer's disease. Numerous neurofibrillary tangles and neuritic plaques that are characteristic of the disease were present in area 38 in the anterior part of the gyrus and in area 22 more posteriorly, but the primary auditory cortex, area 41, was virtually unaffected by these pathological changes. Findings support the suggestion that the distribution of pathological changes in Alzheimer's disease has an anatomical basis due to spread of the disease process along certain well-defined sets of cortical fiber connections.

85. Esiri, Margaret M. & Williams, R. J. (1986). **Comments on an olfactory source for an environmental influence and possible involvement of aluminum in the development of Alzheimer's disease.** Special Issue: Controversial topics on Alzheimer's disease: Intersecting crossroads. *Neurobiology of Aging,* 7(6), 582–583.
Comments on 3 aspects of E. Roberts's (1986) review by discussing the proposed toxic effects of aluminosilicates transported from nose to brain; the nature of the deposits of aluminum and silicon in plaques; and the way in which aluminum and silicon, if they were to reach the brain in soluble rather than particulate form, might bring about the pathological changes described in Alzheimer's disease.

86. Esiri, Margaret M. & Wilcock, G. K. (1986). **Cerebral amyloid angiopathy in dementia and old age.** *Journal of Neurology, Neurosurgery & Psychiatry,* 49(11), 1221–1226.
Conducted a necropsy study of 82 demented and 67 nondemented elderly patients (45 with Alzheimer's disease [AD]) to investigate the relationship of cerebral amyloid angiopathy (CAA) to AD cerebrovascular disease, cerebral infarction, and aging. There was an 82% incidence of CAA in AD patients. Among demented and nondemented Ss, the incidence of CAA was a little over 30% and remained constant for the ages (60–102 yrs) studied.

87. Fine, Alan. (1986). **Peptides and Alzheimer's disease.** *Nature,* 319(6054), 537–538.
Recent research indicates that the neurochemical pathology of Alzheimer's disease (AD) is not restricted to cholinergic pathways and that corticotropin-releasing factor (CRF) is reduced in several brain areas of AD patients. There is evidence that CRF can modulate cholinergic behavioral effects and cortical somatostatin release in rats. Findings indicate that effective therapy for AD patients must involve peptidergic or alpha-adrenergic agonists and that cholinergic deafferentation of the cortex (including the hippocampus) contributes to the cognitive impairments of AD. (26 ref).

88. Fliers, E.; Swaab, Dick F.; Pool, Chr. W. & Verwer, R. W. (1985). **The vasopressin and oxytocin neurons in the human supraoptic and paraventricular nucleus: Changes with aging and in senile dementia.** *Brain Research,* 342(1), 45–53.
Investigated possible age-related changes in the human hypothalamo-neurohypophyseal system (HNS) by analyzing morphometrically immunocytochemically identified neuropeptides vasopressin (AVP) and oxytocin (OXT) in the paraventricular and supraoptic nucleus in 32 10–93 yr old Ss, 3 of whom were patients with senile dementia of the Alzheimer type (SDAT). Cell size was used as a parameter for peptide production. Mean profile area of OXT cells did not show any significant changes with increasing age. Mean profile area of AVP cells, however, showed an initial decrease up to the 6th decade of life, after which a gradual increase was

observed. Size of AVP and OXT cell nuclei did not change significantly with aging. Observations in brains from Ss with SDAT were within the range for their age group. Results do not support degeneration or diminished function of the HNS in senescence or SDAT, as generally presumed in the literature, but suggest an activation of AVP cells after age 80 yrs. The activation of AVP cells in senescence is in accordance with previous findings in the aged Wistar rat found by D. F. Swaab and colleagues (in press). (45 ref).

89. Flood, Dorothy G.; Buell, Stephen J.; Horwitz, Gary J. & Coleman, Paul D. (1987). **Dendritic extent in human dentate gyrus granule cells in normal aging and senile dementia.** *Brain Research,* 402(2), 205–216.
Investigated dendritic extent (DE) of granule cells in hippocampal gyrii by examining autopsy materials from the brains of 17 cognitively normal Ss (aged 43–95 yrs) and 5 patients (aged 70–81 yrs) with senile dementia of the Alzheimer's type (SDAT). DE increased between middle age (50s) and early old age (70s) in normals, was greatly reduced in SDAT patients in their 70s, and slightly reduced in middle age. Very old normals and SDAT patients (90s) showed similar DE decreases, suggesting that the deficits associated with SDAT cannot be explained solely by DE status of single neurons.

90. Folstein, Marshal F. (1986). **Genetics and Alzheimer's disease: Promises and caveats.** Special Issue: Controversial topics on Alzheimer's disease: Intersecting crossroads. *Neurobiology of Aging,* 7(6), 482.
In commenting on the article by P. Davies (1986), the author advances the view that as research continues to clarify the genetic role in Alzheimer's disease (AD), advances in genetic research can be expected, including the emergence of a field of specialty—geriatric genetics. This, in turn, will present additional ethical problems to the medical profession. Whether the risk to relatives of AD patients is consistent with the risk predicted by a genetic model and what proportions of all cases are genetic probands are discussed.

91. Folstein, Marshal F. & Powell, Diane. (1984). **Is Alzheimer's Disease inherited? A methodologic review.** *Integrative Psychiatry,* 2(5), 163–170.
Contends, on the basis of a critical analysis of the world literature on genetic studies of Alzheimer's disease, that although there is a consensus on clinical and pathologic criteria for diagnosis, these criteria have seldom been applied to family studies. All studies indicate that the disorder is familial, and there is evidence from isolated pedigrees that it is an autosomal dominant disorder with age-dependent expression. Suggested clinical standards for future research include (1) criteria for the dementia syndrome that would begin with amnesia and eventually include apraxia and aphasia; (2) criteria for the pathology that would be specified as greater than 12 plaques or multiple tangles per field; (3) classification as familial or nonfamilial; and (4) appropriate survival analysis for familial cases. (5 ref).

92. Foster, Norman L. et al. (1983). **Alzheimer's disease: Focal cortical changes shown by positron emission tomography.** *Neurology,* 33(8), 961–965.
Estimated local rates of cortical glucose metabolism by positron emission tomography in 13 48–69 yr old right-handed patients with Alzheimer's disease. Ss with disproportionate failure of language function had markedly diminished metabolism in the left-frontal, temporal, and parietal regions. Ss with predominant visuoconstructive dysfunction evidenced a hypometabolic focus in the right parietal cortex. Ss with memory failure as the most apparent feature had no significant metabolic asymmetry in cortical regions. In all Ss, verbal competency generally correlated with metabolic activity in the left-frontal and temporal areas, while visuoconstructive test performance was linked to glucose utilization in the right

parietal lobe. Results indicate that Alzheimer patients with specific preponderant cognitive deficits have a focal, as well as a generalized, reduction in cerebral glucose metabolism. (20 ref).

93. Fox, Jacob H. et al. (1985). **Pathological diagnosis in clinically typical Alzheimer's disease.** *New England Journal of Medicine,* 313(22), 1419–1420.
Conducted a pathological examination (left frontal cortical biopsy) of 11 patients (mean age 64.9 yrs) with a clinical diagnosis of mild or moderate Alzheimer's disease with typical manifestations. The unexpected pathological verification of Alzheimer's disease in all cases underscores accuracy of the clinical diagnosis. It is suggested that the early presence of fixed pathologic changes in the neocortex suggests that treatment attempts may have to be made earlier than is currently believed. (8 ref).

94. Francis, Paul T. et al. (1984). **Somatostatin-like immunoreactivity in lumbar cerebrospinal fluid from neurohistologically examined demented patients.** *Neurobiology of Aging,* 5(3), 183–186.
Measured the concentration of somatostatinlike immunoreactivity (SLI) in the lumbar CSF of 26 Ss (mean age 63.2 yrs) with presenile Alzheimer's dementia (AD), 9 Ss (mean age 79.3 yrs) with senile AD, 5 Ss (mean age 54.4 yrs) with suspected AD or Pick's disease, and 34 22–73 yr old controls. No correlation was found between SLI concentration and age in controls. Compared to controls, SLI was slightly reduced in Ss with presenile AD and in Ss with suspected AD or Pick's disease. Findings support the idea that AD can be divided into early- and late-onset types. (29 ref).

95. Francis, Paul T. et al. (1985). **Neurochemical studies of early-onset Alzheimer's disease: Possible influence on treatment.** *New England Journal of Medicine,* 313(1), 7–11.
Analyzed the relationship between the direct measurement of acetylcholine synthesis from [U-^{14}C] glucose and a rating of cognitive impairment in 17 patients (mean age 56 yrs) with Alzheimer's disease and compared differences in autopsy samples of neurochemical markers of cholinergic, serotoninergic, and noradrenergic neurons. Findings show that synthesis of acetylcholine was significantly correlated with cognitive impairment. These results are consistent with the view that the deficit in the presynaptic cholinergic system is a relatively early change in the development of the clinical features of the disease. It is suggested that other alterations in noradrenergic cells, some cortical neurons, postsynaptic receptors, and serotoninergic cells may not be closely associated with Alzheimer's disease. (38 ref).

96. Fujiyoshi, Kenji; Suga, Hirofumi; Okamoto, Koichi; Nakamura, Shigenobu et al. (1987). **Reduction of arginine-vasopressin in the cerebral cortex in Alzheimer type senile dementia.** *Journal of Neurology, Neurosurgery & Psychiatry,* 50(7), 929–932.
Measured arginine-vasopressin (AVP) concentrations in 5 cortical areas postmortem in 9 patients with senile dementia of Alzheimer's type (SDAT) and compared them with a control group of 19 Ss of comparable ages. In SDAT patients, AVP was significantly reduced in Brodmann Areas 4, 7, and 10. In Areas 17 and 22, the detectability and the mean concentrations of AVP were also lower than those of control patients, although not significantly. The clinical use of AVP is discussed.

97. Gajdusek, D. Carleton. (1986). **Calcium aluminum silicon deposits in neurons lead to paired helical filaments identical to those of AD and Down's patients.** Special Issue: Controversial topics on Alzheimer's disease: Intersecting crossroads. *Neurobiology of Aging,* 7(6), 555–556.

In response to D. R. Crapper McLachlan's (1986) article, the author cites recent evidence that shows that calcium aluminum silicate deposits in neurons lead to the early appearance of neurofibrillary tangles in Western Pacific foci of high incidence amyotrophic lateral sclerosis/Parkinsonism dementia (ALS/PD). Moreover, the N-terminal sequence of the paired helical filament (PHF) in Guamanian PD appears identical to that of the PHF, amyloid plaque core, and vascular amyloid of Alzheimer's disease (AD) and Down's syndrome, reported by others. cDNA clones for the precursor protein of the amyloid demonstrate that the gene lies on chromosome 21.

98. Gajdusek, D. Carleton. (1986). **On the uniform source of amyloid in plaques, tangles and vascular deposits.** Special Issue: Controversial topics on Alzheimer's disease: Intersecting crossroads. *Neurobiology of Aging,* 7(6), 453–454.
In response to D. J. Selkoe (1986), the author contends that a series of studies (e.g., D. Guiroy et al, 1987) involving isolation, sequencing, and cloning of a precursor protein of amyloid of Alzheimer's disease, as well as in aging and Guamanian amyotropic lateral sclerosis/Parkinsonian-dementia syndrome, confirms the unifying hypothesis that the amyloid of paired helical filaments, amyloid plaque cores, and vascular amyloid are of one source. The gene for the precursor protein of this brain amyloid is on chromosome 21.

99. Gambert, Steven R. (1984). **"Is Alzheimer's Disease inherited? A methodologic review": Commentary.** *Integrative Psychiatry,* 2(5), 175–176.
Comments on the hypothesis of M. F. Folstein and D. Powell (1984) that most Alzheimer's disease (AD) is transmitted as an autosomal-dominant age-dependent disorder. It is suggested that if AD is found to be universally inherited, research efforts should be focused on early genetic detection and gene manipulation, rather than on the development of pharmacologic agents to slow progression of the disease. It is emphasized that not all dementia is due to AD, and in the absence of brain biopsy or postmortem autopsy, diagnosis can be made only by excluding other causes of dementia.

100. Gambert, Steven R. (1987). **"Pathological similarities between Alzheimer's disease and Down's syndrome: Is there a genetic link?": Commentary.** *Integrative Psychiatry,* 5(3), 169–170.
In response to M. J. Ball (1987), it is noted that although Alzheimer's disease may be familial, the majority of cases are sporadic, and neuropathological studies comparing Alzheimer's disease with Down's syndrome are few and contain large standard deviations.

101. Gambetti, P. (1986). **Role of aluminum in experimental encephalopathy and in Alzheimer disease: A simple view.** Special Issue: Controversial topics on Alzheimer's disease: Intersecting crossroads. *Neurobiology of Aging,* 7(6), 548–550.
Discusses D. R. Crapper McLachlan's (1986) article by reviewing aluminum (AL) effects on neuronal cytoskeleton and identifying several areas of high priority research. These include the (a) effect of AL on synthesis, assembly, and post-translational modifications of neuronal cytoskeleton, (b) mechanism of tolerance to AL intoxication, (c) intracellular presence of AL in dialysis encephalopathy, and (d) specificity of AL accumulation in neurons bearing neurofibrillary tangles of Alzheimer type.

102. Gambetti, P.; Perry, G. & Autilio-Gambetti, L. (1986). **Paired helical filaments: Do they contain neurofilament epitopes?** Special Issue: Controversial topics on Alzheimer's disease: Intersecting crossroads. *Neurobiology of Aging,* 7(6), 451–452.

Discusses the presence of neurofilament epitopes in paired helical filaments associated with Alzheimer's disease (AD) in view of findings showing no cross-reaction between at least one monoclonal antibody to neurofilament and tau protein. Reference is made to D. J. Selkoe's (1986) views on neurofibrillary tangles and neuritic plaques in AD.

103. Geddes, James W. & Cotman, Carl W. (1986). **Plasticity in hippocampal excitatory amino acid receptors in Alzheimer's disease.** *Neuroscience Research,* 3(6), 672–678.
Used quantitative autoradiography to examine the density and distribution of N-methyl-dextro-aspartate (NMDA) and kainic acid (KA) receptors in human hippocampuses obtained postmortem from 5 Alzheimer's disease patients (61–84 yrs old) and from 5 age-matched controls. In Alzheimer's disease, there was an expanded distribution of the KA receptor field in the dentate gyrus, indicative of sprouting of the commissural and associational fibers. No significant change was observed in the density or distribution of NMDA receptors. The distribution of these receptors did, however, correlate with the predilection for neurofibrillary tangles and neuritic plaques in hippocampal subfields.

104. Ghetti, B. & Bugiani, O. (1986). **"Aluminum's disease" and Alzheimer's disease.** Special Issue: Controversial topics on Alzheimer's disease: Intersecting crossroads. *Neurobiology of Aging,* 7(6), 536–537.
Asserts that although the review of D. R. Crapper McLachlan (1986) contributes to clarifying and strengthening the evidence that aluminum is a powerful neurotoxic substance, at this time the proof that aluminum plays a role in the etiology or pathogenesis of Alzheimer's disease remains elusive.

105. Gibson, Candace J.; Logue, Mary & Growdon, John H. (1985). **CSF monoamine metabolite levels in Alzheimer's and Parkinson's disease.** *Archives of Neurology,* 42(5), 489–492.
Assessed the lumbar CSF of 21 patients with Parkinson's disease (PD) and 32 patients with Alzheimer's disease (AD) with regard to levels of homovanillic acid (HVA), 5-hydroxyindoleacetic acid (5-HIAA), and 3-methoxy-4-hydroxyphenylglycol (MHPG). The lumbar CSF of 17 PD and 20 AD Ss was assessed for these 3 substances following 1 day of probenecid (100 mg/kg) administration. Baseline CSF metabolite values did not differ significantly between the 2 groups. Levels of the 3 metabolites increased in AD and PD Ss after probenecid, but HVA levels were higher in AD than in PD Ss. (44 ref).

106. Gilbert, Avery N. (1986). **The neuropsychology of olfaction in Alzheimer's disease.** Special Issue: Controversial topics on Alzheimer's disease: Intersecting crossroads. *Neurobiology of Aging,* 7(6), 578–579.
Contends that E. Roberts's (1986) proposal of a nasal route of entry for an Alzheimer's disease (AD) pathogen leads to a prediction of olfactory dysfunction in AD patients. Recent studies suggesting the presence of olfactory deficits are reviewed, with special attention given to problems in examining olfactory function in demented patients.

107. Glenner, George G. (1986). **Marching backwards into the future.** Special Issue: Controversial topics on Alzheimer's disease: Intersecting crossroads. *Neurobiology of Aging,* 7(6), 439–441.
Contends that Alzheimer's disease (AD) and its characteristic pathologic lesions are not the fate of all humans as they age, as suggested by D. J. Selkoe (1986). Continuing clues as to the nature and pathogenesis of the amyloid fibrillary component of AD have not arisen stochastically, but have derived from a testable hypothesis. It is proposed that the presence of plaques, tangles, and cerebrovascular amyloid in most cases of adult Down's syndrome is of interest in the potential solution of the nature and pathogenesis of AD.

108. Glenner, George G. (1986). **On primal causes in Alzheimer's disease.** Special Issue: Controversial topics on Alzheimer's disease: Intersecting crossroads. *Neurobiology of Aging,* 7(6), 506–508.
Comments on the article by J. A. Hardy et al (1986) in which they combine various theories to define the pathogenesis of Alzheimer's disease (AD). The present author considers Hardy and colleagues' failure to describe primal causative mechanisms in AD as the most important defect in their theory. A pathogenetic sequence in AD that starts with a gene defect and leads to neuritic plaque formation is postulated.

109. Godderis, J. (1985). **Overzicht van de recente opvattingen betreffende de etiologie en pathogenese van de ziekte van Alzheimer (AD). / Dementia of the Alzheimer type: An overview of recent advances in our understanding of the etiology and pathogenesis of the disease.** *Tijdschrift voor Psychiatrie,* 27(1), 39–55.
Reviews recent studies on the etiology and pathogenesis of Alzheimer's disease (AD), a serious and debilitating disease that accounts for about 50% of autopsied cases of dementia. Although this form of dementia is a surprisingly common disorder that destroys certain vital brain cells, its etiology and pathogenesis remain undetermined. However, evidence suggests that genetic, viral (slow-virus hypothesis), immunologic, and toxic factors may play an important role. It remains unclear whether AD should be considered a single disease, 2 major diseases (presenile and senile), or a heterogeneous group of disorders with similar clinical and pathologic characteristics. Recent neuroanatomical and biochemical studies provide growing support for clinical and pathologic heterogeneity in this so-called primary degenerative brain disease. (English abstract).

110. Godridge, H.; Reynolds, G. P.; Czudek, C.; Calcutt, N. A. et al. (1987). **Alzheimer-like neurotransmitter deficits in adult Down's syndrome brain tissue.** *Journal of Neurology, Neurosurgery & Psychiatry,* 50(6), 775–778.
Analyzed brain tissue taken at necropsy from 5 cases of Down syndrome and 6 controls for changes in neurotransmitter markers. Concentrations of noradrenaline (NA), dopamine and its major metabolite homovanillic acid, and 5-hydroxytryptamine (5-HT) and its metabolite 5-hydroxyindoleacetic acid were determined by high pressure liquid chromatography, while choline acetyltransferase (ChAT) was measured by a radiochemical technique. Significant reductions in NA, 5-HT and ChAT were found in most cortical and subcortical regions of the Down syndrome tissue. Neuropathological lesions were also assessed. Results indicate profound transmitter deficits and neuropathological abnormalities in adult patients with Down syndrome that closely resemble those of Alzheimer's disease.

111. Gomez, S.; Davous, P.; Rondot, P.; Faivre-Bauman, A. et al. (1986). **Somatostatin-like immunoreactivity and acetylcholinesterase activities in cerebrospinal fluid of patients with Alzheimer disease and senile dementia of the Alzheimer type.** *Psychoneuroendocrinology,* 11(1), 69–73.
Measured somatostatinlike immunoreactivity (SLI) and acetylcholinesterase (AchE) activities in the cerebrospinal fluid (CSF) of 13 53–73 yr old patients with probable Alzheimer's disease (AD), 12 73–91 yr old patients with senile dementia of the Alzheimer type (SDAT), and 11 controls. Both SLI levels and AchE activities were reduced in the CSF of SDAT and AD Ss. The SLI levels and AchE activities were not correlated with the duration and the dementia score. However, in 2 AD Ss, the CSF SLI concentration was in agreement with the SLI levels in the frontal cortex obtained by biopsy. Findings suggest that CSF SLI may be a good index of cortical SLI activities. (19 ref).

112. Gomez, S.; Puymirat, J.; Ualade, P.; Davous, P. et al. (1986). **Patients with Alzheimer's disease show an increased content of 15Kdalton somatostatin precursor and a lowered level of tetradecapeptide in their cerebrospinal fluid.** *Life Sciences,* 39(7), 623–627.
Evaluated the proportions of both somatostatin-14 and its precursors somatostatin-28 and the 15Kdalton prosomatostatin in the cerebrospinal fluid of 5 patients (aged 59–78 yrs) with Alzheimer's disease. Relative to 4 normal 72–99 yr olds, Alzheimer's Ss had a lowered content of the tetradecapeptide somatostatin and a significant increase in the unprocessed 15Kdalton precursor. Results indicate that Alzheimer's patients possess impaired processing mechanisms that may be responsible for lowered somatostatin-14.

113. Gottfries, C. G. (1986). **Is Alzheimer's a homogeneous disease, are plaques critical and does the blood brain barrier really contribute?** Special Issue: Controversial topics on Alzheimer's disease: Intersecting crossroads. *Neurobiology of Aging,* 7(6), 510–511.
Proposes that several problems exist with the speculative hypothesis presented by J. A. Hardy et al (1986) on the nature and pathogenesis of Alzheimer's disease (AD). The relationship between neuritic plaques and clinical symptoms is not well established and is further complicated by the likely existence of multiple subforms of AD. It is further argued that direct support for changes in the blood brain barrier with AD is lacking, and the available circumstantial evidence argues against it having an important role in the pathogenesis of the disease.

114. Gottfries, C. G. (1985). **Alzheimer's disease and senile dementia: Biochemical characteristics and aspects of treatment.** *Psychopharmacology,* 86(3), 245–252.
A literature review suggests that although Alzheimer's disease (AD) and senile dementia (SD) are often classified together, there are genetic, biochemical, neuropathological, and clinical arguments for separating them. The Alzheimer lesions in the brains of patients with AD and SD are described, as is the loss of neurons in the locus coeruleus. White-matter changes in brains of patients with dementia are also discussed. Biochemical changes in brains of AD and SD patients include reduced activity of acetylcholinesterase and choline-acetyltransferase, indicating reduced activity in the acetylcholinergic system. There is also, however, reduced activity in the dopamine (DA), noradrenaline (NA), and 5-hydroxytryptamine (5-HT) system. Monoamine oxidase (MAO) B is also increased in AD and SD patients. Disturbances in the acetylcholinergic system may explain memory disturbances, disturbances in the DA system may explain parkinsonlike symptoms, and disturbances in the NA and 5-HT systems may explain mood disturbances and emotional symptoms in the disorder. The biochemical changes may also suggest a line of treatment. At present, several attempts have been made to activate the neurotransmitter systems, but the progress of these studies has not been encouraging. (56 ref).

115. Gottfries, C. G. (1985). **Transmitter deficits in Alzheimer's disease.** *Neurochemistry International,* 7(4), 565–566.
Comments on the review by J. Hardy et al (1985) and presents evidence that offers more support for the assumption that Alzheimer's disease and senile dementia are 2 different disorders than for the assumption that they are etiologically the same disorder. It is concluded that the present delimitation of dementia disorders is insufficient. (8 ref).

116. Gottfries, C. G. et al. (1974). **Cerebrospinal fluid pH and monoamine and glucolytic metabolites in Alzheimer's disease.** *British Journal of Psychiatry,* 124, 280–287.
Chemical analysis of cerebrospinal fluid from 15 inpatients with Alzheimer's disease, which causes degenerative changes in the cortex and limbic system, confirmed prior findings of impaired metabolism. It is noted that cellular hypoxia may be present in this disease. Dementia, measured by rating scales, correlated with the homovanillic acid, lactate, and pH content of the fluid samples. (33 ref).

117. Gottfries, Carl-Gerhard et al. (1983). **Biochemical changes in dementia disorders of Alzheimer type (AD/SDAT).** *Neurobiology of Aging,* 4(4), 261–271.
In postmortem examinations, the brain weights of 14 67–85 yr old AD/SDAT patients were significantly reduced relative to those of 16 age-matched controls. In the brains of AD/SDAT Ss, decreases in concentrations of 5-HT, noradrenaline, dopamine, and ganglioside and in choline acetyltransferase activity were found, while increases were noted in MAO B activity and 3-methoxy-4-hydroxyphenylglycol concentration. Intellectual impairment and biochemical disturbances were greater among Ss with early- than late-onset dementia. (71 ref).

118. Gottfries, Carl-Gerhard; Bartfai, Tamas; Carlsson, Arvid; Eckernäs, Sven-Ake et al. (1986). **Multiple biochemical deficits in both gray and white matter of Alzheimer's brains.** *Progress in Neuro-Psychopharmacology & Biological Psychiatry,* 10(3–5), 405–413.
Conducted a postmortem biochemical investigation of 21 brains from patients (mean age 79.3 yrs) with dementia of Alzheimer type (DAT) and 22 brains from controls (mean age 75.6 yrs). It is concluded that in brains from Ss with DAT there were multiple biochemical deficits in gray as well as in white matter. The changes in white matter may be of pathogenetic importance in subgroups of patients with DAT.

119. Greenamyre, J. Timothy. (1986). **The role of glutamate in neurotransmission and in neurologic disease.** *Archives of Neurology,* 43(10), 1058–1063.
Reviews the recent body of physiologic and biochemical evidence that suggests that glutamate is a major excitatory neurotransmitter in the central nervous system (CNS). Glutamate as a neurotoxin and its role in Huntington's disease, epilepsy, hypoxia/ischemia, olivopontocerebellar atrophy, hypoglycemic brain damage, and Alzheimer's disease are discussed. It is suggested that manipulation of the glutamatergic system may be of use in the treatment or prevention of such diseases.

120. Gusella, James F. (1986). **The molecular genetic approach to familial Alzheimer's disease.** Special Issue: Controversial topics on Alzheimer's disease: Intersecting crossroads. *Neurobiology of Aging,* 7(6), 472–473.
Concurs with P. Davies (1986) that there is a strong case to be made for locating the genetic defect underlying at least some proportion of Alzheimer's disease (AD) cases. A strategy involving linkage analysis with DNA markers has already been implemented and has good prospects for success. The ultimate identification of a linked marker could, however, be hastened by the identification, documentation, sampling, and banking of additional large kindreds in which AD appears to inherit as an autosomal dominant defect.

121. Guth, Lloyd. (1986). **Commentary on the speculations that Alzheimer's disease may begin in the nose and may be caused by aluminosilicates.** Special Issue: Controversial topics on Alzheimer's disease: Intersecting crossroads. *Neurobiology of Aging,* 7(6), 572.
Critiques E. Roberts's (1986) comprehensive explanation of the pathogenesis of Alzheimer's disease (AD), suggesting that it represents a potentially new principle of neuropathogenesis that can be applied to various neurological disorders. The olfactory cells are considered a likely site for AD to begin because those neurons are deprived of the more extensive physiological protections (e.g., blood-brain barrier) and are vulnerable to toxic substances (e.g., aluminosilicates) in the air.

122. Haberland, Catherine (1969). **Alzheimer's disease in Down syndrome: Clinical-neuropathological observations.** *Acta Neurologica et Psychiatrica Belgica,* 69(6), 369–380.
The histopathologic features of Alzheimer's disease were presented in 6 persons with Down's syndrome (aged 34–74 yrs). Chromosomal study in 1 S showed a G-trisomy karyotype. The onset of Alzheimer's disease was conspicuous in 2 cases. Convulsive disorder was present in 3 of the Ss. There was an increase in severity and multiformity of senile cerebral pathology with increasing age of the patients. (French & German summaries).

123. Hachinski, Vladimir C.; Potter, Paul & Merskey, Harold. (1987). **Leuko-araiosis.** *Archives of Neurology,* 44(1), 21–23.
Proposes the term leuko-araiosis to define changes in brain-deep white matter for use in clinical and imaging descriptions. Evidence associating white matter changes with cognitive impairment is discussed, and connections between such changes and Binswanger's disease are refuted. The possible etiology of white matter changes as well as their relationship to Alzheimer's disease are explored.

124. Hardy, John A.; Mann, David M.; Wester, P. & Winblad, B. (1986). **"An integrative hypothesis concerning the pathogenesis and progression of Alzheimer's disease": Authors' response to commentaries.** Special Issue: Controversial topics on Alzheimer's disease: Intersecting crossroads. *Neurobiology of Aging,* 7(6), 520–522.
The authors (1986) respond to a series of commentary papers by C. B. Saper, H. M. Wisniewski et al, C. G. Rasool, G. G. Glenner, R. Katzman, C. G. Gottfries, T. Miyakawa, S. H. Appel and J. L. McManaman, F. Hefti, C. L. Masters, P. J. Whitehouse and J. R. Unnerstall, and J. Rogers (1986) concerning their discussion of blood brain barrier function in Alzheimer's disease.

125. Hardy, John A.; Mann, David M.; Wester, P. & Winblad, B. (1986). **An integrative hypothesis concerning the pathogenesis and progression of Alzheimer's disease.** Special Issue: Controversial topics on Alzheimer's disease: Intersecting crossroads. *Neurobiology of Aging,* 7(6), 489–502.
Presents a hypothesis to explain the pathogenesis and progression of Alzheimer's disease (AD), drawing together observations on the pattern of nerve cell damage and loss; the pathology, microchemistry and immunology of senile plaques and neurofibrillary tangles; and alterations in blood vessels. At the heart of this hypothesis lies a defect in blood brain barrier (BBB) function and/or structure within the cerebral cortex; this defect may cause the cerebral vessel amyloidosis common in many AD patients. Age-related alterations in BBB allow for damage to nerve terminals and limited formation of senile plaques within cerebral cortex; neurofibrillary tangles are formed within cortical and subcortical nerve cells that project to or near damaged vessels/senile plaques. Loss of cells in cortically projecting areas of subcortex causes further BBB dysfunction, new plaque formation, and continued cell loss in cortex and subcortex. Clinical dementia results once a threshold of nerve cell damage and loss is reached.

126. Hardy, John et al. (1985). **Transmitter deficits in Alzheimer's disease.** *Neurochemistry International,* 7(4), 545–563.
A review of the pattern of neurotransmitter pathway losses in Alzheimer's disease reveals deficits of the cholinergic pathway from the nucleus basalis, the noradrenergic pathway from the locus coeruleus, and the serotoninergic pathway from the raphe nuclei. Damage to the cortical somatostatin interneurons, dopaminergic neurons, and other neuronal systems, particularly in the hippocampus and temporal cortex, has also been found. A hypothesis is offered that suggests that the basis of the selective neuronal degeneration is due to (1)

chronic attack on nerve endings, (2) the fact that nerve endings with long projections are least able to withstand such attack, and (3) a likely site for this attack is the innervation of the brain blood vessels. (5½ p ref).

127. Haugh, M. C.; Probst, A.; Ulrich, J.; Kahn, J. et al. (1986). **Alzheimer neurofibrillary tangles contain phosphorylated and hidden neurofilament epitopes.** *Journal of Neurology, Neurosurgery & Psychiatry,* 49(11), 1213–1220.
Examined the specificity to phosphorylated epitopes of 3 monoclonal antibodies to neurofilaments: RT97 and BF10, which also recognize neurofibrillary tangles (associated with senile dementia of the Alzheimer type), and antibody 147. Treatment of cerebral cortex, hippocampus, and cerebellum sections with alkaline phosphatase prior to immunostaining resulted in reduction of axonal neurofilament staining with all 3 antibodies. Antibody 147 was found to recognize some neurofibrillary tangles following alkaline phosphatase treatment. Results indicate the presence of structurally abnormal but phosphorylated neurofilaments in neurofibrillary tangles.

128. Haxby, James V.; Grady, Cheryl L.; Duara, Ranjan; Schlageter, Nicholas et al. (1986). **Neocortical metabolic abnormalities precede nonmemory cognitive defects in early Alzheimer's-type dementia.** *Archives of Neurology,* 43(9), 882–885.
Studied 10 patients (mean age 63.7 yrs) with mild dementia of the Alzheimer's type (DAT), 12 patients (mean age 66.7 yrs) with moderate DAT, 25 psychological testing controls (mean age 62.9 yrs), and 29 positron-emission tomography patients (mean age 63.5 yrs). Results for DAT Ss demonstrated parietotemporal reductions and left–right asymmetries in resting neocortical regional cerebral metabolic rates for glucose (rCMRglc) patterns. Significant language and visuoconstructive deficits in moderate DAT Ss were related to left–right asymmetry of rCMRglc in the association cortices.

129. Haxby, James V. & Rapoport, Stanley I. (1986). **Abnormalities of regional brain metabolism in Alzheimer's disease and their relation to functional impairment.** *Progress in Neuro-Psychopharmacology & Biological Psychiatry,* 10(3–5), 427–438.
This review of the literature covers neuropsychological changes in Alzheimer's disease (AD), changing patterns of neuropsychological deficits due to disease progression, individual variations in patterns of neuropsychological deficits, measurement of cerebral blood flow (CBF) and metabolism, global CBF, regional CBF, positron emission tomography (PET), the relation of regional cerebral metabolic rate for glucose and neuropsychological asymmetries in AD, and correlations of metabolic and neuropsychological asymmetries. It is concluded that resting brain metabolism in patients with AD has been demonstrated to be reduced, and the magnitude of the reduction is related to the severity of dementia. PET, which provides regional metabolic rates for glucose in cross-sectional slices of brain, has demonstrated 3 alterations in AD that are related to functional deficits.

130. Hefti, F. (1986). **On the pathogenesis of Alzheimer's disease.** Special Issue: Controversial topics on Alzheimer's disease: Intersecting crossroads. *Neurobiology of Aging,* 7(6), 514–515.
Comments on the article by J. A. Hardy et al (1986) and suggests that recent findings have revealed that Alzheimer's disease (AD) is associated with degenerative changes in many neurotransmitter systems. However, these changes do not explain the existence of neuritic plaques and neurofibrillary tangles. Deficits in cholinergic and catecholaminergic systems might be responsible for some of the typical behavioral deficits associated with AD. Malfunction of the blood brain

14

barrier (BBB) represents one of the hypothetical mechanisms postulated to play a crucial role in the pathogenesis of AD. To support this hypothesis, it has to be shown that BBB changes precede the behavioral manifestations of AD.

131. Henderson, Victor W. (1986). **Non-genetic factors in Alzheimer's disease pathogenesis.** Special Issue: Controversial topics on Alzheimer's disease: Intersecting crossroads. *Neurobiology of Aging,* 7(6), 585–587.
Argues that incomplete and insufficient data fail to distinguish between genetic and environmental hypotheses of Alzheimer's disease (AD) pathogenesis. It is suggested that theories such as those proposed by E. Roberts (1986) that implicate aluminosilicates in AD pathogenesis and that emphasize nongenetic mechanisms offer greater opportunity for prevention and cure than do those that assume AD to be genetically determined.

132. Henderson, Victor W. (1986). **Ambiguities in Alzheimer's disease diagnosis: Implications for genetic research.** Special Issue: Controversial topics on Alzheimer's disease: Intersecting crossroads. *Neurobiology of Aging,* 7(6), 469–471.
In commenting on P. Davies's (1986) article, the present author suggests that genetic studies of Alzheimer's disease (AD) are currently limited by clinical and neuropathologic diagnostic uncertainties. A part of the problem is the clinical-pathological overlap between AD and other disorders (e.g., AD with coincidental infarction is difficult to distinguish from multi-infarct dementia without AD changes). AD may be less amenable to modern techniques of genetic analysis than other disorders in which diagnosis is more straightforward and heritability more clearly established.

133. Hershey, Linda A.; Hershey, Charles O. & Varnes, Arthur W. (1984). **CSF silicon in dementia: A prospective study.** *Neurology,* 34(9), 1197–1201.
Designed a prospective study to determine whether CSF silicon elevation is specific for Alzheimer-type dementia (ATD) and whether it is related to the severity of cognitive or functional impairment. Findings show elevated CSF silicon in 30% of 23 52–84 yr old ATD patients but in only 1 of 23 age-matched nondemented controls. In all ATD patients with elevated CSF silicon, symptoms began after age 65 yrs; 34% of 29 44–86 yr old patients with other types of dementia also had elevated CSF silicon. It is concluded that elevated CSF silicon concentrations are not specific for ATD, but they correlate with age and severity of functional impairment in late-onset ATD. (25 ref).

134. Heston, L. L. & White, June. (1978). **Pedigrees of 30 families with Alzheimer disease: Associations with defective organization of microfilaments and microtubules.** *Behavior Genetics,* 8(4), 315–331.
A study of 30 families located through a proband with Alzheimer disease revealed highly significant excesses of Down's syndrome and immunocytic cancer. A genetic disorder of immune function mediated by microtubules and microfilaments is suggested by the data. The pedigrees of the Alzheimer families are presented. (25 ref).

135. Heston, Leonard L. (1988). **Morbid risk in first-degree relatives of persons with Alzheimer's disease.** *Archives of General Psychiatry,* 45(1), 97–98.
Discusses 2 methodological reasons for doubting the conclusions of R. C. Mohs et al (1987) regarding the morbid risk of 1st-degree relatives of persons with Alzheimer's disease.

136. Hiller, Jacob M.; Itzhak, Yossef & Simon, Eric J. (1987). **Selective changes in μ, δ and χ opioid receptor binding in certain limbic regions of the brain in Alzheimer's disease patients.** *Brain Research,* 406(1–2), 17–23.
Measured total opioid binding and levels of the 3 major types of opioid binding sites in homogenates of various limbic structures from postmortem brains of 7 Alzheimer's disease (AD) patients (aged 58–68 yrs) and 5 age-matched controls. The most consistent finding in AD brains was an increase in chi binding in all 6 areas of the limbic system examined. The AD putamen showed a significantly higher level of total binding. The amygdala of AD Ss exhibited significantly lower levels of mu and delta binding.

137. Hinton, David R.; Sadun, Alfredo A.; Blanks, Janet C. & Miller, Carol A. (1986). **Optic-nerve degeneration in Alzheimer's disease.** *New England Journal of Medicine,* 315(8), 485–487.
In postmortem studies, widespread axonal degeneration was found in the optic nerves of 8 of 10 patients (aged 73–89 yrs) with Alzheimer's disease. The retinas of 4 Ss were also examined histologically, and 3 had a reduction in the number of ganglion cells and in the thickness of the nerve-fiber layer. There was no retinal neurofibrillary degeneration or amyloid angiopathy, both of which are typically seen in the brains of patients with Alzheimer's disease. The changes observed in the Alzheimer's disease Ss were clearly distinguishable from the findings in 10 age-matched nondemented controls.

138. Horwitz, Barry; Grady, Cheryl L.; Schlageter, N. L.; Duara, Ranjan et al. (1987). **Intercorrelations of regional cerebral glucose metabolic rates in Alzheimer's disease.** *Brain Research,* 407(2), 294–306.
Compared patterns of cerebral metabolic correlations between 21 Alzheimer's disease (AD) patients (aged 45–80 yrs) and 21 healthy age-matched controls in the resting state, using positron emission tomography. Partial correlation coefficients were evaluated between pairs of regional glucose metabolic rates in 59 brain regions. Compared with controls, the AD Ss had significantly fewer reliable partial correlation coefficients between frontal and parietal lobe regions and more reliable correlations between the cerebellum and temporal lobe. The number of reliable correlations between many bilaterally symmetric brain regions was reduced in the AD Ss compared with controls. Results suggest that in the early stages of AD, there is a breakdown of the organized functional activity between the 2 cerebral hemispheres and between parietal and frontal lobe structures.

139. Hoyer, Siegfried. (1986). **Senile dementia and Alzheimer's disease: Brain blood flow and metabolism.** *Progress in Neuro-Psychopharmacology & Biological Psychiatry,* 10(3–5), 447–478.
This review of the literature concerning senile dementia and Alzheimer's disease considers the normally aged brain, global cerebral blood flow, global oxidative metabolism, blood flow in cerebral gray and white matter, and oxidative metabolism in cerebral gray and white matter. Brain blood flow and oxidative metabolism have been found to be reduced in patients with Alzheimer's disease.

140. Hubler, Donn W. (1985). **The relationship between volumetric measurements of cerebral atrophy and neuropsychological test results in Alzheimer's disease.** *Dissertation Abstracts International,* 46(4-B), 1374.

141. Inzitari, Domenico; Diaz, Fernando; Fox, Allan J.; Hachinski, Vladimir C. et al. (1987). **Vascular risk factors and leuko-araiosis.** *Archives of Neurology,* 44(1), 42–47.
Studied (1) the risk factors and events that correlate with leuko-araiosis (LA), (2) the extent to which LA is linked with dementia, and (3) the relationship between LA and the types of dementia, and the ischemic scale. 140 patients (mean age 71.8 yrs) referred for dementia and 110 mentally normal controls (mean age 71.3 yrs) served as Ss. Findings show that 49 of the patients and 12 of the controls had LA; 31 of the 95 patients with Alzheimer's type dementia had LA; a history

of stroke was 4 times more likely in those with LA than in those without; and mean systolic blood pressure was associated with LA.

142. Iqbal, Khalid. (1986). **Biology of Alzheimer's disease through biochemistry of tangles and plaques.** Special Issue: Controversial topics on Alzheimer's disease: Intersecting crossroads. *Neurobiology of Aging,* 7(6), 434–437.
Responds to the article by D. J. Selkoe (1986), by maintaining that recent advances on identification of the polypeptides making the paired helical filaments of Alzheimer neurofibrillary tangles and the neuritic (senile) plaque amyloid have provided a new insight into the pathogenesis of Alzheimer's disease (AD). Major breakthroughs toward establishing the underlying primary defect in AD are now in sight. The strength of various data toward identification of the polypeptides of tangles and plaques and the role of these proteins in the biology of AD are discussed.

143. Jolkkonen, J. T.; Sonininen, H. S. & Riekkinen, P. J. (1985). **The effect of ACTH4-9 analog (Org 2766) on some cerebrospinal fluid parameters in patients with Alzheimer's disease.** *Life Sciences,* 37(7), 585–590.
Assessed the central nervous system (CNS) effects of an adrenocorticotropic (ACTH)4-9 analog, Org 2766 (40 mg/day), in Alzheimer's disease by measuring cerebrospinal fluid (CSF) parameters in 75 patients (aged 58–90 yrs) during treatment for 6 mo. Results show that somatostatinlike immunoreactivity and cholinesterase activity did not change during treatment, and dopamine-beta-hydroxylase and homovanillic acid levels remained static. Results suggest that Org 2766 did not interact with the transmitter systems that are thought to be disturbed in Alzheimer's disease. (38 ref).

144. Jope, Richard S. (1986). **Aluminum toxicity: Transport and sites of action.** Special Issue: Controversial topics on Alzheimer's disease: Intersecting crossroads. *Neurobiology of Aging,* 7(6), 541–542.
Responds to D. R. Crapper McLachlan's (1986) review of the role of aluminum (AL) in Alzheimer's disease, by suggesting that emphasis should be placed on 2 aspects of AL neurotoxicity—mechanisms mediating the transport of AL, including peripheral absorption, entry into the central nervous system (CNS), and neuronal uptake—and identification of sites in the CNS that are highly susceptible to the presence of AL.

145. Kang, Jie; Lemaire, Hans-Georg; Unterbeck, Axel; Salbaum, J. Michael et al. (1987). **The precursor of Alzheimer's disease amyloid A4 protein resembles a cell-surface receptor.** *Nature,* 325(6106), 733–736.
Identified the precursor of the A4 protein associated with the formation of neurofibrillary tangles and extracellular plaques in Alzheimer's disease (AD) patients. The precursor DNA sequence contains features characteristic of glycosylated cell-surface receptors. This sequence, together with the localization of its gene on chromosome 21, suggests that the cerebral amyloid deposited in AD, as well as in aged Down syndrome, is caused by aberrant catabolism of a cell-surface receptor.

146. Karlinsky, Harry. (1986). **Alzheimer's disease in Down's syndrome: A review.** *Journal of the American Geriatrics Society,* 34(10), 728–734.
Summarizes the evidence of an association between Alzheimer's disease (AD) and Down's syndrome (DS) and reviews hypotheses that attempt to account for the relationship. The presence of neurofibrillary tangles and senile plaques in both AD and DS and the prevalence of dementia in DS patients are discussed. Hypotheses citing common chromosomal abnormalities and pathogenesis are presented.

147. Katzman, Robert. (1986). **Role of neuritic plaques and blood brain barrier in pathogenesis of Alzheimer's disease.** Special Issue: Controversial topics on Alzheimer's disease: Intersecting crossroads. *Neurobiology of Aging,* 7(6), 508–509.
Reviews the article on Alzheimer's disease (AD) by J. A. Hardy et al (1986) in which they suggest primary roles for the neuritic plaque and a breakdown in the blood brain barrier in AD. It is argued that although the role of the plaque seems reasonable and empirically justified, the hypothesized role for changes in the blood brain barrier as put forward by Hardy et al remains in doubt.

148. Katzman, Robert. (1986). **Alzheimer's disease.** *Trends in Neurosciences,* 9(10), 522–525.
Reviews neurological and neuropsychological research on Alzheimer's disease (AD). Cognitive deficits, cell loss, and cell changes (particularly the neurofibrillary tangle and neuritic plaque) are considered. The chemical structure, source, and pathogenesis of the fibrous proteins characterizing AD are discussed.

149. Kay, Arthur D.; Milstien, Sheldon; Kaufman, Seymour; Creasey, Helen et al. (1986). **Cerebrospinal fluid biopterin is decreased in Alzheimer's disease.** *Archives of Neurology,* 43(10), 996–999.
Assayed cerebrospinal fluid (CSF) and plasma for biopterin in 30 Alzheimer's disease (AD) patients (aged 45–84 yrs) and in 19 healthy controls (aged 20–85 yrs), and correlated the results with CSF concentrations of 5-hydroxyindoleacetic acid, homovanillic acid (HVA), norepinephrine, and 3-methoxy-4-hydroxyphenylglycol. CSF concentration of biopterin was significantly less in the AD group than in age-matched controls. CSF biopterin concentration correlated significantly with CSF HVA.

150. Kay, D. W. (1987). **Heterogeneity in Alzheimer's disease: Epidemiological and family studies.** *Trends in Neurosciences,* 10(5), 194–195.
Discusses recent epidemiological and family studies that have supported both single gene and multifactorial etiologies in Alzheimer's disease (AD). The present author maintains that both hypotheses may be correct, but more data on the incidence of AD at very advanced ages would help to discriminate between them. Advances in molecular biology and the occurrence of AD in Down's syndrome offer additional opportunities of studying the genetic basis of AD.

151. Kellar, Kenneth J.; Whitehouse, Peter J.; Martino-Barrows, Andrea M.; Marcus, Kendall et al. (1987). **Muscarinic and nicotinic cholinergic binding sites in Alzheimer's disease cerebral cortex.** *Brain Research,* 436(1), 62–68.
Measured the total population of muscarinic receptors and a subpopulation of muscarinic receptors with high affinity for agonists with [³H]quinuclidinyl benzilate and [³H]acetylcholine in homogenates of cerebral cortex from control and Alzheimer's disease brains (ADBs). No significant differences between control and ADBs were found. However, when nicotinic cholinergic receptors labeled by [³H]acetylcholine were measured in homogenates and by autoradiography in the same brain areas, binding to nicotinic sites was markedly decreased in ADBs.

152. Khachaturian, Z. S. (1986). **Aluminum toxicity among other views on the etiology of Alzheimer disease.** Special Issue: Controversial topics on Alzheimer's disease: Intersecting crossroads. *Neurobiology of Aging,* 7(6), 537–539.
In response to D. R. Crapper McLachlan (1986), the present author proposes that aluminum (AL) toxicity must be viewed as only one among several co-factors in the etiology of Alzheimer's disease (AD). A brief overview of the major clusters of studies concerned with identifying the cause(s) of AD is

provided. The present author also suggests that AL's role needs to be examined in the broader context of other ideas concerning the etiology of AD (e.g., genetics, metabolic disorders, blood-brain barrier changes, neurochemical deficits).

153. Knesevich, John W. et al. (1982). **Birth order and maternal age effect in dementia of the Alzheimer type.** *Psychiatry Research,* 7(3), 345–350.
Birth order and maternal age were unrelated to dementia of the Alzheimer type (DAT) in a study of 42 probands with clinically diagnosed DAT and 42 age-matched control Ss. Mean birth order in both groups did not differ significantly from the general population. The mean maternal age for the DAT probands was neither significantly different from that for the controls nor from that for the 1920 US Caucasian population. Since the diagnostic criteria for the DAT group were only clinical, an additional 14 probands with DAT confirmed by autopsy were studied. Mean maternal age did not differ significantly in this group from the controls, the general population, or the clinically diagnosed DAT group. It is concluded that maternal age and birth order bear no special relationship to DAT in this sample. (18 ref).

154. Kolata, Gina. (1986). **Researchers hunt for Alzheimer's disease gene.** *Science,* 232(4749), 448–450.
Indicates that at least some cases of Alzheimer's disease appear to be inherited as though there were a dominant gene, leading researchers to believe that they can find a gene that causes the disease.

155. Kolata, Gina. (1985). **Down syndrome–Alzheimer's linked.** *Science,* 230(4730), 1152–1153.
Discusses studies of the parallels between Down syndrome and Alzheimer's disease. It is indicated that Down syndrome adults over age 30 develop brain lesions that are typical of Alzheimer's disease. In both cases, the brain tissue contains extensive plaques and tangles—lesions that appear to be concentrated in the hippocampus, the area of the brain that plays a selective role in learning and memory. However, only 25–40% of Down syndrome adults actually become demented.

156. Kopelman, Michael D. (1986). **The cholinergic neurotransmitter system in human memory and dementia: A review.** Special Issue: Human memory. *Quarterly Journal of Experimental Psychology: Human Experimental Psychology,* 38(4-A), 535–573.
Reviews 3 types of evidence implicating the role of acetylcholine in human memory and dementia: (1) neuropathological evidence that the cholinergic transmitter system is depleted in Alzheimer-type dementia; (2) psychopharmacological studies that have employed cholinergic blockade as a model of cholinergic depletion; and (3) clinical studies of cholinergic "replacement" therapy in Alzheimer-type dementia. Evidence that the cholinergic system is depleted in Alzheimer-type dementia has been complemented by the finding that cholinergic blockade in healthy Ss causes a substantial learning deficit in episodic memory. Studies of replacement therapy have generally been disappointing, and the role of the cholinergic system remains to be elucidated.

157. Koss, Elisabeth; Friedland, Robert P.; Ober, Beth A. & Jagust, William J. (1985). **Differences in lateral hemispheric asymmetries of glucose utilization between early- and late-onset Alzheimer-type dementia.** *American Journal of Psychiatry,* 142(5), 638–640.
Performed positron emission tomography on 18 55–75 yr old patients who met DSM-III criteria for primary degenerative dementia. Each S received iv injections of 5–10 mCi of [^{18}F]fluorodeoxyglucose. Results indicate greater right- than left-hemispheric impairment of cortical glucose metabolism in the Ss with probable Alzheimer's disease who were younger than 65 yrs but not in Ss over 65 yrs of age. This asymmetry was related to poor visuospatial performance. (10 ref).

158. Kral, V. A. (1976). **On the etiology of senile dementia.** *Psychiatric Journal of the University of Ottawa,* 1(1-2), 31–34.
Discusses the etiology of senile dementia. Emphasis is placed on the following points: (a) Senile dementia and Alzheimer's presenile dementia are one disease. It occurs in only a relatively small proportion of the population. (b) A genetic factor appears to operate in the etiology of Alzheimer's dementia. (c) Alzheimer patients have an increased sensitivity to stress, such that stress seems to be at least a contributing etiological factor. It is proposed that the genetic factor (or factors) involve primarily a weakness of the stress resisting mechanism, particularly the hypothalamic portion. (21 ref).

159. Kulmala, Henrik K. & Hutton, J. Thomas. (1985). **Role of the senile plaque in neuropeptide deficits of Alzheimer's disease.** Eighth Annual Meeting of the Canadian College of Neuropsychopharmacology: Perspectives in Canadian neuro-psychopharmacology (1985, London, Canada). *Progress in Neuro-Psychopharmacology & Biological Psychiatry,* 9(5–6), 625–628.
Examined postmortem brain tissue of 7 controls and 13 patients with Alzheimer's disease (AD) to investigate the formation of senile plaques (SPs). Results show that SPs participated in a cropping of the dendritic tree of enkephalinergic dentate granule cells and hl and subicular pyramidal cells. Somatostatin-containing pyramidal neurons were lost in AD, whereas nonpyramidal somatostatin neurons were less affected. Fibers containing somatostatin penetrated immature, but not end-stage, SPs. Findings suggest that SPs may precipitate much of the hippocampal denervation seen in AD. (8 ref).

160. Lal, S. et al. (1984). **CSF acetylcholinesterase in dementia and in sequential samples of lumbar CSF.** *Neurobiology of Aging,* 5(4), 269–274.
Measured acetylcholinesterase (AchE) activity (nmol/ml/min) in lumbar CSF from 11 56–89 yr old patients with dementia of the Alzheimer type (DAT), 8 53–74 yr old patients with Korsakoff psychosis, and 33 20–78 yr old patients with low back pain who were undergoing myelography (controls). There was no significant difference in enzyme activity between the 3 groups, nor was there a significant correlation between age and AchE activity. AchE was also measured in 20 2-ml samples of CSF collected sequentially by lumbar puncture in 2 neurosurgical patients (aged 63 and 79 yrs) who had been recumbent for at least 8 hrs. Variations in AchE between samples were small. In neither patient was there an increase in AchE activity with progressive sampling. These data indicate the following: (1) AchE is unchanged in Korsakoff psychosis. (2) Decreases in brain AchE that are found in DAT are not readily reflected in lumbar CSF. (3) AchE in lumbar CSF has a diffuse origin, including spinal cord. (4) CSF AchE activity is unlikely to be a useful clinical marker for DAT. (28 ref).

161. Leverenz, James & Sumi, S. Mark. (1986). **Parkinson's disease in patients with Alzheimer's disease.** *Archives of Neurology,* 43(7), 662–664.
Studied the substantia nigra of 40 cases of pathologically confirmed Alzheimer's disease for changes caused by Parkinson's disease. Pathological confirmation of Alzheimer's disease in 25 men and 15 women was followed by examination for neuronal loss, Lewy bodies, or neurofibrillary tangles. 13 Ss had clinical signs of Parkinson's disease; 11 of these revealed pathological signs. These Ss ranged in age from 48 to 92 yrs, with most being 80 yrs old. 18 Ss overall had abnormalities in the substantia nigra, 14 Ss had Lewy bodies, 1 S had neurofibrillary tangles, and 3 Ss had significant cell loss without other signs. In comparison with the incidence expected in the population, these Ss had a 2.5 to 3.6 greater prevalence of Parkinson's disease, indicating that Alzheimer's patients have an increased risk for Parkinson's disease.

162. Lewis, D. A. & Bloom, F. E. (1987). **Clinical perspectives on neuropeptides.** *Annual Review of Medicine,* 38, 143–148.
Reviews the neuropeptide data on 2 degenerative neurologic disorders—Huntington's disease and Alzheimer's disease—to illustrate the ways in which neuropeptide changes have been correlated with disease states. Reported alterations in multiple neuropeptide systems in these diseases may help define the primary pathologic change and lead to new therapeutic strategies. Understanding the pathophysiological significance of these findings requires considering them in the context of the neural circuits involved.

163. Liss, Leopold & Thornton, David J. (1986). **The rationale for aluminum absorption control in early stages of Alzheimer disease.** Special Issue: Controversial topics on Alzheimer's disease: Intersecting crossroads. *Neurobiology of Aging,* 7(6), 552–554.
Comments on D. R. Crapper McLachlan's (1986) article by reporting that the role of aluminum (AL) as a link in the chain of events leading to progressive degeneration of the brain and dementia has been tested by lowering the postprandial AL peak in the serum. The progression of symptoms has been slowed down, indicating that AL plays a role in the multifactorial etiology of Alzheimer disease.

164. Liston, Edward H.; Jarvik, Lissy F. & Gerson, Sylvia. (1987). **Depression in Alzheimer's disease: An overview of adrenergic and cholinergic mechanisms.** *Comprehensive Psychiatry,* 28(5), 444–457.
Depression is frequently associated with Alzheimer's disease and has traditionally been viewed as either a psychological reaction to the dementia or a coincidental phenomenon. However, recent studies suggest that neuroanatomic and neurochemical interrelationships between Alzheimer's disease and depression may exist. That is, the loss of ascending noradrenergic and cholinergic cortical projections due to neuronal degeneration in the nucleus locus coeruleus and the nucleus basalis of Meynert may have implications for the development of depressive disorder in this primary degenerative dementia. These issues are reviewed, related brain-behavior hypotheses are explored, and research strategies and questions for further investigation are suggested.

165. Luxenberg, J. S.; Haxby, James V.; Creasey, H.; Sundaram, M. et al. (1987). **Rate of ventricular enlargement in dementia of the Alzheimer type correlates with rate of neuropsychological deterioration.** *Neurology,* 37(7), 1135–1140.
Studied 12 men (mean age 62.8 yrs) and 6 women (mean age 70.8 yrs) with dementia of the Alzheimer type (DAT) and 12 healthy men as controls (mean age 65.1 yrs) at intervals of 6 mo to 5 yrs. In the male DAT Ss, mean computerized tomography (CT) rates of enlargement of 3rd ventricle and of total lateral ventricular volumes differed significantly from zero and exceeded respective control values. The rate of neuropsychological decline correlated with rates of enlargement of the 3rd ventricle or right lateral ventricle. Women with DAT also had significant rates of enlargement of the 3rd and total lateral ventricles. The rate of lateral ventricular dilatation discriminated DAT Ss from controls.

166. Lynch, Gary & Baudry, Michel. (1987). **Brain spectrin, calpain and long-term changes in synaptic efficacy.** Sixteenth Annual Meeting of the Society for Neuroscience: Brain spectrum: Structure, location, and function (1986, Washington, DC). *Brain Research Bulletin,* 18(6), 809–815.
Discusses the possibility that proteolytic digestion of cytoskeletal proteins, in particular spectrin, is part of the mechanisms through which physiological activity elicits structural and chemical changes in brain synapses. The possibility is discussed that excessive activation of this biochemical process is responsible for some instances of neuropathology, including Alzheimer's disease and age-related neuronal degeneration, and implications for the neurological bases of learning and memory are noted.

167. Maire, Jean-Claude E. & Wurtman, Richard J. (1984). **Choline production from choline-containing phospholipids: A hypothetical role in Alzheimer's disease and aging.** Proceedings of the 7th Annual Meeting of the Canadian College of Neuro-Psychopharmacology: Perspectives in Canadian neuro-psychopharmacology (1984, Halifax, Canada). *Progress in Neuro-Psychopharmacology & Biological Psychiatry,* 8(4–6), 637–642.
Deficits in certain long-axon cholinergic brain neurons have been demonstrated both in senile dementia of the Alzheimer type (SDAT) and, to a lesser degree, in association with the cognitive and memory impairments sometimes observed with normal aging. A brief overview is given of studies that support a hypothesis concerning the selective vulnerability of these neurons: The use of choline (especially for the release of acetylcholine) originating from the breakdown of membrane phospholipids (PLs) may result in an impoverishment in certain PLs. Since only cholinergic neurons use their membrane PLs as a reservoir for their neurotransmitter's precursor, this relationship might explain the major deficits in long-axon cholinergic nerve terminals observed in SDAT and other age-related memory disorders. (19 ref).

168. Malone, Michael J. & Szoke, Maria C. (1985). **Neurochemical changes in white matter: Aged human brain and Alzheimer's disease.** *Archives of Neurology,* 42(11), 1063–1066.
Examined the white matter in the postmortem brains of 6 patients (64–86 yrs old) who died from nonneurologic diseases and 4 patients with a diagnosis of senile dementia of the Alzheimer type. Total myelin yields were decreased in the subcortical areas of the anterior temporal lobe, cingulum, superior frontal gyrus, and in the subcortex of the precentral gyrus. Increased desaturation or unsaturation of the longest lipid acyl changes in the myelin was also found and appeared to be related to age but not to the Alzheimer process. (36 ref).

169. Mann, D. M.; Yates, P. O. & Marcyniuk, B. (1986). **A comparison of nerve cell loss in cortical and subcortical structures in Alzheimer's disease.** *Journal of Neurology, Neurosurgery & Psychiatry,* 49(3), 310–312.
Examined the extent of cell loss from the temporal cortex, hippocampus, nucleus basalis of Meynert, and locus ceruleus measured at necropsy from 32 patients (aged 48–92 yrs) with Alzheimer's disease. Findings indicate that cortical nerve cells were damaged just as severely as those in the subcortex. It is suggested that the pathological relationship between the 2 regions may be primary or secondary or may even coexist. In the latter context it is possible that, because both cortical and subcortical neuron types show a similar neurofibrillary degeneration, a common and fundamental abnormality in all 4 cell types may underlie the pathogenesis of Alzheimer's disease. (27 ref).

170. Mann, David M.; Eaves, Nigel R.; Marcyniuk, Borys & Yates, Peter O. (1986). **Quantitative changes in cerebral cortical microvasculature in ageing and dementia.** *Neurobiology of Aging,* 7(5), 321–330.
Examined brains obtained postmortem from 25 mentally normal patients aged 26–96 yrs and from 3 patients with Alzheimer's disease. It is concluded that the extent of the capillary network in the cerebral cortex alters to match the number and activity of functioning nerve cells; changes in quantity of capillary occurring with age or Alzheimer's disease may, therefore, secondarily reflect a primary loss of nerve cells and do not form, per se, part of the degenerative process.

171. Mann, David M. & Hardy, John A. (1986). **The importance of altered structural proteins in the pathogenesis of Alzheimer's disease.** Special Issue: Controversial topics on Alzheimer's disease: Intersecting crossroads. *Neurobiology of Aging,* 7(6), 444–446.
Responds to D. J. Selkoe's (1986) article, by maintaining that the senile plaque and the neurofibrillary tangle probably represent the fundamental pathological substrate of Alzheimer's disease. Plaques mark the site of nerve terminal damage, and tangle marks the neuronal response to such injury. It is proposed that the key to therapy is a strategy that prevents their formation or promotes their dissolution. Such will come from understanding their molecular structure and knowledge of how they relate to each other, to normal structural proteins, and to changes that occur in blood vessels.

172. Maragos, William F.; Greenamyre, J. Timothy; Penney, John B. & Young, Anne B. (1987). **Glutamate dysfunction in Alzheimer's disease: An hypothesis.** *Trends in Neurosciences,* 10(2), 65–68.
Presents evidence of an involvement of glutamate (GM) in the pathophysiology of Alzheimer's type dementia (AZD). Animal studies show that GM (namely a GM receptor, *N*-methyl-dextroaspartate) may function in learning and memory impairment. Studies of AZD patients show a profound loss of glutamate receptors, decreased GM binding, and a correspondence between anatomical localization of plaques and tangles and the terminal of proposed GM pathways. Increasing declines in cognitive test scores of AZD patients correlate with the GM level in cerebrospinal fluid (CSF). GM-ergic inputs to cortical association and hippocampal pyramidal neurons become hyperactive leading to impaired energy stores and an inability to maintain normal neurofilament structure. This leads to cell loss in which GM receptors would be preferentially lost as they are concentrated on the spinous process of distal dendrites of pyramidal neurons, which leads to the prominent memory and learning deficits of AZD.

173. Marazita, Mary L.; Spence, M. Anne & Heyman, Albert. (1987). **Tests for genetic heterogeneity among 18 families with Alzheimer's disease.** *Neurology,* 37(10), 1678–1679.
Performed 2 tests for genetic heterogeneity within the framework of linkage analysis among 18 families with Alzheimer's disease (AD) for each of 27 phenotypic markers. Both tests were performed twice, first assuming that individuals with Down's syndrome were also affected with AD and then assuming that they were not. No significant heterogeneity was found under either test, regardless of the affected status assumption. However, trends in the data were consistent with heterogeneous etiology between families with both AD and Down's syndrome vs families with AD only.

174. Marotta, Charles A. (1986). **Both genetic and non-genetic risk factors of Alzheimer's disease must continue to be evaluated.** Special Issue: Controversial topics on Alzheimer's disease: Intersecting crossroads. *Neurobiology of Aging,* 7(6), 481–482.
Maintains that although a genetic role of Alzheimer's disease (AD) remains an intriguing, but unproven possibility, attempts to map gene defects and to define aberrant genetic control elements will likely provide important information in the future. It is suggested, however, that the study of non-genetic risk factors should be incorporated into current research and thinking concerned with potential genetic factors. Reference is made to P. Davies's (1986) review of studies on the genetics of AD.

175. Marquis, Judith K. (1986). **Chronic aluminum toxicity: Effects of aluminum on neurotransmitters.** Special Issue: Controversial topics on Alzheimer's disease: Intersecting crossroads. *Neurobiology of Aging,* 7(6), 547–548.
In response to D. R. Crapper McLachlan's (1986) discussion of the role of aluminum (AL) in Alzheimer's disease, the present author notes that available data suggest that chronic neurotoxicity may be associated with repeated dietary exposure to extremely low concentrations of AL in susceptible populations. Adverse effects of AL on central neurotransmitter function in the mammalian central nervous system (CNS) have been demonstrated both in vivo and in vitro with several different AL salts.

176. Marquis, Judith K. et al. (1985). **Cholinesterase activity in plasma, erythrocytes, and cerebrospinal fluid of patients with dementia of the Alzheimer type.** *Biological Psychiatry,* 20(6), 605–610.
Conducted 2 studies to examine the relationship of cholinesterase (ChE) activities in Ss with dementia of the Alzheimer type (DAT) and comparison Ss. ChE activity was measured in plasma, erythrocytes, and cerebrospinal fluid (CSF) from DAT patients and compared with ChE activity in normal controls and patients with diagnoses other than DAT. Study 1, which measured ChE levels in cerebrospinal fluid (CSF), involved 14 presenile and senile DAT patients, 10 parkinsonian patients, 7 alcoholics, and 12 controls. Study 2, which measured ChE levels in plasma and erythrocytes, involved 14 presenile and senile DAT patients, 4 cerebrovascular accident victims, 3 multiple sclerosis patients, and 9 controls. Results indicate that no significant differences in total enzyme activity were observed in any of the comparisons. Calculations of acetylcholinesterase and butyrylcholinesterase ratios in CSF also provided no significant indication of any changes in ChE activities in DAT Ss. It is suggested that measurements of total AChE or BChE activity in these biological materials do not provide a useful index of alterations in central cholinergic function in patients with DAT. (15 ref).

177. Marx, Jean L. (1986). **Nerve growth factor acts in brain.** *Science,* 232(4756), 1341–1342.
Recent research by neurobiologists has indicated that nerve growth factor (NGF) is active in the brain and not on peripheral nerve cells as previously thought. It has been shown that NGF acts on cholinergic neurons, which use the neurotransmitter acetylcholine. Research on NGF could lead to a better understanding of Alzheimer's and Huntington's diseases, which are caused by progressive degeneration of brain neurons.

178. Masters, Colin L. (1986). **Disordered innervation of cerebral vasculature as a cause of Alzheimer's disease plaques and tangles.** Special Issue: Controversial topics on Alzheimer's disease: Intersecting crossroads. *Neurobiology of Aging,* 7(6), 516.
Critiques the article on Alzheimer's disease (AD) by J. A. Hardy et al (1986) and argues that although the authors integrate certain important concepts with novel ideas, they fail to support the idea that a breakdown in the blood brain barrier occurs in AD, or how it would produce the specific pathology that characterizes the disease. The present author supports hypotheses on the pathogenesis of the neurofibrillary tangle that suggest that a neuronally derived protein is responsible for amyloid deposition in AD.

179. Masters, Colin L. (1986). **Amyloid proteins in Alzheimer's disease.** Special Issue: Controversial topics on Alzheimer's disease: Intersecting crossroads. *Neurobiology of Aging,* 7(6), 441–443.
Asserts that much of the controversy concerning the protein deposits found in Alzheimer's disease (AD) brain tissue will diminish as the biochemical properties of the amyloid proteins are more clearly defined, and as application of molecular biology techniques helps identify precursor molecule(s)

and the gene sequence of the abnormal proteins. The present author concurs with D. J. Selkoe's (1986) view that the neurofibrillary tangle and Alzheimer plaque core are pathognomic for AD.

180. Masters, Colin L. & Beyreuther, Konrad. (1986). **The structure of amyloid filaments in Alzheimer's disease and the unconventional virus infections of the nervous system.** *Psychological Medicine,* 16(4), 735–737.
Reviews recent data in which 2 or more important classes of cerebral amyloid proteins have been identified at the molecular level—those in Alzheimer's disease and those in the unconventional virus diseases (scrapie, kuru, and Creutzfeldt-Jakob disease). A series of studies indicates that the structures of amyloid filaments in these disorders are based on the polymerization of small protein subunits.

181. Matsuyama, Steven S. & Jarvik, Lissy F. (1984). **"Is Alzheimer's Disease inherited? A methodologic review": Commentary.** *Integrative Psychiatry,* 2(5), 174–175.
Reviews the literature on Alzheimer's disease in order to comment on a similar review by M. F. Folstein and D. Powell (1984). The present authors disagree with Folstein and Powell's conclusion that the disorder is familial and with their hypothesis that most Alzheimer's disease is transmitted as an autosomal-dominant age-dependent disorder. It is concluded that there is an urgent need for follow-up studies of children of patients with this disorder. (8 ref).

182. May, C.; Rapoport, S. I.; Tomai, T. P.; Chrousos, G. P. et al. (1987). **Cerebrospinal fluid concentrations of corticotropin-releasing hormone (CRH) and corticotropin (ACTH) are reduced in patients with Alzheimer's disease.** *Neurology,* 37(3), 535–538.
Examined CRH immunoreactivity (CRH-LI) and corticotropin (ACTH) levels in the cerebrospinal fluid (CSF) of 33 patients (mean age 67 yrs) with presumptive Alzheimer's disease (AD) and 13 healthy, age-matched controls. Results show that the mean CRH-LI and ACTH levels of the AD patients were significantly less than controls. Despite these reductions, none of the Ss had evidence of pituitary-adrenal dysfunction. It is suggested that a disorder of extrahypothalamic CRH may be involved in the pathophysiology of AD.

183. Mayor, G. H. (1986). **Aluminum and Alzheimer's disease: New directions.** Special Issue: Controversial topics on Alzheimer's disease: Intersecting crossroads. *Neurobiology of Aging,* 7(6), 542–543.
Responds to D. R. Crapper McLachlan (1986), by maintaining that while the evidence for the physiological toxicity of aluminum (AL) is now well-established, the possible role it plays in Alzheimer's disease (AD) continues to be an interesting but unproven possibility. It is suggested that future studies might directly compare clinical, neuropathologic, and non-neurological changes in AD patients with those characterized in other clinical conditions that have a more firmly established AL etiology. Information from such studies might help finally establish a clearer relationship between AL toxicity and AD.

184. Mazurek, Michael F.; Beal, M. Flint; Bird, Edward D. & Martin, Joseph B. (1987). **Oxytocin in Alzheimer's disease: Postmortem brain levels.** *Neurology,* 37(6), 1001–1003.
Studied oxytocin (OXY) immunoreactivity in postmortem brain tissue from 12 patients (aged 62–90 yrs) with histologically confirmed Alzheimer's disease (AD) and 13 controls (aged 36–87 yrs) with no history of neurologic or psychiatric disease. OXY concentration was increased 33% in the hippocampus and temporal cortex of AD brains but normal in all other regions examined. Results suggest that elevated hippocampal OXY levels may contribute to the memory disturbance associated with AD.

185. Mazurek, Michael F.; Growdon, John H.; Beal, M. Flint & Martin, Joseph B. (1986). **CSF vasopressin concentration is reduced in Alzheimer's disease.** *Neurology,* 36(8), 1133–1137.
Measured the concentration of arginine vasopressin (AVP) in the cerebrospinal fluid (CSF) of 44 Alzheimer's disease patients (56–78 yrs old), 12 Huntington's disease patients, 8 patients with normal-pressure hydrocephalus, 25 patients with vertebral disk herniation, 9 with neuropathy, 11 with myelopathy, 16 with aseptic meningitis, 11 with multiple sclerosis, and 51 controls. Levels of CSF AVP were reduced by 37% in Alzheimer's disease but were normal in other neurologic disorders. Low CSF levels of AVP may assist in the identification of demented patients who are not likely to benefit from ventricular shunting.

186. McGeer, Edith G.; Singh, Edith A. & McGeer, Patrick L. (1987). **Sodium-dependent glutamate binding in senile dementia.** *Neurobiology of Aging,* 8(3), 219–223.
Investigated sodium-dependent glutamate binding as a possible index of the integrity of glutamate/aspartate nerve endings in 7 cortical areas from postmortem brains of 15 persons with senile dementia of the Alzheimer type (SDAT); 10 controls matched for age, sex, and postmortem delay (PMD); and single cases of Down's syndrome and Parkinson dementia. Results show that binding affinities were variable from brain to brain. Specific binding site densities showed overall a significant negative correlation with PMD, a significant decrease in SDAT, and a significant correlation in the SDAT samples with choline acetyltransferase activities.

187. McKinney, Michael. (1983). **Cholinergic innervation of the mammalian cerebral cortex and hippocampus by the basal forebrain: Implications for senile dementia of the Alzheimer type.** *Dissertation Abstracts International,* 43(9-B), 2873.

188. Meier-Ruge, W.; Ulrich, J. & Stähelin, H. B. (1985). **Morphometric investigation of nerve cells, neuropil and senile plaques in senile dementia of the Alzheimer type.** *Archives of Gerontology & Geriatrics,* 4(3), 219–229.
Evaluated 8 brains from patients (aged 85–95 yrs) showing neuropathological manifestations of senile dementia of the Alzheimer type and 6 control brains from Ss (aged 85–95 yrs) who were mentally normal or who had minimal senile impairment of memory. Stereological measurements were made of the size and number of senile plaques, nerve cell area, capillary diameter and length, and intercapillary distance. Findings suggest that nerve cell shrinkage may be a characteristic indicator of senile dementia and that neuropil atrophy may be of secondary importance. (25 ref).

189. Meyer, John S. et al. (1980). **Regional changes in cerebral blood flow during standard behavioral activation in patients with disorders of speech and mentation compared to normal volunteers.** *Brain & Language,* 9(1), 61–77.
Reviews results obtained from over 2,000 measurements made in Ss aged 15–91 yrs. Discussed are the reproducibility of regional cerebral blood flow (rCBF) measurements in normal Ss; changes in rCBF during arousal, relaxation, sleep, and behavioral activation; behavioral activation by standard multiple psychophysiological activation; results of behavioral activation in normal Ss and in Ss with speech disorders due to infarction of the speech dominant hemisphere; multi-infarct dementia; and dementia due to Alzheimer's disease. (26 ref).

190. Miller, Bruce L. (1986). **Aluminum in Alzheimer's disease: A testable hypothesis.** Special Issue: Controversial topics on Alzheimer's disease: Intersecting crossroads. *Neurobiology of Aging,* 7(6), 570–571.

Comments on the article by E. Roberts (1986), which suggests that Alzheimer's disease (AD) might be caused by the entrance of aluminosilicates into the aging nasal mucosa. The present author argues that while the article is speculative it offers a testable hypothesis with experiments that could be carried out to prove or disprove the theory.

191. Miller, Christopher; Haugh, Margaret; Kahn, Jacob & Anderton, Brian. (1986). **The cytoskeleton and neurofibrillary tangles in Alzheimer's disease.** *Trends in Neurosciences,* 9(2), 76–81.
Reviews research concerning the cytoskeleton and neurofibrillary tangles in Alzheimer's disease. Tangles in the hippocampus are localized to neurons that connect the hippocampus to other areas of the cortex, basal forebrain, thalamus, and hypothalamus, thus implicating tangles in a local pathology which may account for the memory disorder of Alzheimer's disease.

192. Miyakawa, Taihei. (1986). **Commentary on the pathogenesis of Alzheimer's disease.** Special Issue: Controversial topics on Alzheimer's disease: Intersecting crossroads. *Neurobiology of Aging,* 7(6), 511–512.
Concurs with J. A. Hardy et al (1986) that a dysfunction of the blood brain barrier and degeneration of the blood vessels in the cortex of the brain seem to be fundamental to the pathogenesis of Alzheimer's disease (AD). It is speculated that the degeneration of blood vessels is caused by some agents affecting the aged blood vessel. The present author cites evidence that shows that senile plaque is a more important finding than neurofibrillary tangles for the pathogenesis of AD.

193. Mohs, Richard C.; Breitner, John C.; Silverman, Jeremy M. & Davis, Kenneth L. (1988). **"Morbid risk in first-degree relatives of persons with Alzheimer's disease": Reply.** *Archives of General Psychiatry,* 45(1), 98.
Responds to comments by L. L. Heston (1988) regarding the methods and conclusions of the present authors' (1987) report concerning the morbid risk among 1st-degree relatives of patients with Alzheimer's disease.

194. Mölsä, Pekka K.; Säkö, E.; Paljärvi, L.; Rinne, J. O. et al. (1987). **Alzheimer's disease: Neuropathological correlates of cognitive and motor disorders.** *Acta Neurologica Scandinavica,* 75(6), 376–384.
Investigated correlations between clinical symptoms and neuropathology in 34 patients (aged 69–88 yrs) with Alzheimer's disease and 17 controls (aged 73–88 yrs). Patients were originally found in a community survey of dementia and were followed up until death. A significant correlation emerged between the severity of dementia and the number of plaques and tangles in the brain material as a whole. Low brain weight correlated with many clinical symptoms and signs and the severity of dementia. Dyskinetic movements were associated with damage of brain areas, suggesting a multiple etiology.

195. Moore, Deborah K. (1985). **Genetic studies of Alzheimer's type dementia.** *Dissertation Abstracts International,* 46(5-B), 1448.

196. Morimatsu, Mitsunori; Hirai, Shunsaku; Muramatsu, Atsushi & Yoshikawa, Masaki. (1975). **Senile degenerative brain lesions and dementia.** *Journal of the American Geriatrics Society,* 23(9), 390–406.
Results of a study of brain lesions—including Alzheimer's neurofibrillary changes, senile plaques, and amyloid angiopathy—show that the incidence and quantity of neurofibrillary changes and senile plaques rose with age and that an approximate positive correlation in quantity was noted among the 3 kinds of degenerative change. The cause of dementia was studied retrospectively, and findings are presented. (46 ref).

197. Morita, Kotaro; Kaiya, Hisanobu; Ikeda, Tsuneko & Namba, Masuyuki. (1987). **Presenile dementia combined with amyotrophy: A review of 34 Japanese cases.** Eric K. Fernström Foundation Symposium: Frontal lobe degeneration of non-Alzheimer type (1986, Lund, Sweden). *Archives of Gerontology & Geriatrics,* 6(3), 263–277.
Reviews 34 cases of presenile dementia combined with amyotrophy and presents 4 case reports. The clinical feature of dementia was generally unspecific and could not be clearly diagnosed as Pick's disease or Alzheimer's disease. Neuropathological features simulated a combination of progressive subcortical gliosis and spinal progressive muscular atrophy. It is concluded that amyotrophy-dementia complex (ADC) might be a new kind of multisystemic degeneration. It is possible that there is a transitional form even among ADCs.

198. Morley, John E. (1986). **Neuropeptides, behavior, and aging.** *Journal of the American Geriatrics Society,* 34(1), 52–62.
Discusses research findings regarding the role of neuropeptides in the behavioral changes associated with the aging process. The role of neuropeptide change in the aging process is examined in relation to the role of opioids in decreased analgesia and the role of neuropeptides in anorexic behavior, memory loss, and central nervous system (CNS) disease. Specific alterations in neuropeptide concentration in Alzheimer's, Parkinson's, Huntington's, and psychiatric diseases are described. (167 ref).

199. Moroni, Flavio; Lombardi, G.; Robitaille, Y. & Etienne, P. (1986). **Senile dementia and Alzheimer's disease: Lack of changes of the cortical content of quinolinic acid.** *Neurobiology of Aging,* 7(4), 249–253.
The content of quinolinic acid (QUIN) was fragmentographically measured in the frontal, parietal, and temporal cortex obtained at autopsy from 8 60–90 yr old patients affected by Alzheimer's disease/senile dementia Alzheimer type (AD/SDAT) and 7 matched controls. In the 3 cortical areas studied, the content of QUIN was similar in AD/SDAT Ss and in the controls. Findings do not support the possibility that an accumulation of QUIN plays a role in the neuronal degeneration occurring in the cortex of AD/SDAT patients.

200. Morrison, John H.; Lewis, David A.; Campbell, Michael J.; Huntley, George W. et al. (1987). **A monoclonal antibody to non-phosphorylated neurofilament protein marks the vulnerable cortical neurons in Alzheimer's disease.** *Brain Research,* 416(2), 331–336.
Various cytoskeletal proteins have been implicated in the formation of neurofibrillary tangles in Alzheimer's disease (AD). A monoclonal antibody to nonphosphorylated neurofilament protein labels a distinct subset of pyramidal cells in the normal human cortex that have a distribution similar to that of neurofibrillary tangles in brains from patients with AD. In addition, regions and layers that normally contain a high density of such cells, in AD, have large numbers of neurofibrillary tangles and few remaining immunoreactive cells.

201. Mortimer, James A. & Pirozzolo, Francis J. (1985). **Remote effects of head trauma.** *Developmental Neuropsychology,* 1(3), 215–229.
Suggests that new neuropsychological deficits may emerge months or years after an episode of head trauma. Head injury has been suggested as a risk factor for several degenerative neurological conditions, including the punch-drunk syndrome, Alzheimer's disease, Pick's disease, Parkinson's disease, and Creutzfeldt-Jacob disease. The evidence for an etiologic role of head trauma in these conditions is reviewed, and possible mechanisms for the production of delayed neuropsychological deficits are considered.

202. Mountjoy, C. Q.; Roth, M.; Evans, N. J. & Evans, H. M. (1983). **Cortical neuronal counts in normal elderly controls and demented patients.** *Neurobiology of Aging,* 4(1), 1–11.
Investigated whether there is significant neuronal loss in dementia, and if so, whether it is general or localized, and examined the relationship between neuronal counts, senile plaques, and neurofibrillary change. Neuronal counts were made in 9 cortical areas in the postmortem brains of 25 patients with senile dementia of the Alzheimer type and 25 age-matched controls. Results indicate that the size of the neuronal population in Ss with Alzheimer's disease was not identical to that observed in well-preserved aged controls. (22 ref).

203. Nakamura, Shinichi & Vincent, Steven R. (1986). **Somatostatin- and neuropeptide Y-immunoreactive neurons in the neocortex in senile dementia of Alzheimer's type.** *Brain Research,* 370(1), 11–20.
Studied morphological changes in neocortical somatostatin (STN)- and neuropeptide-Y (NPY)-immunoreactivity cells in senile dementia of the Alzheimer type (SDAT) in 3 male Ss (aged 81–88) and 3 controls (aged 75–91), using light-microscopic immunohistochemical methods. The density of STN-immunoreactive cells in the neocortex did not decrease in cases of SDAT compared with controls, although many STN-positive fibers were abnormally swollen and bulbous in shape and were often within senile plaques. Similar fiber abnormalities were observed in sections stained with antibodies to NPY. STN- and NPY-positive cells in aged normal Ss were distributed from layer II through to the subcortical white matter. It is suggested that a primary degenerative process might begin at the fiber terminals of the STN neuronal system in the neocortex in SDAT.

204. Naugle, Richard I. (1987). **Catastrophic minor head trauma.** *Archives of Clinical Neuropsychology,* 2(1), 93–100.
Describes the case of a 39-yr-old man who tested positive for the human T-lymphatropic virus Type III (HTLV-III) associated with acquired immune deficiency syndrome (AIDS) and AIDS-related complex and who suffered a closed-head injury as a consequence of a physical assault. His course was rapid and his symptomatology more profound than would be expected on the basis of his injury alone. The assault is regarded as a second, catalytic injury and is presumed to derive its pronounced effect from the ongoing neurologic disorder resulting from or associated with the HTLV-III virus. Relevant contributions from sports medicine literature and Alzheimer's disease research are reviewed.

205. Naugle, Richard I.; Cullum, C. Munro; Bigler, Erin D. & Massman, Paul J. (1987). **Handedness and dementia.** *Perceptual & Motor Skills,* 65(1), 207–210.
Examined the speculation that left-hand dominance is more prevalent among patients suffering from dementia of the Alzheimer's type that began prior to age 65 yrs and that in these patients the disease runs a more rapid course. Seven left-handed and 7 right-handed dementia patients (aged 56–79 yrs), matched on the basis of age and years of education, were compared on neuropsychological compromise. The difference between the groups was not significant.

206. Neary, D.; Snowden, J. S.; Mann, D. M.; Bowen, D. M. et al. (1986). **Alzheimer's disease: A correlative study.** *Journal of Neurology, Neurosurgery & Psychiatry,* 49(3), 229–237.
Examined psychological, pathological, and chemical measures of disorder, using 17 Alzheimer's patients (mean age 59 yrs). Studied were severity of dementia, pathological change in large cortical neurons, cortical senile plaque and neurofibrillary tangle frequency reduction in acetylcholine synthesis, cell loss, reductions in nuclear and nucleolar volume and cytoplasmic RNA content, and reduction in choline acetyltransferase activity. Findings suggest that the dementia of Alzheimer's disease is a reflection of the state of large cortical neurons and that abnormalities in the latter may not be directly related to primary loss of cholinergic neurons in the subcortex. (31 ref).

207. Nee, L. E.; Eldridge, R.; Sunderland, T.; Thomas, C. B. et al. (1987). **Dementia of the Alzheimer type: Clinical and family study of 22 twin pairs.** *Neurology,* 37(3), 359–363.
Studied 22 twin pairs (aged 57–85 yrs) in which one or both twins had dementia of the Alzheimer type (DAT). Results show that in 4 twins, diagnosis was confirmed by autopsy. Seven monozygotic (MZ) pairs were concordant for DAT; 10 MZ pairs were discordant. Two dizygotic (DZ) pairs were concordant for DAT and 3 DZ pairs were discordant. The current concordance rate was 41% for MZ twins and 40% for DZ twins. Results support the belief that, etiologically, DAT cannot be entirely accounted for by a single autosomal dominant gene. Data suggest that in certain genetic circumstances, disease expression may be delayed in females.

208. Nicoll, Roger A. (1985). **The septo-hippocampal projection: A model cholinergic pathway.** *Trends in Neurosciences,* 8(12), 533–536.
Discusses electrophysiological research with regard to the establishment of acetylcholine (ACh) as a transmitter in the septo-hippocampal projection and to indications that the action of this pathway differs from that described for classical synaptic transmission. It is noted that there is a selective and profound loss of ACh in patients with Alzheimer's disease and that these cholinergic systems are implicated in the higher cognitive systems, such as memory.

209. Nieto-Sampedro, Manuel. (1987). **Astrocyte mitogenic activity in aged normal and Alzheimer's human brain.** *Neurobiology of Aging,* 8(3), 249–252.
Measured astrocyte mitogenic activity in the cortex of human beings, 2 aged 30–55 yrs, 8 aged 75–85 yrs, and 8 aged 70–91 yrs who had Alzheimer's disease (AD), using purified cultures of neonatal rat cortex astrocytes. Findings show that human brain mitogenic activity was 2- to 4-fold that found in comparable extracts from rat brain. A 1.3-fold increase in specific mitogenic activity was observed in extracts from AD cortex when compared with normal aged or adult tissue.

210. Nyberg, P. et al. (1985). **Catecholamine topochemistry in human basal ganglia: Comparison between normal and Alzheimer brains.** *Brain Research,* 333(1), 139–142.
A postmortem analysis of catecholamine levels in 6 human control and 4 Alzheimer brains (mean age 64.7 and 70.8 yrs) revealed lower mean concentrations of noradrenaline, but not dopamine, in the nucleus caudatus, putamen, and globus pallidus, but not in the hippocampus, of the Alzheimer brains. Generally, noradrenaline levels were higher in the more posterior parts of nucleus caudatus and putamen in the control brains, whereas such gradients were absent in the Alzheimer brains. (20 ref).

211. Oliver, C. & Holland, A. J. (1986). **Down's Syndrome and Alzheimer's disease: A review.** *Psychological Medicine,* 16(2), 307–322.
Reviews studies concerning similarities between the neuropathological change found in Down's syndrome (DS) individuals over the age of 35 yrs and that found in Alzheimer's disease (AD) patients. Studies that have investigated cognitive deficits are also reviewed, but the extent to which dementia occurs as a result of the reported neuropathological change is unclear. Theories put forward to explain the association between these 2 disorders and their possible significance to the understanding of the etiology of AD are discussed. It is concluded that neuropathological and clinical evidence points to a link between DS and AD. However, although a high proportion of DS individuals develop neuropathologic

changes similar to those found in AD, only a portion develop definite signs of deterioration.

212. Op Den Velde, W. & Stam, F. C. (1976). **Some cerebral proteins and enzyme systems in Alzheimer's presenile and senile dementia.** *Journal of the American Geriatrics Society,* 24(1), 12–16.
Autopsy findings in cases of Alzheimer's presenile and senile dementia, Pick's disease, and cerebral arteriosclerosis show that profiles of cerebral gray-matter proteins were normal. In the patients with advanced dementia, the enzyme patterns usually were abnormal. Particularly in Alzheimer's disease, the activity of malate dehydrogenase was markedly increased. (32 ref).

213. Oyanagi, Kiyomitsu; Takahashi, Hitoshi; Wakabayashi, Koichi & Ikuta, Fusahiro. (1987). **Selective involvement of large neurons in the neostriatum of Alzheimer's disease and senile dementia: A morphometric investigation.** *Brain Research,* 411(2), 205–211.
Evaluated the quantitative changes in the neostriatum in Alzheimer's disease (AD) and senile dementia of Alzheimer type (SDAT). Sections of the caudate head (CN) and putamen (PT) from 4 AD/SDAT patients aged (59–79 yrs) and 6 age-matched controls were stained with Klüver-Barrera, and the cell body and nuclear areas of the neurons were measured. Results show a significant decrease in the number of large neurons and good preservation of the number of small neurons in the CN and PT of AD/SDAT patients.

214. Palmer, A. M.; Francis, P. T.; Bowen, D. M.; Benton, J. S. et al. (1987). **Catecholaminergic neurones assessed antemortem in Alzheimer's disease.** *Brain Research,* 414(2), 365–375.
Investigated the possible relationship between neurotransmitter abnormalities and the impairment of memory and intellect in Alzheimer's disease. Indices of dopaminergic and noradrenergic varicosities were assayed in neocortical tissue obtained at diagnostic craniotomy from patients with Alzheimer's disease. Noradrenergic markers were significantly reduced in the temporal cortex, and release of endogenous serotonin was significantly reduced in the frontal cortex. Presynaptic cholinergic and serotonergic markers correlated with severity of disease.

215. Palmer, Alan M.; Wilcock, Gordon K.; Esiri, Margaret M.; Francis, Paul T. et al. (1987). **Monoaminergic innervation of the frontal and temporal lobes in Alzheimer's disease.** *Brain Research,* 401(2), 231–238.
In the postmortem brains of 46 Alzheimer's disease patients, noradrenaline and serotonin concentrations were significantly reduced in the frontal and temporal cortex relative to the values observed in 34 control brains. Severely demented Ss had evidence of generalized neuronal loss, whereas those with moderate dementia showed significant loss of only choline acetyltransferase activity. In Alzheimer Ss, a significant inverse relationship was found between 5-hydroxyindoleacetic acid concentration and the number of neurofibrillary tangles.

216. Parnetti, L.; Gottfries, J.; Karlsson, I.; Långström, G. et al. (1987). **Monoamines and their metabolites in cerebrospinal fluid of patients with senile dementia of Alzheimer type using high performance liquid chromatography and gas chromatography-mass spectrometry.** *Acta Psychiatrica Scandinavica,* 75(5), 542–548.
Measured monoamines and their main metabolites in cerebrospinal fluid (CSF) from 12 age-matched elderly inpatients (aged 77–90 yrs) affected with senile dementia of Alzheimer type and chronic schizophrenia. Results show a clear psychobehavioral and neurochemical differentiation of the 2 patient groups. Four-hydroxy-3-methoxyphenylacetic acid and 5-hydroxyindole-3-acetic acid levels were significantly lower in Alzheimer's patients and showed a trend toward negative correlation with the degree of dementia.

217. Paula-Barbosa, M. M.; Saraiva, A.; Tavares, M. A.; Borges, M. M. et al. (1986). **Alzheimer's disease: Maintenance of neuronal and synaptic densities in frontal cortical layers II and III.** *Acta Neurologica Scandinavica,* 74(5), 404–408.
In frontal cortex biopsic material from 9 patients (aged 50–62 yrs) with Alzheimer's disease (AD), the numerical densities of neurons and synapses were not significantly different from 9 16–70 yr old non-AD controls, suggesting that changes in the highest cognitive functions might not depend on a generalized loss of neurons and synapses and that quantitative morphological differences may exist between AD and senile dementia of the Alzheimer type.

218. Pearlson, Godfrey D. & Tune, Larry E. (1986). **Cerebral ventricular size and cerebrospinal fluid acetylcholinesterase levels in senile dementia of the Alzheimer type.** *Psychiatry Research,* 17(1), 23–29.
Computed tomography (CT) was performed in 16 patients (mean age 72.2 yrs) with a diagnosis of senile dementia of the Alzheimer type. CT scans were rated without knowledge of clinical and laboratory data, and lateral ventricle-brain ratios (VBRs) were calculated. Cerebrospinal fluid (CSF) acetylcholinesterase (AChE) activity was measured by radioenzymatic assay in all Ss, and degree of dementia was quantified using the Mini-Mental State Examination (MMSE). There were significant correlations between cerebral atrophy as assessed by VBR and CSF AChE activity. Cognitive impairment on MMSE also correlated significantly with VBR. These correlations were not accounted for by age, dilutional effects, or duration of illness. The relationship between VBR and AChE activity demonstrates an association between 2 independently determined premortem measures of illness. (29 ref).

219. Perdahl-Wallace, Eva B. (1986). **Biochemical changes in the brain in chronic alcoholism: A comparison with dementia conditions.** *Dissertation Abstracts International,* 46(12-B, Pt 1), 4180.

220. Perl, Daniel P. (1986). **The aluminum hypothesis of Alzheimer's disease: A personal view based on microprobe analysis.** Special Issue: Controversial topics on Alzheimer's disease: Intersecting crossroads. *Neurobiology of Aging,* 7(6), 550–552.
Responds to D. R. Crapper McLachlan's (1986) article by arguing that although bulk aluminum (AL) analyses have produced conflicting results, microprobe analyses have demonstrated focal accumulations within the neurofibrillary tangle-bearing neurons associated with Alzheimer's disease. Similar accumulations have been identified within the numerous tangle-bearing neurons encountered in the brains of the indigenous natives of the island of Guam who suffer from amyotrophic lateral sclerosis and parkinsonism with dementia. These findings are discussed in relationship to environmental factors and the inherent integrity of barrier systems that insure isolation of the central nervous system (CNS) from those environmental sources of AL.

221. Perry, E. (1988). **Acetylcholine and Alzheimer's disease.** *British Journal of Psychiatry,* 152, 737–740.
Contends that the hypothesis that cognitive impairment in Alzheimer's disease is related to cholinergic degeneration in the brain is still subject to critical evaluation, rests largely on evidence of neurochemical pathology in affected tissue, but still depends on effective therapy for its ultimate validation. A number of key questions specifically relating to the cholinergic involvement in Alzheimer's disease are considered: (1) What is the functional significance of the cholinergic

deficit? (2) What is the relevance of other neuronal involvements? (3) What are the prospects for cholinergic treatment? (4) What is the role of acetylcholine in memory? (5) What are the possible origins of cholinoneurodegeneration? It is concluded that these questions are already being answered both within and, as so often in the history of biological psychiatry, outside the immediate area of investigation.

222. Perry, E. K.; Perry, R. H.; Smith, C. J.; Dick, D. J. et al. (1987). **Nicotinic receptor abnormalities in Alzheimer's and Parkinson's diseases.** *Journal of Neurology, Neurosurgery & Psychiatry,* 50(6), 806–809.
Quantified the nicotinic receptor using the binding of (^{3}H)nicotine to washed hippocampal membranes, prepared postmortem from patients with Alzheimer's (*n* = 8), Parkinson's (4 demented, 7 nondemented), and Huntington's (*n* = 4) diseases. Group mean ages ranged from 67 to 76 yrs. Findings indicate substantial reductions of hippocampal nicotine (i.e., high affinity nicotine) binding, occurring in conjunction with decreased choline acetyltransferase, in both Alzheimer's and Parkinson's but not Huntington's diseases.

223. Perry, Elaine K. et al. (1985). **Cholinergic correlates of cognitive impairment in Parkinson's disease: Comparisons with Alzheimer's disease.** *Journal of Neurology, Neurosurgery & Psychiatry,* 48(5), 413–421.
Dementia in Parkinson's disease has previously been attributed to the presence in the cerebral cortex of Alzheimer-type neuropathological abnormalities. Evidence resulting from a study by R. H. Perry et al (1983) suggests that dementia in this disease usually occurs in the absence of substantial Alzheimer-type changes in the cortex and may be related to abnormalities in the cortical cholinergic system. The present postmortem study of 8 controls with no neurological or psychiatric symptoms (aged 63–89 yrs), 14 Parkinson's patients (aged 62–80 yrs), and 8 Alzheimer's patients (aged 73–92 yrs) showed that in Parkinsonian patients with dementia there were extensive reductions of choline acetyltransferase and less extensive reduction of acetylcholinesterase in all 4 cortical lobes. Choline acetyltransferase reductions in temporal neocortex correlated with the degree of mental impairment that had been assessed by a memory and information test but not with the extent of plaque or tangle formation. In Parkinson's but not Alzheimer's patients, the decrease in neocortical (particularly temporal) choline acetyltransferase correlated with the number of neurons in the nucleus of Meynert, suggesting that primary degeneration of these cholinergic neurons may be related to declining cognitive function in Parkinson's disease. (30 ref).

224. Perry, Elaine K. et al. (1983). **Decreased imipramine binding in the brains of patients with depressive illness.** *British Journal of Psychiatry,* 142, 188–192.
The binding of tritiated imipramine was significantly reduced in the hippocampus and occipital cortex from 16 patients with depressive illness (mean age 78 yrs) compared with 14 age-matched patients with no psychiatric disorder. In contrast, there was no change in imipramine binding in 13 established cases of senile dementia of Alzheimer type. Scatchard analysis indicated normal binding affinity but a reduction in the number of imipramine binding sites in depression. These observations parallel previous findings of decreased binding sites in platelets from depressed patients and suggest that there may be an abnormality in the uptake mechanism for serotonin in depression. (18 ref).

225. Perry, Elaine K. & Perry, Robert H. (1982). **The cholinergic system in Alzheimer's disease.** *Trends in Neurosciences,* 5(8), 261–262.
Discusses the cholinergic abnormality in Alzheimer's disease, which has aroused new interest in the neurochemical pathology of this disorder. The connection between the loss of cholinergic activities in the brain and the classical neuropathological features of the disease—neocortical senile plaques and neurofibrillary tangles—is far from clear. P. G. Whitehouse et al (1982) suggest that a critical neuropathological abnormality may be a loss of the neurons from the basal nucleus of Meynert, a subcortical nucleus that supplies the neocortex with cholinergic afferent processes. This research may also prove useful in the identification of key changes in the brains of people with deficient memory function, which may help identify the actual mechanism of human memory. (13 ref).

226. Perry, Elaine K. & Perry, Robert H. (1985). **New insights into the nature of senile (Alzheimer-type) plaques.** *Trends in Neurosciences,* 8(7), 301–303.
The present authors discuss 3 apparently unconnected lines of investigation that have identified novel plaque constituents: microscopic analyses of neurotransmitter systems, protein analysis of plaque amyloid, and inorganic chemical analysis. Advances in these areas suggest new approaches to determining the origin of plaques and possibly of Alzheimer's disease itself. (30 ref).

227. Perry, Elaine K. & Perry, Robert H. (1986). **Unfolding the nature of senile plaque amyloid.** Special Issue: Controversial topics on Alzheimer's disease: Intersecting crossroads. *Neurobiology of Aging,* 7(6), 437–439.
Argues that D. J. Selkoe (1986) presents a convincing case for considering senile plaque amyloid, as opposed to the paired helical filaments of the tangle, as a distinct or specific feature of Alzheimer type but not other cerebral degenerative diseases. While the precise nature and origin of the amyloid are still elusive, it is suggested that some of the evidence indicative of a vascular origin favored by Selkoe is open to question.

228. Pettegrew, Jay W. (1986). **Aluminum and Alzheimer's disease: An evolving understanding.** Special Issue: Controversial topics on Alzheimer's disease: Intersecting crossroads. *Neurobiology of Aging,* 7(6), 539–540.
In response to D. R. Crapper McLachlan (1986), the present author acknowledges that aluminum (AL) has been demonstrated to accumulate in the grey matter in Alzheimer's disease (AD) neurofibrillary degeneration. However, it is argued that since the structures that contain AL are metabolically inert (neurofibrillary tangles, nuclear heterochromatin, amyloid core of neuritic plaques), the presence of AL in these structures may simply reflect a final repository of AL due to the availability of phosphate groups which can strongly complex AL.

229. Preobrazhenskaya, N. S. (1985). **Some quantitative characteristics of the pathological architectonics of the brain cortex in Pick's disease and Alzheimer's disease.** *Zhurnal Nevropatologii i Psikhiatrii,* 85(7), 969–973.
Studied the pathological architectonics of brain hemispheres from Ss with Pick's or Alzheimer's disease. Changes in the size of hemispheric surfaces and individual areas were determined. The findings indicate that the degenerative, atrophic process in both types of presenile dementia involves the whole brain cortex. No correlation was found between the degree of macroscopic atrophy of convolutions and the severity of pathological architectonic changes in cortical formations. (English abstract).

230. Price, Donald L. et al. (1982). **Alzheimer's disease and Down's syndrome.** *Annals of the New York Academy of Sciences,* 396, 145–164.
Reviews clinical and pathological similarities between Alzheimer's disease (AD) and the dementia of Down's syndrome (DS) relative to the (1) cholinergic systems in the basal forebrain in AD; (2) neuropathological and neurochemical changes in the brains of DS patients; and (3) anatomy, neurochemistry, and physiology of cholinergic systems in the

basal forebrain. It is suggested that the cholinergic deficiency in AD may be partly responsible for the cognitive behavioral disturbances in AD patients and possibly in the dementia of DS patients. (145 ref).

231. Price, Donald L.; Altschuler, Richard J.; Struble, Robert G.; Casanova, Manuel F. et al. (1986). **Sequestration of tubulin in neurons in Alzheimer's disease.** *Brain Research,* 385(2), 305–310.
Examined whether granulovacuolar degeneration represents a type of cytoskeletal abnormality similar to the formation of neurofibrillary tangles, neurites, and Hirano bodies found in Alzheimer's disease (AD) patients. The sequestration of tubulin in granules in hippocampal pyramidal neurons from 8 AD patients (aged 52–87 yrs) is consistent with the concept that abnormalities of the neuronal cytoskeleton are an important part of the cellular pathology of AD.

232. Prusiner, Stanley B. (1987). **Prions causing degenerative neurological diseases.** *Annual Review of Medicine,* 38, 381–398.
Discusses research on the unique biological particles called prions that cause degenerative neurological diseases—scrapie in animals and Creutzfeldt-Jakob disease (CJD) in humans. The studies described clearly demonstrate that knowledge about scrapie is relevant to understanding CJD in humans. The significance of prior research for understanding nontransmissible degenerative disorders such as Alzheimer's disease is unknown.

233. Prusiner, Stanley & McKinley, Michael P. (1986). **Relationship of aluminosilicates to CNS degenerative disorders.** Special Issue: Controversial topics on Alzheimer's disease: Intersecting crossroads. *Neurobiology of Aging,* 7(6), 573.
Comments on E. Roberts's (1986) hypothesis, by noting that the ubiquity of aluminum and silicon makes the study of these elements in Alzheimer's disease all the more difficult. Research is cited indicating that aluminosilicates may play a central role in the pathogenesis of a variety of central nervous system (CNS) degenerative disorders (e.g., amyotrophic lateral sclerosis, Parkinson's disease).

234. Rabins, Peter; Pearlson, Godfrey; Jayaram, Geetha; Steele, Cynthia et al. (1987). **Increased ventricle-to-brain ratio in late-onset schizophrenia.** 139th Annual Meeting of the American Psychiatric Association (1986, Washington, DC). *American Journal of Psychiatry,* 144(9), 1216–1218.
For 29 patients (mean age 73 yrs) with schizophrenia that began after age 44 yrs, the mean ventricle-to-brain ratio was significantly higher than for 23 age-matched normal Ss (mean age 72.1 yrs) but significantly smaller than for 23 patients (mean age 71.9 yrs) with Alzheimer's disease and hallucinations or delusions.

235. Raskind, Murray A. et al. (1986). **Cerebrospinal fluid vasopressin, oxytocin, somatostatin, and β-endorphin in Alzheimer's disease.** *Archives of General Psychiatry,* 43(4), 382–388.
Measured cerebrospinal fluid (CSF) concentrations of arginine vasopressin, somatostatin, oxytocin, and beta-endorphin in 10 males (mean age 67 yrs) with Alzheimer's disease (AD), 9 normal elderly males (mean age 68 yrs), and 15 normal young males (mean age 25 yrs). Results show lower CSF arginine vasopressin levels in AD Ss than in normal elderly Ss, which suggests an arginine vasopressin deficiency in AD. A deficit in the CSF concentration of somatostatin in AD was also confirmed. (76 ref).

236. Rasool, C. G. (1986). **Pathogenesis and progression of Alzheimer's disease: A new hypothesis!** Special Issue: Controversial topics on Alzheimer's disease: Intersecting crossroads. *Neurobiology of Aging,* 7(6), 505–506.

Notes that based on impairment of the blood brain barrier (BBB), several theories, including the proposal of J. A. Hardy et al (1986), have been put forward for the pathogenesis of Alzheimer's disease (AD). It is argued, however, that the cause and the existence of BBB breakdown are still unresolved questions in AD. An alternate hypothesis without the involvement of an impaired BBB is proposed for the etiology of AD.

237. Rasool, Chaudri G. & Selkoe, Dennis J. (1984). **Alzheimer's disease: Exposure of neurofilament immunoreactivity in SDS-insoluble paired helical filaments.** *Brain Research,* 322(1), 194–198.
Isolated neurofibrillary tangles (NFTs) prepared from 4 59–74 yr old Alzheimer's disease patients were examined by the indirect peroxidase method for their reactivities with several antibodies. Isolated NFTs, initially unreactive with monoclonal RT97, apparently developed exposed antigenic sites following incubation under denaturing conditions. Results suggest that at least 1 neurofilament epitope is buried in the sodium dodecyl sulfate-insoluble paired helical filaments (PHFs) fiber and that conformational changes in PHF proteins allow its exposure. (12 ref).

238. Ravid, R.; Swaab, D. F.; Fliers, E. & Hoogendijk, J. E. (1986). **Verhoogde vasopressine-produktie gedurende ouderdom en dementie. / Increased vasopressin production in senescence and dementia.** *Tijdschrift voor Gerontologie en Geriatrie,* 17(4), 136–140.
Discusses the present authors' research on changes in vasopressin-containing neurons in the human supraoptic, paraventricular, and suprachiasmatic brain nuclei in senescence and senile dementia and age-related changes in renal vasopressin binding sites in rats. (English abstract).

239. Reinikainen, K. J.; Riekkinen, P. J.; Jolkkonen, J.; Kosma, V.-M. et al. (1987). **Decreased somatostatin-like immunoreactivity in cerebral cortex and cerebrospinal fluid in Alzheimer's disease.** *Brain Research,* 402(1), 103–108.
Determined the somatostatinlike immunoreactivity in postmortem brain tissue of 6 histopathologically confirmed Alzheimer's disease (AD) patients (aged 79–92 yrs) and 11 control patients (aged 66–87 yrs) and in the cerebrospinal fluid (CSF) of 75 probable AD patients (aged 58–90 yrs). Results confirm the involvement of somatostatinergic neurons in AD and suggest that this involvement may be related to the progression of dementia symptoms.

240. Reisberg, Barry. (1984). **"Is Alzheimer's Disease inherited? A methodologic review": Commentary.** *Integrative Psychiatry,* 2(5), 171–173.
Comments on the hypothesis of M. F. Folstein and D. Powell (1984) that most Alzheimer's disease is transmitted as an autosomal-dominant age-dependent disorder. It is argued that although lack of consistent clinical and pathologic criteria for diagnosis was noted by Folstein and Powell, absence of controls, lack of rigor in the collection of pedigree data, bias in recall of poorly defined illness processes, and overinclusive diagnostic criteria were not examined. The present author suggests that Alzheimer's disease is a global clinical process that can be described in terms of either concentration and calculation ability, recent memory, remote memory, orientation, or functioning and self-care. (7 ref).

241. Renvoize, E. B.; Mindham, R. H.; Stewart, M.; McDonald, R. et al. (1986). **Identical twins discordant for presenile dementia of the Alzheimer type.** *British Journal of Psychiatry,* 149, 509–512.

Presents the case of genetically proven identical female twins, discordant for presenile dementia of the Alzheimer type, in which the affected twin began to dement at the age of 49 and died 15 yrs later. However, the surviving twin remains clinically unaffected 20 yrs after the onset of dementia in her sister. Environmental etiological factors are postulated to account for this discordance.

242. Reyes, Patricio F.; Golden, Gregory T.; Fagel, Pantaleon L.; Fariello, Ruggero G. et al. (1987). **The prepiriform cortex in dementia of the Alzheimer type.** *Archives of Neurology,* 44(6), 644–645.
Examined the prepiriform cortex (PPC) of 4 deceased Ss who had clinical and pathological diagnosis of dementia of the Alzheimer type (DAT). Results were compared with those of age- and sex-matched controls who died of nonneurologic diseases. Neuropathological findings indicate that for these Ss, DAT was accompanied by morphological changes in the PPC, an area that has connections with structures concerned with cognitive and behavioral functions.

243. Rinne, J. O. et al. (1985). **Brain muscarinic receptors in senile dementia.** *Brain Research,* 336(1), 19–25.
Analyzed muscarinic receptors in postmortem brain samples of 39 patients (mean age 79 yrs) with different types of dementia and of 30 age-matched controls by the specific binding of 1-quinuclidinyl[phenyl-4-^{3}H]benzilate (QPB). Results show that the binding of QPB was significantly decreased in the hippocampus, amygdala, and nucleus accumbens in Ss with Alzheimer's disease (AD) and with combined type of dementia (CD), whereas in Ss with multi-infarct dementia (MID) the binding was not significantly decreased in the limbic areas but only in the caudate nucleus. Of the clinical variables, orofacial dyskinesias in Ss with AD but not with MID correlated with low brain weight and with the decreased QPB binding in the striatum and frontal cortex. Changes in muscarinic receptor binding show that the cholinergic neurons in the limbic system are especially vulnerable in Ss with AD and CD. (34 ref).

244. Risberg, Jarl. (1987). **Frontal lobe degeneration of non-Alzheimer type: III. Regional cerebral blood flow.** Eric K. Fernström Foundation Symposium: Frontal lobe degeneration of non-Alzheimer type (1986, Lund, Sweden). *Archives of Gerontology & Geriatrics,* 6(3), 225–233.
Results from measurements of regional cerebral blood flow (rCBF) by ^{133}Xe inhalation are presented for 18 neuropathologically proven cases of frontal lobe degeneration of non-Alzheimer type, Pick's disease, Alzheimer's and Creutzfeldt-Jakob's diseases with frontal predominance, and 1 case of bilateral thalamic infarction. It is concluded that the extent and localization of cerebral dysfunction in patients with organic dementing disorders can be described by means of rCBF measurements.

245. Rissler, Klaus; Cramer, Hinrich; Schaudt, Dieter; Strubei, Denise et al. (1986). **Molecular size distribution of somatostatin-like immunoreactivity in the cerebrospinal fluid of patients with degenerative brain disease.** *Neuroscience Research,* 3(3), 213–225.
Investigated somatostatinlike immunoreactivity (SLI) in the cerebrospinal fluid (CSF) of 32 Ss with senile dementia of the Alzheimer type (SDAT [mean age 84 yrs]), 17 Ss with multi-infarct dementia (MID [mean age 79 yrs]), 5 Ss with normal pressure hydrocephalus (NPH [mean age 71 yrs]), 14 paranoid schizophrenics (mean age 36 yrs), and 13 controls (mean age 83.5 yrs). Controls and schizophrenics exhibited an SLI distribution pattern consisting mainly of 2 pronounced peaks, the 1st eluting with the void volume of the column, the 2nd being compatible with a peptide of N-terminally extended somatostatin-14. SLI from the CSF of Ss with SDAT, MID, and NPH showed the same 2 peaks and a 3rd co-eluting with somatostatin-14.

246. Roberts, Eugene. (1986). **Alzheimer's disease may begin in the nose and may be caused by aluminosilicates.** Special Issue: Controversial topics on Alzheimer's disease: Intersecting crossroads. *Neurobiology of Aging,* 7(6), 561–567.
Suggests that genetic factors may interact with aging changes in the nasal mucociliary apparatus to increase the probability that ubiquitously occurring aluminosilicates may enter sensory neurons of the olfactory epithelium and spread transneuronally to several olfactory-related areas of the brain, thereby initiating changes that eventually result in neuronal damage typical of Alzheimer's disease. A speculative sequence of events is suggested by which neuronally contained aluminosilicates might cleave or otherwise alter a normal cellular protein in such a manner that aggregates would arise that could interfere with cellular function and that also could act in a pseudoinfective manner, relaxing translational and transcriptional controls in the synthesis of the native protein. Some relevant experiments and potential therapies arising from the hypothesis presented are discussed.

247. Roberts, Eugene. (1986). **Author's response to commentaries.** Special Issue: Controversial topics on Alzheimer's disease: Intersecting crossroads. *Neurobiology of Aging,* 7(6), 587–590.
The author (1986) responds to commentary papers by H. Baker and F. L. Margolis, R. D. Terry, B. L. Miller, L. Guth, S. Prusiner and M. P. McKinley, C. D. Ward, K. A. Ansari, S. S. Schiffman, A. N. Gilbert, J. Corwin et al, M. M. Esiri and R. J. Williams, R. E. Wimer, and V. W. Henderson (1986) concerning his hypothesis that Alzheimer's disease may begin in the nose and be caused by aluminosilicates.

248. Roberts, Gareth W. (1987). **Herpesvirus in Alzheimer's disease: A refutation.** *Archives of Neurology,* 44(1), 12.
Refutes the hypothesis that herpes simplex virus is involved in the etiology of Alzheimer's disease (AD) by noting that, although the herpes simplex virus has a predilection for the temporal lobe (the main site of pathology in AD) and that recovered encephalitis cases display amnesiac syndromes similar to those found in AD, immunocytochemical, neuropathological, and animal model studies have failed to detect active or latent viral infections in the majority of AD cases.

249. Rogers, Joseph. (1986). **Key concepts in a modern view of Alzheimer's pathogenesis.** Special Issue: Controversial topics on Alzheimer's disease: Intersecting crossroads. *Neurobiology of Aging,* 7(6), 518–520.
Suggests that recent research has prompted a welcome evolution of theory in Alzheimer's disease (AD) and that some of these new ideas are well set out and incorporated in the work of J. A. Hardy et al (1986). They include the reemerging consensus that AD has a distinct neuroanatomical distribution, that it has a primary cortical and limbic basis, which involves subcortical structures, that the classic pathology of AD is indeed pathologic, and that no single neurotransmitter can alone account for Alzheimer's pathogenesis.

250. Roher, Alex. (1987). **"Pathological similarities between Alzheimer's disease and Down's syndrome: Is there a genetic link?": Commentary.** *Integrative Psychiatry,* 5(3), 166–167.
Responding to M. J. Ball (1987), it is noted that the genes apparently responsible for the amyloid protein found in Down's syndrome (DS) and Alzheimer's disease (AD) have been localized on Chromosome 21 and that that the decreasing cognitive capacity found in AD may be due to an as yet undetected biochemical mechanism that is not as active in DS.

251. Roses, Allen D. (1986). **Alzheimer's disease: New genetic research strategies.** Special Issue: Controversial topics on Alzheimer's disease: Intersecting crossroads. *Neurobiology of Aging,* 7(6), 466–468.
Describes molecular genetic strategies focused at Alzheimer's disease (AD), which include both sib-pair linkage testing as well as standard likelihood (LOD score) methods. Reference is made to the article by P. Davies (1986), which points out some of the problems in studying the genetics of AD using LOD and linkage analysis methods. The present author outlines techniques for testing candidate genes. Strategies using subtraction cDNA libraries to determine disease-specific, brain-region-specific, and chromosome-specific mRNAs are presented.

252. Rossor, M. N. (1985). **Transmitter deficits in Alzheimer's disease.** *Neurochemistry International,* 7(4), 567–570.
Comments on the review of the transmitter deficits in Alzheimer's disease reported by J. Hardy et al (1985), focusing on the relationship of neurotransmitter changes to cortical histopathology. The rejection by Hardy et al of the hypothesis that Alzheimer's disease is due to a specific loss of cholinergic neurons is supported, and it is suggested that the importance of individual neurotransmitter changes in Alzheimer's disease currently offers the best model for general therapeutic strategies. (30 ref).

253. Rubenstein, Richard; Kascsak, Richard J.; Merz, Patricia A.; Wisniewski, Henryk M. et al. (1986). **Paired helical filaments associated with Alzheimer disease are readily soluble structures.** *Brain Research,* 372(1), 80–88.
Notes that considerable controversy exists concerning the origin and composition of Alzheimer neurofibrillary tangles (ANTs) and of paired helical filaments (PHFs), the abnormal cytoplasmic fibers that are the major components of ANTs. Thus far, the unusual solubility properties of PHFs have hindered the analysis of ANTs. The present authors report a new procedure for isolating purified PHFs that are soluble in the presence of sodium dodecyl sulfate. The purification protocol involves differential and rate zonal centrifugation treatment with the detergents sarcosyl and sulfobetain 3-14 and sonication. The isolated PHFs from Alzheimer disease/senile dementia of the Alzheimer type (7 cases) and Down's syndrome (1 case) were characterized structurally, biochemically, and immunologically. Distinct polypeptides were shown to be associated with this structure and not seen in preparation from young and age-matched normal brains.

254. Sadovnick, A. D. (1987). **"Pathological similarities between Alzheimer's disease and Down's syndrome: Is there a genetic link?": Commentary.** *Integrative Psychiatry,* 5(3), 164–165.
Responding to M. J. Ball (1987), it is noted that with a greater life expectancy for individuals with Down's syndrome, there should be a greater incidence of reportable dementia, and it is urged that studies of correlation between Down's syndrome and Alzheimer's disease need to account for the mother's age at the birth of the Down's syndrome infant.

255. Sagvolden, Terje. (1985). **Biologiske årsaker til dårligere hukommelse i forbindelse med aldring—fellestrekk av demens av Alzheimers type. / Biological correlates to memory problems in old age and in dementia disorders of Alzheimer's type.** *Tidsskrift for Norsk Psykologforening,* 22(11), 632–635.
Discusses similarities between memory disorders in old age and in Alzheimer-type dementia disorders in which similar structural and neurochemical changes occur. Neurochemical changes are most striking in the cholinergic system originating in the (1) magnocellular olivary nucleus and projecting to the neocortex and (2) medial septal nucleus (MSN) and projecting to the hippocampus. Memory for spatial maps is poor following hippocampal dysfunction. Lesions of the MSN cause a decrease in the level of hippocampal acetylcholine, which is correlated with classical-conditioning impairments. It is argued that these impairments may explain some spatial-memory deficits. It is assumed that memory problems accompanying normal aging are less pronounced in intellectually active than inactive persons. (English abstract).

256. Sakamoto, Noboru; Michel, Jean-Philippe; Kiyama, Hiroshi; Tohyama, Masaya et al. (1986). **Neurotensin immunoreactivity in the human cingulate gyrus, hippocampal subiculum and mammillary bodies: Its potential role in memory processing.** *Brain Research,* 375(2), 351–356.
Mapped the distribution of neurons immunoreactive for neurotensin (NT) in 3 human infant brains. Results show that NT immunoreactive neurons comprise the majority of large perikarya in the human subiculum and project axons to the alveus, fimbria, fornix, and neuropil of the mammillary bodies. Since these regions are prominently involved in conditions such as Wernicke's and Alzheimer's disease in which memory is impaired, it is suggested that NT has potential significance as a peptide in a human brain circuit, which may serve a role in memory processing.

257. Saper, C. B. (1986). **Which came first, the neuritic plaque or the neurofibrillary tangle?** Special Issue: Controversial topics on Alzheimer's disease: Intersecting crossroads. *Neurobiology of Aging,* 7(6), 502–503.
Argues that while J. A. Hardy et al (1986) emphasize the relationship of the vascular amyloid and the neuronal pathology in Alzheimer's disease, at times they try too hard to fit incomplete and sometimes not entirely germane data into their hypothesis. Despite the fact that there are several pieces still missing in this puzzle, the proposed hypothesis should direct research into important and hitherto overlooked directions.

258. Saper, Clifford B.; German, Dwight C. & White, Charles L. (1985). **Neuronal pathology in the nucleus basalis and associated cell groups in senile dementia of the Alzheimer's type: Possible role in cell loss.** *Neurology,* 35(8), 1089–1095.
The loss of cortical cholinergic innervation in senile dementia of the Alzheimer's type (SDAT) is associated with cell loss in the nucleus basalis and related cell groups (magnocellular basal nucleus [MBN]). The authors examined the MBN in 2 cases of SDAT and in 4 control brains after autopsy. Senile plaques were easily demonstrated in the MBN, and most MBN neurons showed neurofibrillary degeneration as an early change. Cell loss appeared to be due to maturation of neurofibrillary tangles, displacing normal cellular contents. It is suggested that the MBN neuronal perikarya may be involved by the same primary processes as cortical neurons. (48 ref).

259. Schapiro, Mark B. & Rapoport, Stanley I. (1987). **"Pathological similarities between Alzheimer's disease and Down's syndrome: Is there a genetic link?": Commentary.** *Integrative Psychiatry,* 5(3), 167–169.
Responding to M. J. Ball (1987), the author cites evidence in support of a genetic hypothesis relating Alzheimer's disease (AD) to Down's syndrome (DS) and describes studies showing neuropathological similarities between AD and DS.

260. Schauss, Alexander G. (1987). **Advances in Alzheimer's disease research: Recent reports on the entry, source, and cellular activity of aluminum and aluminosilicates.** *International Journal of Biosocial Research,* 9(1), 31–34.
Discusses 3 studies on the entry, source, and cellular mechanism of aluminum and silicon in characteristic senile dendritic-neuritic plaques related to Alzheimer's disease: D. P. Perl and P. F. Good (1987), A. M. Coriat and R. D.

Gillard (1986), and T. L. MacDonald et al (1987). The role of the nasal-olfactory mucosa as primary entry site, the leaching of aluminum from cooking vessels, and competition between magnesium and aluminum near microtubules are examined.

261. Schiffman, Susan S. (1986). **The nose as a port of entry for aluminosilicates and other pollutants: Possible role in Alzheimer's disease.** Special Issue: Controversial topics on Alzheimer's disease: Intersecting crossroads. *Neurobiology of Aging,* 7(6), 576–578.
Contends that considerably more research is necessary to evaluate the possible role of aluminosilicates in the brain pathology of Alzheimer's disease (AD) and that other environmental pollutants could be equally responsible for the neurodegeneration and olfactory deficits reviewed by E. Roberts (1986). Animal studies could be useful in determining which chemicals might actually invade the central nervous system (CNS) through the nose and produce the pattern of neurodegeneration characteristic of AD.

262. Schneider, Edward L. & Emr, Marian. (1985). **Research highlights.** Special Issue: Alzheimer's disease. *Geriatric Nursing,* 6(3), 136–138.
Describes areas of research on Alzheimer's disease (AZD) and discusses the disease in relation to the increase of life expectancy that Americans have experienced. One problem encountered in studying AZD is separating the experimental from the control population—the diagnosis of AZD during life is made by excluding other disorders. Research, however, has produced added knowledge about the pathophysiology of AZD and the specific neurotransmitters involved in AZD. The brain's cholinergic system seems to be the most severely afflicted. The enzyme involved in the synthesis of acetylcholine, a neurotransmitter important to learning and memory, is diminished in AZD brains. Recent research has revealed that somatostatin and other brain neurotransmitters are also diminished in AZD. Other research has discovered that in AZD brains the cells' protein-synthesizing mechanisms are decreased because of increased levels of ribonuclease, which is no longer inhibited properly. The relationship of genetics and genetic technology to AZD is also discussed.

263. Schweber, Miriam. (1985). **A possible unitary genetic hypothesis for Alzheimer's disease and Down syndrome.** Symposium of the National Down Syndrome Society: Molecular structure of the number 21 chromosome and Down syndrome (1984, New York, New York). *Annals of the New York Academy of Sciences,* 450, 223–238.
Postulates that Alzheimer's disease (AD) and Down's syndrome (DS) form a continuum. The genesis of AD could involve a tripling of only a subsection of the critical segment of DNA present in DS. As a result, all DS patients would eventually develop AD, but AD could occur without DS. Familial AD would be ascribable to inheritance of the triple amount of the subsection, while sporadic AD would be associated with de novo formation (through a variety of possible mechanisms). Interrelationships between DS and AD are discussed in terms of epidemiologic data, neuroanatomy, biochemical data, and psychosocial level. Current evidence suggests that all older persons with DS develop the neuroanatomy and biochemical changes associated with AD and that the great majority undergo mental decline of some sort with advancing age. Pathophysiological considerations suggest that there may be a similar pattern of molecular effects operative in the expression of both AD and DS, perhaps affecting some type of general genetic regulatory control function. (29 ref).

264. Seeldrayers, P. et al. (1985). **CSF levels of neurotransmitters in Alzheimer-type dementia: Effects of ergoloid mesylate.** *Acta Neurologica Scandinavica,* 71(5), 411–414.
Determined the cerebrospinal fluid (CSF) level of homovanillic acid (HVA), 5-hydroxyindoleacetic acid (5-HIAA), and 3 methoxy-4-hydroxyphenylglycol (MHPG) twice at a 12–15 day interval among 23 51–88 yr olds with Alzheimer-type dementia (ATD). No correlation was found with the degree of dementia as assessed by psychometric testing. Neurotransmitter levels were relatively stable in most Ss. The observation of a decrease in the concentration of HVA but not of 5-HIAA or MHPG in 10 out of 12 Ss treated with ergoloid mesylate may be of interest in elucidating the mechanism of action of this drug in ATD. (16 ref).

265. Selkoe, Dennis J. (1986). **"Altered structural proteins in plaques and tangles: What do they tell us about the biology of Alzheimer's disease?" Author's response to commentaries.** Special Issue: Controversial topics on Alzheimer's disease: Intersecting crossroads. *Neurobiology of Aging,* 7(6), 454–456.
The author (1986) responds to a series of commentaries by S.-H. Yen, K. Iqbal, E. K. Perry and R. H. Perry, G. G. Glenner, C. L. Masters, B. A. Anderton, D. M. Mann and J. Hardy, H. M. Wisniewski and D. L. Miller, M. L. Shelanski, D. A. Drachman, P. Gambetti et al, and D. C. Gajdusek (1986) concerning his review of the role of altered structural proteins in the plaques and tangles associated with Alzheimer's disease.

266. Selkoe, Dennis J. (1987). **Deciphering Alzheimer's disease: The pace quickens.** *Trends in Neurosciences,* 10(5), 181–184.
Discusses several subjects that have drawn special interest in the pathogenesis of Alzheimer's disease (AD), including amyloidogenic proteins and the genes that encode them, alterations of neuronal cytoskeletal proteins in AD, and cytoarchitectural disorganization in the cerebral cortex. The present author maintains that the rough outlines of a pathogenetic sequence that could explain cortical degeneration in AD have emerged, and understanding the cellular and molecular mechanisms of amyloid deposition and neuritic plaque formation may lead to an elucidation of the etiology of the disease.

267. Selkoe, Dennis J. (1986). **Altered structural proteins in plaques and tangles: What do they tell us about the biology of Alzheimer's disease?** Special Issue: Controversial topics on Alzheimer's disease: Intersecting crossroads. *Neurobiology of Aging,* 7(6), 425–432.
Asserts that the progressive dysfunction and loss of neurons in Alzheimer's disease (AD) is accompanied by structural changes in neuronal cell bodies and neurites, particularly in limbic and association cortices. Paired helical filaments (PHF) and antigenically related straight filaments accumulate in perikaryal tangles and the neurites of neuritic plaques. Recent studies indicate that altered forms of the microtubule-associated phosphoprotein, tau, are important constituents of PHF. Other neuronal cytoskeletal proteins, particularly microtubule-associated protein 2 and neurofilament, have been associated with PHF. It is suggested that the widespread neuritic and perikaryal alterations in brain tissue are likely to represent, at least in part, the morphological substrate of cortical dysfunction in AD.

268. Seltzer, Benjamin. (1984). **"Is Alzheimer's Disease inherited? A methodologic review": Commentary.** *Integrative Psychiatry,* 2(5), 170–171.
Comments on the hypothesis of M. F. Folstein and D. Powell (1984) that most Alzheimer's disease is transmitted as an autosomal-dominant age-dependent disorder. 65 males with primary degenerative dementia of the Alzheimer type (PDDAT) were divided into 2 groups on the basis of age of onset and compared on clinical features said to distinguish the groups by using the Boston Diagnostic Aphasia Examina-

tion. Results show that early onset Ss fell short of reaching their life expectancy and had a high prevalance of left-handedness. It is hypothesized that there are 2 different forms of PDDAT. (12 ref).

269. Serby, Michael et al. (1984). **CSF somatostatin in Alzheimer's disease.** *Neurobiology of Aging,* 5(3), 187–189.
10 nondepressed Alzheimer's disease Ss (mean age 73.2 yrs) had significantly lower CSF somatostatin levels than did 9 Ss (mean age 65.9 yrs) with other neurological disorders. An S with Parkinson's disease and dementia had a level in the range of the AD group, while a nondemented Parkinson's disease S had a level above this range. It is suggested that CSF somatostatin may be useful in differentiating dementias in cases in which depression has been ruled out. (17 ref).

270. Shalat, Stuart L.; Seltzer, Benjamin; Pidcock, Candace & Baker, Edward L. (1987). **Risk factors for Alzheimer's disease: A case-control study.** *Neurology,* 37(10), 1630–1633.
Conducted a case-control study to assess personal and family medical history and the appearance of Alzheimer's disease (AD). 98 male patients with clinically diagnosed AD were compared with 162 controls, matched by sex, year of birth, and town of residence. Family history of dementia and personal history of depression were more frequent in patients. The number of cigarettes smoked was also greater in AD cases.

271. Sharman, Melanie G.; Watt, D. C.; Janota, I. & Carrasco, L. H. (1979). **Alzheimer's disease in a mother and identical twin sons.** *Psychological Medicine,* 9(4), 771–774.
Alzheimer's disease confirmed by histological examination is described for the 1st time in identical twin brothers who both died at the age of 38 yrs. Their mother died of a dementing illness at the age of 42 yrs, and her brain was atrophied at postmortem. (5 ref).

272. Shefer, V. F. (1984). **Correlation between the severity of dementia and the degree of pathomorphological changes in the cerebral cortex in senile dementia and Alzheimer's disease.** *Zhurnal Nevropatologii i Psikhiatrii,* 84(7), 1004–1006.
Obtained medical histories and examined the temporal poles of 169 patients with senile dementia and Alzheimer's disease—in addition to counting Ss' senile plaques, neurofibrillar nodes, and neurofibrillar skeletons—to examine the correlation between severity of dementia and degree of pathomorphological changes in Ss' cerebral cortexes. The degree of pathomorphological changes was scored. Results indicate a marked correlation between severity of Ss' dementia and degree of pathomorphological changes in the cortex of the temporal pole. (English abstract) (7 ref).

273. Shelanski, Michael L. (1986). **The proteins of plaques and tangles: How much do they tell us about the biology of Alzheimer's disease?** Special Issue: Controversial topics on Alzheimer's disease: Intersecting crossroads. *Neurobiology of Aging,* 7(6), 448–449.
Asserts that D. J. Selkoe (1986) has prepared a comprehensive review of the status of knowledge of the chemistry of the morphological hallmarks of Alzheimer's disease (AD)—the neurofibrillary tangle and the senile plaque. The present author expands on issues concerning the role of the tau protein and intracellular changes and questions whether the key to understanding AD is primarily hidden in plaques and tangles, or even within the brain.

274. Silverman, Jeremy M.; Breitner, John C.; Mohs, Richard C. & Davis, Kenneth L. (1986). **Reliability of the family history method in genetic studies of Alzheimer's disease and related dementias.** *American Journal of Psychiatry,* 143(10), 1279–1282.

Examined 27 families of Alzheimer's disease probands (aged 50–85 yrs) and 22 control families of nondemented Ss (aged 46–79 yrs) to assess the reliability of the family history method in the study of late-onset dementing illness. Results indicate that family history data obtained from multiple informants with standardized instruments are consistent across informants. The rate of Alzheimer's disease in the families studied was similar to rates found in previous studies. (11 ref).

275. Simpson, James; Boyd, Janice M.; Yates, Celia M.; Christie, Janice E. et al. (1986). **Autoantibodies to Alzheimer and normal brain structures from virus-transformed lymphocytes.** *Journal of Neuroimmunology,* 13(1), 1–8.
Investigated the role of immune mechanisms in the pathogenesis of Alzheimer-type dementia and the possibility of generating senile plaque and neurofibrillary tangle antibodies. B-lymphocytes from 2 female patients (aged 60 and 63 yrs) with Alzheimer's disease and 1 healthy 62-yr-old female were transformed into lymphoblastoid cells by exposure to Epstein-Barr virus. 30% of the resulting IgM antibodies from each S recognized brain components (neurons, astrocytes, nuclei, nucleoli) and Alzheimer plaques and neurofibrillary tangles.

276. Sims, N. R.; Finegan, J. M.; Blass, John P.; Bowen, D. M. et al. (1987). **Mitochondrial function in brain tissue in primary degenerative dementia.** *Brain Research,* 436(1), 30–38.
Examined in vitro oxygen uptake by homogenates of fresh samples of frontal neocortex from 7 adult patients with dementia and with neurosurgical controls as a measure of energy-related metabolism and mitochondrial function. Maximal respiratory rates were similar for 7 controls, 5 patients with Alzheimer's disease, and 2 patients with Pick's disease. However, under some conditions producing submaximal metabolic activity, oxygen uptake rates were elevated in the dementia group. Results indicate that metabolic changes may be relevant to the pathogenesis of Alzheimer's disease and related dementias.

277. Sinex, F. Marott & Myers, Richard H. (1982). **Alzheimer's disease, Down's syndrome, and aging: The genetic approach.** *Annals of the New York Academy of Sciences,* 396, 3–13.
Presents evidence that Alzheimer's disease (AD) is inherited and that penetrance in a particular family is a function of aging. The stages, pathology, and genetics of AD are discussed. Implications for counseling are considered in terms of reassuring adults whose parents have late-onset AD that their chances of not getting the disease are good, and of allowing the appropriate preparation by persons at risk for developing AD. (17 ref).

278. Skullerud, Kari. (1985). **Variations in the size of the human brain: Influence of age, sex, body length, body mass index, alcoholism, Alzheimer changes, and cerebral atherosclerosis.** *Acta Neurologica Scandinavica,* 71(102, Suppl), 94 p.
Investigated the factors that determined brain weight (BW) and lateral ventricle volume (LVV) in 467 autopsy cases (64 males and 17 females between 45 and 50 yrs of age and 196 males and 190 females between 70 and 79 yrs of age). Tissue samples were taken from standard levels of the cerebral cortex and hippocampus. BW and LVV were correlated with age, sex, body length, body weight, cerebral atherosclerosis, Alzheimer changes, and alcoholism. Results show a significant correlation between the weight of supra- and infratentorial parts and between LVV and the weight of cerebral hemispheres in normal brains. Females had smaller brains and smaller lateral ventricles proportionate to their hemispheres. Severe Alzheimer changes were found to cause an increase in LVV in both males and females and suggested a slow progression in symptom onset. Severe Alzheimer cases demonstrated an even distribution of lesions, whereas mild cases reflected an uneven distribution. Alcoholism was found to cause a

clear decline in the weight of the cerebral hemispheres and of the cerebellum and brain stem. No indication was found to suggest that cerebral atherosclerosis leads to generalized brain atrophy. (80 ref).

279. Smith, C. C. et al. (1985). **Putative amino acid transmitters in lumbar cerebrospinal fluid of patients with histologically verified Alzheimer's dementia.** *Journal of Neurology, Neurosurgery & Psychiatry,* 48(5), 469–471.
Concentrations of individual free amino acids were determined in lumbar cerebrospinal fluid (CSF) from 11 53–69 yr old patients with various complaints including histologically verified Alzheimer's dementia. Glycine and glutamine in the CSF of Alzheimer's dementia samples were lower than that of 23 23–71 yr old controls. The concentration of glutamic acid in Alzheimer's dementia patients correlated with psychological measures (e.g., Token test, reaction-time measures, IQ). (17 ref).

280. Smith, D. A. & Lantos, P. L. (1983). **A case of combined Pick's disease and Alzheimer's disease.** *Journal of Neurology, Neurosurgery & Psychiatry,* 46(7), 675–677.
Describes the case of a male in his 60's with presenile dementia in which the histological changes of Pick's disease and Alzheimer's disease were mingled. When S died at age 66, the brain showed no focal atrophy, but the Pick changes were most numerous in the hippocampus and in the temporal lobe. An antibody against the 155 kilodalton component of neurofilaments demonstrated not only neurofibrillary tangles and components of senile plaques, but also Pick's inclusions. (11 ref).

281. Soininen, Hikka; Pitkänen, Asla; Halonen, Toivo & Riekkinen, Paavo J. (1984). **Dopamine-β-hydroxylase and acetylcholinesterase activities of cerebrospinal fluid in Alzheimer's disease.** *Acta Neurologica Scandinavica,* 70(1), 29–34.
Measured dopamine-beta-hydroxylase (DBH) activity in the CSF from 60 Alzheimer patients (aged 57–86 yrs) and 20 controls (aged 57–82 yrs). The DBH activity of the CSF from Alzheimer patients did not differ significantly from those for the controls. DBH activity was not correlated with severity of dementia. The activity of acetylcholinesterase was reduced in the CSF of Alzheimer patients. Interestingly, DBH activity was correlated with acetylcholinesterase activity in both Alzheimer patients and the control group. (23 ref).

282. Sorbi, Sandro; Fani, Carla; Piacentini, Silvia; Giannini, Emiliana et al. (1986). **Energy metabolism in demented brain.** *Progress in Neuro-Psychopharmacology & Biological Psychiatry,* 10(3–5), 591–597.
Reviews the literature regarding changes in cerebral glucose metabolic rate, cerebral oxygen consumption, and cerebral blood flow reported in vivo in demented patients (including those with Alzheimer's disease). Observations of changes in energy metabolism related enzymes and the relationship between these changes and those in neurotransmitter related substances are also reviewed. It is suggested that impairment of oxidative metabolism causes abnormality in nerve cell functioning.

283. Sparks, D. Larry & Slevin, John T. (1985). **Determination of tyrosine, tryptophan and their metabolic derivatives by liquid chromatography-electrochemical detection: Application to post mortem samples from patients with Parkinson's and Alzheimer's disease.** *Life Sciences,* 36(5), 449–457.
Presents the regional distribution of 9 neurochemicals (NCs) from the rat brain and levels of 10 NCs from human brains. Levels of NCs from the caudate and putamen of a 56-yr-old demented patient with Parkinson's disease were variably decreased. Levels of NCs in the caudate and putamen of 3 74–88 yr old patients with Alzheimer's disease (SDAT) were also variably decreased; loss of norepinephrine (NE) was seen only in putamen, and losses of dopamine, homovanillic acid, and serotonin were uniform across both caudate and putamen. The cerebrospinal fluid (CSF) of SDAT Ss showed changes in NE only. (25 ref).

284. Spector, Reynold & Kornberg, Arthur. (1985). **Search for DNA alterations in Alzheimer's disease.** *Neurobiology of Aging,* 6(1), 25–28.
Examined the DNA of brain cortex obtained from autopsy specimens of 8 patients with Alzheimer's disease and 8 controls for content of normal and abnormal bases. DNA, purified by hydroxyapatite chromatography, was hydrolyzed under mild conditions and the deoxynucleosides were measured by high-performance liquid chromatography. No differences in the mole percentages of deoxynucleosides in DNA were detected in Ss with Alzheimer's disease compared to controls, nor were abnormal deoxynucleosides found. Restriction-nuclease digests examined by agarose gel electrophoresis also showed no changes. Thus, diffuse and persistent damage to the DNA in brain in Alzheimer's disease was not detected by these methods. These negative findings do not support the hypothesis that diffuse damage to brain DNA is the basis of Alzheimer's disease. (17 ref).

285. Spence, M. Anne; Heyman, Albert; Marazita, Mary L.; Sparkes, Robert S. et al. (1986). **Genetic linkage studies in Alzheimer's disease.** *Neurology,* 36(4), 581–584.
Studied 18 families with Alzheimer's disease in family members, under the assumption that the disease is due to a single gene with an autosomal dominant form of inheritance. There was no evidence of linkage of Alzheimer's disease with any of 27 phenotypic gene markers analyzed, but close linkage for the Rh and MNS blood group loci was excluded.

286. Spillane, J. A. et al. (1977). **Selective vulnerability of neurones in organic dementia.** *Nature,* 266(5602), 558–559.
In Alzheimer's disease (organic dementia) characteristic nerve cell loss appears, cause unknown, and assessment has been difficult. Whole temporal lobes were analyzed as indices of total neural cell numbers, and it was found that while numbers of glial cells remained unchanged, there was a loss of approximately half the total nerve cell population when compared to age-matched controls. To discover evidence of selective changes in the number or state of specific types of neurons, the concentration of neurotransmitters and their biosynthetic enzymes were measured; and indications of reduced activity of choline acetyltransferase (CAT), a marker of cholinergic neurons, were found. Indications of a similar reduction in activity for glutamic acid decarboxylase (GAD), a marker of gamma-aminobutyric acid-containing neurons, were suspect because of the manner of death of persons from whom samples were taken. To resolve this difficulty, cortical biopsies were examined in 4 Alzheimer cases: Reduced activity was found for CAT but not GAD. The data suggest that at least the presynaptic cholinergic system is selectively affected in Alzheimer's disease. Implications for treatment are discussed. (27 ref).

287. St Clair, David. (1987). **Chromosome 21, Down's syndrome and Alzheimer's disease.** *Journal of Mental Deficiency Research,* 31(2), 213–214.
Suggests that the recent demonstration of a genetic link between Alzheimer's disease (AD) and chromosome 21 should be of interest to researchers into mental handicap. Over the last decade, clinical, neuropathological, and neurochemical evidence had gradually accumulated that the premature dementia found in a high proportion of middle-aged Down's syndrome persons was qualitatively indistinguishable from AD. Such evidence supports the hypothesis that an abnormality on chromosome 21 might be implicated in both conditions.

288. Steingart, Allan; Hachinski, Vladimir C.; Lay, Catherine; Fox, Allan J. et al. (1987). **Cognitive and neurologic findings in demented patients with diffuse white matter lucencies on computed tomographic scan (leuko-araiosis).** *Archives of Neurology,* 44(1), 36–39.
Studied the relationship between the psychometric test performance and neurologic findings in 113 patients (mean age at onset 65.6 yrs) with suspected dementia. Each S underwent a neurologic examination, psychometric testing, a computerized tomography scan, and EEG. 39 Ss were found to have leuko-araiosis (LA [patchy or diffuse lucencies in the white matter]); these Ss also had significantly lower mean scores on the Extended Scale for Dementia (ESD). Ss with clinically diagnosed Alzheimer's disease showed a strong relationship between LA and ESD performance before severe deterioration occurred. LA was also linked with increased age and multi-infarct dementia.

289. Sturt, Elizabeth. (1986). **Application of survival analysis to the inception of dementia.** *Psychological Medicine,* 16(3), 583–593.
Examined the age at onset of dementia of Alzheimer's, Pick's, or senile type in relatives of probands with early onset dementia using survival analytical techniques applied to data collected by T. Sjögren et al. (1952). Female relatives had a higher risk of dementia than males, and there was a deficit of affected brothers compared with fathers of probands. Relatives of probable and definite Pick probands had a higher risk than relatives of probable and definite Alzheimer probands, but the difference was not significant and dementia did not occur at an earlier age to the former group. For the relatives as a whole, and for subgroups of relatives, the risk of dementia increased with age, at least up to age 80 yrs. It is hypothesized that the pattern of the age-related hazard of dementia is due to the nature of the dementing process; that this slow degenerative process is widespread; and that individual differences in the rate of the process are under the influence of genes.

290. Sulkava, Raimo; Erkinjuntti, Timo & Laatikainen, Timo. (1985). **CSF β-endorphin and β-lipotropin in Alzheimer's disease and multi-infarct dementia.** *Neurology,* 35(7), 1057–1058.
In 8 Alzheimer's disease patients and 8 patients with multi-infarct dementia (aged 59–79 yrs), the mean concentration of cerebrospinal fluid (CSF) beta-endorphin was significantly lower in 8 age-matched nondemented controls. Mean beta-lipotropin levels did not differ significantly between demented Ss and controls. The possibility that decreased beta-endorphin concentration is related to the dementia syndrome is discussed. (20 ref).

291. Sunderland, Trey; Rubinow, David R.; Tariot, Pierre N.; Cohen, Robert M. et al. (1987). **CSF somatostatin in patients with Alzheimer's disease, older depressed patients, and age-matched control subjects.** 139th Annual Meeting of the American Psychiatric Association, (1986, Washington DC). *American Journal of Psychiatry,* 144(10), 1313–1316.
Measured somatostatin-like immunoreactivity in the cerebrospinal fluid (CSF) of 12 patients (mean age 61.2 yrs) with Alzheimer's disease, 15 age-matched controls, and 20 depressed Ss (mean age 58.7 yrs). Ss with dementia or depression had lower CSF somatostatin concentrations than controls despite markedly different clinical presentations. Severity of depression was clearly different in all 3 groups but showed no significant correlation with CSF concentration of somatostatin. There was a significant positive correlation between CSF somatostatin-like immunoreactivity and cognitive functioning in all Ss, but this was not statistically significant within individual diagnostic groups. These data raise questions about possible biological links between Alzheimer's disease and depression in older patients.

292. Svendsen, C. N. (1986). **"MPTP-induced neurotoxicity: Clues to the pathophysiology of Parkinson's disease":** Commentary. *Integrative Psychiatry,* 4(2), 92–93.
In response to J. A. Javitch's (1986) article, the present author discusses the role of neurotoxicity in the occurrence of mental disorders. If there is a chronic accumulation of 1-methyl-4-phenyl-1,2,3,6-tetrahydropyridine (MPTP) or a related neurotoxin in the central nervous system (CNS), it may be possible to detect the compound postmortem in human brain tissue. It has been suggested that Parkinson's disease (PD) may involve MPTP accumulation in the brain. Research on the possible neurotoxic etiology of Alzheimer's disease may shed light on the cause and development of PD.

293. Swaab, Dick F.; Fliers, E. & Partiman, T. S. (1985). **The suprachiasmatic nucleus of the human brain in relation to sex, age and senile dementia.** *Brain Research,* 342(1), 37–44.
Investigated the suprachiasmatic nucleus (SCN), which is considered to be the endogenous clock of the brain essential for the ovulation cycle and the temporal organization of sleep-wake patterns, in 12 nondemented males and 16 females and in 1 male and 3 females who suffered from senile dementia of the Alzheimer type (SDAT). Immunocytochemical staining with antivasopressin as a marker permitted a morphometric study of this nucleus in the human brain, which revealed that the shape of the SCN is sexually dimorphic. The shape of the SCN was elongated in women and more spherical in men. In both sexes a decrease in SCN volume and cell number was observed in senescence (80–100 yrs). The latter change was especially pronounced in Ss with SDAT. Results suggest the presence of a structural defect in the SCN that underlies the general disturbance of biological rhythms in senescence and SDAT. (40 ref).

294. Swihart, Andrew A. (1987). **Cerebral cortical somatostatin and cognitive dysfunction in Alzheimer's disease.** *Dissertation Abstracts International,* 47(11-B), 4697.

295. Tagliavini, F. & Pilleri, G. (1984). **Note on the pathology of the basal nucleus of Meynert in degenerative brain disorders.** *Schweizer Archiv für Neurologie, Neurochirurgie und Psychiatrie,* 135(2), 277–280.
Discusses the role of the basal nucleus of Meynert (bnM) in disorders accompanied by cognitive disturbances (e.g., Alzheimer's and Parkinson's diseases). The usefulness of using bnM as an index of the disease's severity is noted. (16 ref).

296. Tago, H.; McGeer, P. L. & McGeer, E. G. (1987). **Acetylcholinesterase fibers and the development of senile plaques.** *Brain Research,* 406(1–2), 363–369.
Applied a new histochemical technique for actylcholinesterase (AChE) to a study of Alzheimer's disease (AD) brain tissue of 6 AD patients (aged 68–83 yrs) and 3 controls (aged 50–75 yrs). Lesion data in rats established the relationship between AChE-positive neocortical axons and medial basal forebrain cholinergic cells. In AD tissue, many degenerating neurons in the basal forebrain were detected by the AChE histochemical stain. Findings provide evidence of an association between the cholinergic system of the basal forebrain and the early formation of senile plaques in the cortex in AD.

297. Tamminga, C. A.; Foster, N. L. & Chase, T. N. (1985). **Reduced brain somatostatin levels in Alzheimer's disease.** *New England Journal of Medicine,* 313(20), 1294–1295.
Analyzed the concentration of somatostatin and the activity of choline acetyltransferase in postmortem brain tissue of 9 patients with Alzheimer's disease and 8 controls in the area of maximal neuronal hypometabolism. Results extend previous reports of a somatostatin deficit in Alzheimer's dementia, suggesting that the loss is greatest in the brain areas most affected in this disorder (e.g., the parietal association cortex). (8 ref).

31

298. Tanzi, Rudolph E.; St George-Hyslop, Peter H.; Haines, Jonathan L.; Polinsky, Ronald J. et al. (1987). **The genetic defect in familial Alzheimer's disease is not tightly linked to the amyloid β-protein gene.** *Nature,* 329(6135), 156–157.
Determined the pattern of segregation of the amyloid betaprotein (AP) gene in familial Alzheimer's disease (FAD) pedigrees using restriction fragment length polymorphisms. The detection of several recombination events with FAD suggests that the AP gene is not the site of the inherited defect underlying this disorder.

299. Taylor, G. R. & Crow, T. J. (1986). **Viruses in human brains: A search for cytomegalovirus and herpes virus 1 DNA in necropsy tissue from normal and neuropsychiatric cases.** *Psychological Medicine,* 16(2), 289–295.
Reports the use of molecular hybridization to screen 79 postmortem human brains for cytomegalovirus and herpes simplex type 1 sequences. The brains were from patients with Alzheimer-type dementia, schizophrenia, Huntington's chorea, or without neurological disease. It is concluded that at the level of sensitivity used, the viruses cannot be regarded as normal residents of the higher central nervous system (CNS) and that at the time of death, they do not appear to have been associated with the neuropsychiatric conditions.

300. Terry, Robert D. (1986). **Does Alzheimer's disease spread, and is it causally related to aluminum?** Special Issue: Controversial topics on Alzheimer's disease: Intersecting crossroads. *Neurobiology of Aging,* 7(6), 570.
Questions views expressed by E. Roberts (1986) concerning lesions in the olfactory cortex associated with Alzheimer's disease (AD), which Roberts believes is an indication of the early involvement of this area, with subsequent spread. The present author contends that degenerative diseases probably do not spread, but rather affect the nervous system according to local vulnerability. (0 ref).

301. Tomlinson, B. E. (1982). **Plaques, tangles and Alzheimer's disease.** *Psychological Medicine,* 12(3), 449–459.
Suggests that to gain total satisfaction with the morphological diagnosis of Alzheimer's disease, both plaques (clusters of abnormal, enlarged nerve processes and terminals surrounding a central mass of amyloid fibrils) and tangles (large clusters of paired helical filaments) must be present in large or considerable numbers in the neocortex. Until the role of tangles and plaques is precisely defined, knowledge of an important area of neuropathology and human aging will be incomplete. (125 ref).

302. Trapp, George A. et al. (1978). **Aluminum levels in brain in Alzheimer's disease.** *Biological Psychiatry,* 13(6), 709–718.
In both human Alzheimer's disease and aluminum encephalopathy of animals, changes are observed in neurofibrillary structures. The present study showed that brains from Alzheimer patients contain approximately 1.4 times the aluminum level found in a control series. Some possible methodological problems are discussed. A plausible chemical mechanism for the changes of aluminum encephalopathy is proposed. (42 ref).

303. Tuček, S.; Doležal, V. & Nedoma, J. (1986). **Cholinergic mechanisms in the brain.** 27th Annual Psychopharmacology Meeting (1985, Jeseník, Czechoslovakia). *Activitas Nervosa Superior,* 28(1), 42–43.
Discusses research on cholinergic neurons and synapses in the brain. Six groups of neurons have been identified as the origins of the main cholinergic ascendant pathways in the brain. Choline acetyltransferase activity is decreased consider-

ably in the cerebral cortex of patients with Alzheimer's disease (AD). It is contended that the impairment of cholinergic mechanisms is of major importance in the pathogenesis of AD.

304. Van Broeckhoven, C.; Genthe, A. M.; Vandenberghe, A.; Horsthemke, B. et al. (1987). **Failure of familial Alzheimer's disease to segregate with the A4-amyloid gene in several European families.** *Nature,* 329(6135), 153–155.
Presents data that indicate that a mutation in the amyloid protein gene is not the primary defect causing familial Alzheimer's disease in all cases and suggest that the amyloid protein gene is closer to the 21q22 Down's syndrome phenotype region than has been previously reported.

305. Vincent, Steven R.; Satoh, Keiji & Fibiger, Hans C. (1986). **The localization of central cholinergic neurons.** *Progress in Neuro-Psychopharmacology & Biological Psychiatry,* 10(3–5), 637–656.
Suggests that interest in central cholinergic neurons has intensified due to the involvement of cholinergic mechanisms in Alzheimer's disease. The distribution of central cholinergic neurons is reviewed, focusing on recent work in experimental animals. The pharmacohistochemical procedure for acetylcholinesterase and the development of antibodies to choline acetyltransferase are 2 major technical advances that have shaped knowledge of the distribution of central cholinergic neurons. The results, advantages, and limitations of both techniques are discussed, as well as the phenomenon of coexistence of acetylcholine with neuroactive peptides in central neurons.

306. Volicer, Ladislav et al. (1985). **Serotonin and 5-hydroxyindoleacetic acid in CSF: Difference in Parkinson's disease and dementia of the Alzheimer's type.** Society for Neuroscience Meeting (1983, Boston, Massachusetts). *Archives of Neurology,* 42(2), 127–129.
Measured 5-hydroxytryptamine (5-HT) and 5-hydroxyindoleacetic acid (5-HIAA) levels in fractions of cerebrospinal fluid (CSF) in 14 patients (mean age 67.1 yrs) with dementia of the Alzheimer's type (DAT), 11 patients (mean age 67.8 yrs) with Parkinson's disease (PD), and 17 neurologically intact controls. 5-HT and 5-HIAA levels in the 20th ml of CSF were positively correlated in the PD Ss and negatively correlated in DAT Ss. In the 7 Ss with senile DAT, 5-HIAA levels in the 20th ml of CSF were higher than in PD Ss. Results suggest differential involvement of the serotonergic system in DAT and PD and indicate possible chemical markers for the diagnosis of DAT. (25 ref).

307. Volicer, Ladislav et al. (1985). **Serotoninergic system in dementia of the Alzheimer type: Abnormal forms of 5-hydroxytryptophan and serotonin in cerebrospinal fluid.** *Archives of Neurology,* 42(12), 1158–1161.
Measured serotonin (5-hydroxytryptamine [5-HT]), 5-hydroxytryptophan (5-HTP), and 5-hydroxyindoleacetic acid in the cerebrospinal fluid (CSF) of 14 patients (67.2 yrs) with a diagnosis of probable Alzheimer's disease (DAI) and in 9 control patients (mean age 64.6 yrs) with normal mental status. It was found that concentrations of 5-HTP, 5-HT, and 5-HIAA were lower in DAT CSF than in a corresponding fraction of control CSF, indicating the involvement of the serotonergic system in DAT. (22 ref).

308. Volk, B. (1982). **Zur Morphologie der Demenz vom Alzheimer-Typ. / Morphological aspects in dementia of the Alzheimer type.** *Zeitschrift für Gerontologie,* 15(6), 199–305.
Senile dementia of the Alzheimer type (SDAT) is a common disease of the nervous system in persons over 65 yrs of age. Histological alterations of SDAT like neurofibrillary tangles and neuritic plaques are described together with experimental work on neurofibrillary changes induced by spindle inhibitors

and aluminum. The role of the cholinergic system deficiency in SDAT is discussed. This deficiency involves the selective loss of cholinergic neurons and the cholinergic innervation of neuritic plaques. (English abstract) (43 ref).

309. Vostrikov, V. M. (1985). **Electron cytochemical examination of microglia in Alzheimer's disease and senile dementia.** *Zhurnal Nevropatologii i Psikhiatrii,* 85(7), 974–976.
Used electron cytochemistry to identify microglial cells in the senile plaques of brains from patients with Alzheimer's disease and senile dementia. A high level of activity of nucleoside diphosphatase was found in the plasma membrane of microglial cells and also in the extracellular substance, which suggests that microglial cells play an important role in the accumulation of amyloid in senile plaques. (English abstract).

310. Wallace, William & Winblad, Bengt. (1986). **Towards a molecular genetic approach to Alzheimer's disease.** *Progress in Neuro-Psychopharmacology & Biological Psychiatry,* 10(3–5), 657–663.
Observations of a familial form of Alzheimer's disease and alterations in the neurochemistry of Alzheimer tissue, including neurotransmitter deficits, paired helical filament, and RNA degradation, suggest that the modification of specific genes may be responsible for the disease. Some basic guidelines are given for using molecular probes to help identify an Alzheimer gene. Preliminary results from the present authors' work in this area are described.

311. Ward, Christopher D. (1986). **Commentary on "Alzheimer's disease may begin in the nose and may be caused by aluminosilicates."** Special Issue: Controversial topics on Alzheimer's disease: Intersecting crossroads. *Neurobiology of Aging,* 7(6), 574–575.
Argues that E. Roberts's (1986) suggestion that the nose is the portal of entry for aluminosilicates is implausible but readily testable. The proposed mode of action of aluminosilicates in triggering changes in the structure and function of cerebral proteins is considered plausible but lacking in convincing data supporting the model.

312. Whalley, L. J. (1986). **Conceptual issues involved with the genetics of Alzheimer's disease.** Special Issue: Controversial topics on Alzheimer's disease: Intersecting crossroads. *Neurobiology of Aging,* 7(6), 473–475.
Asserts that although P. Davies (1986) succinctly discusses the technical issues surrounding a possible genetic role in Alzheimer's disease (AD), important conceptual issues require careful consideration. One involves the general assumption that plaques and tangles represent the critical qualitative variable for defining patients with AD, and the effect that deviations from this assumption will have on genetic studies. Another issue involves the value of research strategies based on single-gene or gene-candidate concepts, given the probable multifactorial characteristic of AD.

313. Whalley, L. J. (1982). **The dementia of Down's syndrome and its relevance to aetiological studies of Alzheimer's disease.** *Annals of the New York Academy of Sciences,* 396, 39–53.
A literature survey of neuropathological studies on Down's syndrome (DS) suggests that in DS, there may be an interaction between genetic and environmental agents or that the pathogenesis of Alzheimer's disease (AD) is influenced by age-related processes that occur precociously in this condition. The strong association between DS and AD also suggests that chromosomal abnormalities may be present in AD. Recent data suggest that, as in DS, increases in parental age may be related to AD. (46 ref).

314. Whalley, Lawrence J. et al. (1982). **A study of familial factors in Alzheimer's disease.** *British Journal of Psychiatry,* 140, 249–256.

Presents data on the families of 74 Ss with autopsy-proven Alzheimer's disease. Data do not support the hypothesis of a familial association between Alzheimer's disease, Down's syndrome, and immunoproliferative disorders. Only the data for immunoproliferative disorders are incompatible with the hypothesis, those for Down's syndrome being too few to be informative. The incidence of presenile dementia among the first-degree relatives of probands was raised, as in many previous studies, and is consistent with a simple polygenic model. (28 ref).

315. White, June A.; McGue, Matthew & Heston, Leonard L. (1986). **Fertility and parental age in Alzheimer disease.** *Journal of Gerontology,* 41(1), 40–43.
Investigated the association of Alzheimer's disease (AD) with reduced fertility and increased parental age at time of birth using data for 126 deceased Ss with AD. Comparison data were collected from AD probands' normal siblings and from 200 age-matched (to AD Ss) individuals. Relative to their normal siblings, maternal age at time of birth of the AD Ss was not significantly increased, nor were AD Ss more likely to be laterborns in their sibships. The percentage of individuals bearing children was 75.7% for AD Ss vs 70.8% for their normal siblings. For those ever bearing children, AD Ss produced slightly more children than their normal siblings. It is concluded that AD is not associated with reduced fertility or increased parental age. (14 ref).

316. Whitehouse, P. J.; Vale, W. W.; Zweig, R. M.; Singer, H. S. et al. (1987). **Reductions in corticotropin releasing factor-like immunoreactivity in cerebral cortex in Alzheimer's disease, Parkinson's disease, and progressive supranuclear palsy.** *Neurology,* 37(6), 905–909.
Examined brain tissue of 9 patients (mean age 75 yrs) with Alzheimer's disease (AD), 7 Ss (mean age 76 yrs) with Parkinson's disease (PD), 4 Ss (mean age 76 yrs) with both AD and PD, and 3 Ss (mean age 74 yrs) with progressive supranuclear palsy. Decreased levels of corticotropin releasing factor (CRF)-like immunoreactivity in the frontal, temporal, and occipital poles of the neocortex were demonstrated in these 3 disorders. Reductions in peptidergic immunoreactivity correlated with reductions in the activity of choline acetyltransferase. It is suggested that the reduction in cortical CRF levels may be due to abnormalities of intrinsic cortical neurons or to dysfunction in neurons that contain CRF and innervate cortex.

317. Whitehouse, Peter J. et al. (1982). **Alzheimer's disease and senile dementia: Loss of neurons in the basal forebrain.** *Science,* 215(4537), 1237–1239.
Results of a study of 5 patients with presumed sporadic Alzheimer's disease and senile dementia of the Alzheimer's type show that neurons of the nucleus basalis of Meynert underwent a profound and selective degeneration in these patients and provided a pathological substrate of the cholinergic deficiency in their brains. Findings represent a significant step in the understanding of the pathophysiology of this neurological disorder.

318. Whitehouse, Peter J. & Au, Kin Sing. (1986). **Cholinergic receptors in aging and Alzheimer's disease.** *Progress in Neuro-Psychopharmacology & Biological Psychiatry,* 10(3–5), 665–676.
Reviews studies of muscarinic cholinergic receptors (MCRs) and nicotinic cholinergic receptors in Alzheimer's disease (AD) and compares the alterations that occur in this disease to those that occur in normal aging. Inconsistent findings with regard to alterations in MCR density may be due to a differential effect of AD on subtypes of MCRs or to the existence of subtypes of AD.

319. Whitehouse, Peter J.; Martino, Andrea M.; Antuono, Piero G.; Lowenstein, Pedro R. et al. (1986). **Nicotinic acetylcholine binding sites in Alzheimer's disease.** *Brain Research,* 371(1), 146–151.
In Alzheimer's disease (AD), there is a loss of presynaptic cholinergic markers in the cerebral cortex, but the nature of cholinergic receptor changes is unclear. In the present study, [^{3}H]acetylcholine and [^{3}H]nicotine were used to label nicotinic cholinergic binding sites in cerebral cortical tissues obtained at autopsy from 19 patients (mean age 72 yrs) with AD and from 13 matched controls (mean age 64 yrs). A consistent and severe loss of nicotinic receptors was found in AD.

320. Whitehouse, Peter J. & Unnerstall, James R. (1986). **The continuing search for the primary event in Alzheimer's disease: A criticism.** Special Issue: Controversial topics on Alzheimer's disease: Intersecting crossroads. *Neurobiology of Aging,* 7(6), 517–518.
Reviews the article on Alzheimer's disease (AD) by J. A. Hardy et al (1986) in which they propose a model of pathogenesis and progression of the neurodegeneration in AD and argues that these authors have created artificial dichotomies in characterizing research in this area. Although they attempt to define the cortex as the primary locus of the lesion, their ultimate conclusions suggest a cyclical process involving both cortical and subcortical involvement.

321. Wietgrefe, S. et al. (1985). **Cloning of a gene whose expression is increased in scrapie and in senile plaques in human brain.** *Science,* 230(4730), 1177–1179.
Constructed a complementary DNA library from messenger RNAs extracted from the brains of Swiss mice infected with the scrapie agent to find clones that might be used as markers of infection and to find clones of genes whose increased expression might be correlated with the pathological changes common to scrapie and Alzheimer's disease. A gene was identified whose expression is increased in scrapie. Findings suggest that increased expression of some cellular RNAs may be common to infection by unconventional agents and to degenerative changes in the aging human brain exemplified by Alzheimer's disease. (24 ref).

322. Wilcock, G. K. & Esiri, M. M. (1987). **Asymmetry of pathology in Alzheimer's disease.** *Journal of Neurology, Neurosurgery & Psychiatry,* 50(10), 1384–1386.
Examined the asymmetry of plaque counts in the brains of 5 Alzheimer's disease (AD) patients (aged 56–81 yrs) and the number of nucleolated pigmented neurons in 10 prospectively assessed undemented Ss (aged 55–102 yrs) and 13 AD patients (aged 55–88 yrs). Results indicate the importance of performing correlative histology and biochemistry on material from the same side of the brain.

323. Wilkins, R. H. & Brody, Irwin A. (1969). **Alzheimer's disease: Neurological classics.** *Archives of Neurology,* 21(1), 109–110.
Presents Alzheimer's translated classic on clinical–pathological correlation applied to presenile dementia, together with comment concerning its applicability today. Investigations subsequent to those of Alzheimer have revealed the same kinds of neurological changes in persons with senile dementia and in elderly persons without dementia.

324. Wimer, Richard E. (1986). **Two topics for further exploration.** Special Issue: Controversial topics on Alzheimer's disease: Intersecting crossroads. *Neurobiology of Aging,* 7(6), 584.

Comments on E. Roberts's (1986) hypothesis, by arguing that information concerning brain regions selectively affected in Alzheimer's disease is still incomplete, and the unique involvement of olfactory regions remains to be demonstrated conclusively. The very high incidence of Alzheimer neuropathology in aging humans with Down's syndrome raises issues concerning the role of aluminosilicates.

325. Winblad, Bengt; Hardy, John; Bäckman, Lars & Nilsson, Lars-Göran. (1985). **Memory function and brain biochemistry in normal aging and in senile dementia.** *Annals of the New York Academy of Sciences,* 444, 255–268.
Reviews the literature on memory function and brain biochemistry in normal aging and in senile dementia, noting that the distinctive feature of this literature is that of interactions between age and type of task. Biochemical changes in normal aging include dopamine depletion in striatal nuclei and noradrenaline reduction in certain limbic regions, the hippocampus, and the hypothalamus. In Alzheimer's disease and senile dementia, however, there is a marked decrease in cholinergic and serotonergic activity. The cortical motor areas are relatively spared from neurodegenerative changes in normal aging, Alzheimer's disease, and senile dementia of the Alzheimer type, and this might provide a neuroanatomical basis for the elderly's and mildly to moderately demented patients' success in memory performance when motor action is involved. The role of dopamine in motor function and its stability with age in the hippocampus may also provide a neurochemical basis for the preservation of memory when the Ss are allowed to act physically during encoding. (108 ref).

326. Wisniewski, Henry M.; Moretz, Roger C. & Iqbal, Khalid. (1986). **No evidence for aluminum in etiology and pathogenesis of Alzheimer's disease.** Special Issue: Controversial topics on Alzheimer's disease: Intersecting crossroads. *Neurobiology of Aging,* 7(6), 532–535.
Contends that the review by D. R. Crapper McLachlan (1986) provides a one-sided view in support of the possible role of aluminum (AL) in Alzheimer's disease (AD) without going into the biology, pathology, and biochemistry of the disease or the disease process. AL has been implicated as a cause or an important factor in AD, amyotrophic lateral sclerosis (ALS), ALS-parkinsonism dementia, and dialysis dementia. It is concluded, however, that outside of the dialysis dementia syndrome, to date there is no evidence that AL has a role in the observed pathological changes, signs, and symptoms in any of these diseases.

327. Wisniewski, Henry M. & Miller, David L. (1986). **Morphology and biochemistry of abnormal fibrous proteins in Alzheimer's disease and senile dementia of the Alzheimer type (AD/SDAT).** Special Issue: Controversial topics on Alzheimer's disease: Intersecting crossroads. *Neurobiology of Aging,* 7(6), 446–447.
Comments on the article by D. J. Selkoe (1986) on Alzheimer's disease (AD) and rates it as a well-written review about biochemistry and immunochemistry of neuronal paired helical filaments (PHF) and nonneuronal (amyloid) fibrous proteins in AD/Senile Dementia of the Alzheimer type. A weakness of the article is considered to be an insufficient description of the ultrastructural morphology of the PHF normal neurofilaments and plaque and vascular amyloid.

328. Wisniewski, Henry M.; Rudelli, R. D.; Iqbal, K. & Merz, G. (1986). **AD/SDAT, plaques, tangles and BBB changes.** Special Issue: Controversial topics on Alzheimer's disease: Intersecting crossroads. *Neurobiology of Aging,* 7(6), 504.

Suggests that although J. A. Hardy et al (1986) correctly point to the role of changed blood brain barrier (BBB) in pathogenesis of Alzheimer's disease/Senile Dementia of the Alzheimer Type (AD/SDAT) pathology, their hypothesized sequence of events leading to BBB changes and plaque and tangle formation is at variance to what is known about the neuropathology and biochemistry of AD/SDAT.

329. Wisniewski, K. E. et al. (1985). **Alzheimer's disease in Down's syndrome: Clinicopathologic studies.** *Neurology,* 35(7), 957–961.
Clinical and neuropathologic evidence points to the development of Alzheimer's disease (AD) in 7 Down's syndrome patients over 40 yrs of age. Dementia was observed in these Ss over 2.5–9.2 yrs. The 1st clinical sign of AD, visual memory loss, was succeeded by impaired learning capacity, decreased occupational and social functioning, and seizures and urinary incontinence. The morphometric observations of Ss' brains showed that the numbers of plaques and tangles exceeded 20 per 1.5×10^6 μm^2 area in both the prefrontal and hippocampal cortices. Plaques and tangles were also evident in the basal ganglia, thalamus, hypothalamus, and midbrain. In addition, 4 of the 7 brains showed small strokes and 5 of the 7 amyloid angiopathy. Findings also indicate that by longitudinal neuropsychological evaluations and lab tests, which exclude other causes of dementia, the diagnosis of AD can be made even in severely and profoundly retarded patients. (29 ref).

330. Wisniewski, K. E.; Rabe, A. & Wisniewski, H. M. (1987). **"Pathological similarities between Alzheimer's disease and Down's syndrome: Is there a genetic link?": Commentary.** *Integrative Psychiatry,* 5(3), 165–166.
In responding to M. J. Ball (1987) concerning the relationship between Down's syndrome (DS) and Alzheimer's disease (AD), the authors reaffirm the possibility of a genetic connection but suggest that more data are needed to substantiate the hypothesis of primary hippocampal involvement in demented elderly persons with DS. It is also suggested that dementia in DS patients may reflect a developmental hippocampal hypoplasia, rather than a dropout of neurons reflecting AD.

331. Wolozin, Benjamin L.; Pruchnicki, Alex; Dickson, Dennis W. & Davies, Peter. (1986). **A neuronal antigen in the brains of Alzheimer patients.** *Science,* 232(4750), 648–650.
A monoclonal antibody was prepared against pooled homogenates of brain tissue taken at autopsy from 4 patients with Alzheimer's disease. This antibody recognized an antigen present in much higher concentration in certain brain regions of Alzheimer patients than in normal brain. The antigen appears to be a protein present in neurons involved in the formation of neuritic plaques and neurofibrillary tangles, and in some morphologically normal neurons in sections from Alzheimer brains.

332. Wright, A. F. & Whalley, Lawrence J. (1984). **Genetics, ageing and dementia.** *British Journal of Psychiatry,* 145, 20–38.
Discusses the contribution of genetic differences to variation in aging and the relationship of aging to certain types of dementia. Neuropathological changes commonly found in the aging brain are present in more severe form in Alzheimer-type dementia, Down's syndrome, multi-infarct dementia, and a substantial number of patients with Parkinson's disease. An increased frequency of aging-associated changes outside the brain have been reported in Alzheimer-type dementia, Down's syndrome, and multi-infarct dementia, although the evidence is generally meager and in many cases requires further corroboration. Genetic studies of Alzheimer-type dementia support the existence of heterogeneity on the basis of family history and age of onset; early onset is associated with greater genetic risk and severity of abnormality. It is suggested that the increasing evidence of an association between

DNA damage, premature aging, and neuronal cell loss may provide insights into the etiology of these and other forms of dementia. (7 p ref).

333. Wurtman, Richard J. (1985). **Alzheimer's disease.** *Scientific American,* 252(1), 62–74, 120.
Notes that the cause of Alzheimer's disease (AD) has not been determined and discusses 6 models—the genetic, abnormal-protein, infectious-agent, toxin, blood-flow, and acetylcholine (AC) models—that underlie current research on AD. The unifying characteristic of all 6 models is that they provide different explanations for the same fundamental symptom of AD: the loss of neurons in the brain, particularly in regions essential to memory and cognition. The AC model has attracted the most interest and resulted in the most attempts at therapy. This model suggests that AC is reduced by as much as 90% in AD patients and proposes explanations for the selective loss of the neurons from which AC is released. Attempts to find a way to restore the AC level are described. Focusing on AC in treatment attempts, however, has a disadvantage: It obscures the fact that, in AD, the brain often exhibits major deficits in other transmitters (e.g., norepinephrine, serotonin). It is suggested that all 6 models may contain some viability and eventually aid in uncovering the essential nature of AD and the key to its successful treatment.

334. Wurtman, Richard J.; Blusztajn, Jan K. & Maire, Jean-Claude. (1985). **"Autocannibalism" of choline-containing membrane phospholipids in the pathogenesis of Alzheimer's disease: A hypothesis.** *Neurochemistry International,* 7(2), 369–372.
Discusses why certain cholinergic brain neurons that characterize Alzheimer's disease are more likely to be damaged than other neurons. It is suggested that their vulnerability may derive from a peculiarity in their metabolic pathways; of all cells, they alone utilize the choline in their membrane phospholipids for 2 purposes—as a structural component and as a reservoir for molecules to be converted to acetylcholine. Observations that are consistent with the autocannibalism hypothesis are listed. (17 ref).

335. Yates, Celia M. (1985). **Transmitter deficits in Alzheimer's disease.** *Neurochemistry International,* 7(4), 571–573.
Reviews the transmitter deficits in Alzheimer's disease, focusing on reductions in choline acetyltransferase (ChAT) activity and reductions in the monoamines noradrenaline, dopamine, and 5-hydroxytryptamine (5-HT). It is asserted that if future studies confirm previous reports of unaltered amino acid transmitters in Alzheimer's disease, it must be concluded that the reduction in ChAT activity remains the major neurotransmitter-related deficit in Alzheimer's disease. (17 ref).

336. Yen, Shu-hui. (1986). **More thoughts on plaques and tangles.** Special Issue: Controversial topics on Alzheimer's disease: Intersecting crossroads. *Neurobiology of Aging,* 7(6), 432–434.
In response to D. J. Selkoe (1986) the present author suggests that Alzheimer neurofibrillary tangles (NFTs) contain unique antigenic determinants and determinants in common with several normal cytoskeletal proteins, including the high molecular weight neurofilament proteins, microtubule associated proteins, and vimentin. The unique determinants are found in nearly all NFTs, whereas the determinants in common with normal cytoskeletal proteins are generally detected only in a fraction of NFTs.

337. Zubenko, George S. et al. (1985). **Cerebrospinal fluid levels of angiotensin-converting enzyme in Alzheimer's disease, Parkinson's disease and progressive supranuclear palsy.** *Brain Research,* 328(2), 215–221.

Angiotensin-converting enzyme (ACE) activity in CSF from 30 adults without known neurologic disorder correlated positively with age of 50–90 yrs. 13 Ss with moderate degrees of senile dementia of the Alzheimer's type and 13 comparably demented patients with Parkinson's disease or progressive supranuclear palsy exhibited mean levels of ACE activity that were decreased 41, 27, and 53%, respectively, compared to the mean level in the age and sex-matched group of neurologically intact Ss. Results raise the possibility that ACE activity in CSF may be an index of neuronal dysfunction in certain central neurodegenerative disorders. (35 ref).

338. Zubenko, George S. (1986). **Hippocampal membrane alteration in Alzheimer's disease. Brain Research,** 385(1), 115–121.
Examined the biophysical properties of hippocampal membrane preparations from 8 patients with Alzheimer's disease and 8 without (Ss' mean age range at death 71.1–73.8 yrs). Results suggest that Alzheimer's disease is associated with a biophysical alteration in superficial regions of brain cell membranes. The biophysical changes did not appear to reflect a loss of neuronal membranes relative to glial membranes or the presence of senile plaques or neurofibrillary tangles.

Animal Research

339. Arendash, Gary W.; Millard, William J.; Dunn, Adrian J. & Meyer, Edwin M. (1987). **Long-term neuropathological and neurochemical effects of nucleus basalis lesions in the rat. Science,** 238(4829), 952–956.
The long-term effects of excitotoxic lesions in the nucleus basalis magnocellularis (NBM) of the rat were found to mimic several neuropathological and chemical changes associated with Alzheimer's disease, in the form of neuritic plaque-like structures, neurofibrillary changes, and neuronal atrophy or loss. It is suggested that NBM-lesioned rats are useful models for studying cholinergic-based dysfunction in Alzheimer's disease.

340. Arnsten, Amy F. & Goldman-Rakic, Patricia S. (1985). **Catecholamines and cognitive decline in aged nonhuman primates. Annals of the New York Academy of Sciences,** 444, 218–234.
Discusses the role of catecholamine loss in the cognitive decline exhibited by aged nonhuman primates whose cognitive deficits resemble those associated with normal aging in humans. The distribution of catecholamines in the cortex of the rodent brain has been known for many years. Dopamine cells project selectively to the prefrontal and anterior cingulate regions, whereas noradrenergic cells project uniformly to all cortical areas. The prefrontal cortex in monkeys is extensively interconnected with the hippocampus, amygdala, dorsomedial thalamus, locus coeruleus, and nucleus basalis. With connections to so many structures implicated in memory function, it is not surprising that several areas of prefrontal cortex are critical foci for normal performance of 2 spatial memory tasks: the spatial delayed response and delayed alternation tasks. The pattern of cognitive impairment that develops in aged monkeys bears a marked resemblance to that produced by lesions to the dorsolateral prefrontal cortex. Implications for the treatment of Alzheimer's disease are discussed. (49 ref).

341. Ball, Melvyn J. et al. (1983). **Paucity of morphological changes in the brains of ageing beagle dogs: Further evidence that Alzheimer lesions are unique for primate central nervous system. Neurobiology of Aging,** 4(2), 127–131.
Studied 12 regions of grey matter from the brains of 25 beagle dogs, varying from 1 to over 16 yrs in age, by serially sectioning and sequentially scanning with a semi-automated sampling stage microscope, in a morphometric search for neuritic plaques, neurofibrillary tangles, and evidence of nerve cell loss. Examination of 227,776 light microscopic fields failed to reveal any senile plaques or neurofibrillary tangles. The neuronal densities, which ranged from 473 to 37,014 nucleolated neurons/mm^3, showed no significant relationship with aging. It is suggested that neuronal lesions of Alzheimer type may be more typical of the human CNS, and physiological evidence for regionally reduced glucose metabolic rate in this animal model may require other structural alterations for its explanation. (32 ref).

342. Barbeau, André; Dallaire, Lise & Poirier, Judes. (1986). **"Animals and experimentation: An evaluation of animal models of Alzheimer's and Parkinson's disease": Commentary. Integrative Psychiatry,** 4(2), 75–78.
Discusses J. H. Kordower and D. M. Gash's (1986) thesis that nonhuman primates constitute the best available model for the study of Alzheimer's disease (AD) and Parkinson's disease (PD). Although it is agreed that any animal model is only an approximation of the human disease being studied, it is argued that the advantages presented by nonhuman primates for pathologic and behavioral paradigms are less evident when the biochemistry, neuropharmacology, or pathophysiology of AD and PD are being investigated. Studies of PD are used to substantiate the premise that the choice of animal species or in-vitro system depends entirely on the questions being asked.

343. Bartus, Raymond T. et al. (1985). **Selective memory loss following nucleus basalis lesions: Long term behavioral recovery despite persistent cholinergic deficiencies. Pharmacology, Biochemistry & Behavior,** 23(1), 125–135.
21 male Sprague-Dawley rats were trained to perform a radial arm maze task and then given either sham or ibotenic acid lesions of the nucleus basalis magnocellularis (NBM), the primary cholinergic projection to the neocortex. Findings indicate that the lesion produced a profound and selective disturbance in memory for recent events. Although the memory deficit persisted for several weeks, a gradual but complete recovery eventually occurred. When these functionally recovered Ss were later tested on a passive avoidance task that is normally sensitive to lesions of the NBM, no deficit was found. Postmortem determinations revealed that the lesions caused marked neurodegeneration of the NBM and decreases in both cortical choline acetyltransferase activity and high affinity choline uptake but had no effect on density of muscarinic receptors. Results support the idea that the cortically projecting cholinergic cells of the NBM normally play an important role in mediating recent memory and demonstrate that any simple relationship between the function of this brain region and the mediation of recent memory is unlikely. Findings highlight issues related to the extent to which degeneration of this brain area may contribute directly to the severe disturbance of cognitive function associated with such neurodegenerative diseases as Alzheimer's, Pick's, and Parkinson's diseases. (78 ref).

344. Bartus, Raymond T. (1986). **"Animals and experimentation: An evaluation of animal models of Alzheimer's and Parkinson's disease": Commentary. Integrative Psychiatry,** 4(2), 74–75.
Discusses J. H. Kordower and D. M. Gash's (1986) paper on the development of animal models for Alzheimer's and Parkinson's diseases. The various perspectives presented on animal models for these diseases are addressed.

345. Björklund, Anders & Gage, Fred H. (1985). **Neural grafting in animal models of neurodegenerative diseases.** Institute for Child Development Research Conference: Hope for a new neurology (1984, New York, New York). **Annals of the New York Academy of Sciences,** 457, 53–81.

Reviews the results obtained by implantation of dopaminergic and cholinergic neurons in animals with lesions of the nigrostriatal or septohippocampal systems (i.e., in conditions that can be said to represent analogous models of Parkinson's and Alzheimer's diseases). It is argued that neural grafting in aged rats may offer new opportunities to study both the factors underlying the age-related decrements in motor and cognitive function and the possibilities of improving the performance of selected brain systems in the aged brain.

346. Boegman, R. J. et al. (1985). **Quinolinic acid neurotoxicity in the nucleus basalis antagonized by kynurenic acid.** *Neurobiology of Aging,* 6(4), 331–336.
When quinolinic acid (QA) was injected unilaterally into the nucleus basalis magnocellularis (NBM) of male Sprague-Dawley rats, neuronal destruction of the basal forebrain occurred. However, no cell loss was observed when kynurenic acid (KA) and QA were co-injected. KA also prevented QA-induced decreases in cortical choline acetyltransferase (CCA), acetylcholinesterase, high-affinity choline uptake, and [^{3}H]-acetylcholine release. A significant decrease in CCA activity was observed 3 mo following QA lesions of the nucleus basalis. Results indicate that QA can be used as an endogenous neurotoxin to produce lesions of the NBM resulting in impaired cortical cholinergic function similar to that seen in Alzheimer's disease. (31 ref).

347. Boylan, Marea K.; Fisher, Robin S.; Hull, Chester D.; Buchwald, Nathaniel A. et al. (1986). **Axonal branching of basal forebrain projections to the neocortex: A double-labeling study in the cat.** *Brain Research,* 375(1), 176–181.
Double-labeling of cat basal forebrain neurons by retrograde axonal transport demonstrated divergent collateralization among undecussated axonal projections to the neocortex, a finding that may be of clinical significance for the neuropathology of Alzheimer's disease. The loss of branched basal forebrain projections to the neocortex may be critical because it removes a common extracortical coordinative input to separated neocortical sites outside the range of local intracortical coupling.

348. Bruce, Moira E. (1984). **Scrapie and Alzheimer's disease.** *Psychological Medicine,* 14(3), 497–500.
Suggests that research on Alzheimer's disease (AD) has been limited by the lack of satisfactory experimental models and discusses the parallels between AD and scrapie, an infectious neurological disease found in sheep and goats. It is argued that, even though attempts to transmit AD to laboratory animals have either failed or have been inconclusive, scrapie still provides valuable models for this type of degenerative pathology. (35 ref).

349. Brufani, M.; Castellano, C.; Marta, M.; Oliverio, A. et al. (1987). **A long-lasting cholinesterase inhibitor affecting neural and behavioral processes.** *Pharmacology, Biochemistry & Behavior,* 26(3), 625–629.
Investigated the inhibitory effects of physostigmine analogs on acetylcholinesterase to find a means of increasing brain acetylcholine to treat Alzheimer's disease. A "heptyl" physostigmine derivative was evaluated for its anticholinesterase activity, acute toxicity, and behavioral effects in 62 male Wistar rats and 526 male DBA$_2$ mice. The heptyl antagonized the stimulating effect of scopolamine on locomotor activity and facilitated memory consolidation. At active doses, the heptyl was significantly less toxic than physostigmine.

350. Cuello, A. C.; Stephens, P. H.; Tagari, P. C.; Sofroniew, M. V. et al. (1986). **Retrograde changes in the nucleus basalis of the rat, caused by cortical damage, are prevented by exogenous ganglioside GM$_1$.** *Brain Research,* 376(2), 373–377.

In male Wistar rats with extensive unilateral cortical damage, retrograde effects on the cholinergic cells of the basal nucleus were observed. Cells of the basal nucleus stained immunocytochemically for choline acetyltransferase were shrunken, and choline acetyltransferase enzymatic activity in that region was reduced. Both these effects could be prevented by the administration of the ganglioside GM$_1$. Implications are noted for the study of neurodegenerative diseases, including Alzheimer-type dementia.

351. Decker, Michael W. & Gallagher, Michela. (1987). **Scopolamine-disruption of radial arm maze performance: Modification by noradrenergic depletion.** *Brain Research,* 417(1), 59–69.
Administration of 6-hydroxydopamine into the dorsal noradrenergic (NA) bundle did not by itself alter the performance of rats on a radial maze working memory task. In Exp I, scopolamine, a muscarinic antagonist, impaired the performance of the NA-depleted Ss more than that of Ss in an operated control group. This result was again observed in Exp II, but here a lesion by order of dose administration interaction provided evidence for recovery from the effects of NA depletion. In Exp III, NA denervation did not alter the functional status of basal forebrain cholinergic neurons. Results suggest that an age-related decline in brain NA neurons, as well as further deterioration in this system in some cases of Alzheimer's disease, may contribute to the cognitive and memory deficits more typically ascribed to cholinergic dysfunction.

352. Egan, Terry M. & North, R. Alan. (1986). **Acetylcholine hyperpolarizes central neurones by acting on an M$_2$ muscarinic receptor.** *Nature,* 319(6052), 405–407.
Intracellular recordings were made from neurons in the rat nucleus parabrachialis, a group of neurons in the upper pons some of which themselves synthesize acetylcholine (ACh). ACh and muscarine caused a membrane hyperpolarization that resulted from an increase in the membrane conductance to potassium ions. The muscarinic receptor subtype was characterized by determining the dissociation equilibrium constant (K_D) for pirenzepine during the intracellular recording; the value of –600 nM indicated a receptor in the M$_2$ class. This muscarinic receptor is different from those that bring about a decrease in potassium conductance in other neurons, which have a pirenzepine K_D of –10 nM (M$_1$ receptors). Results suggest that antagonist selective for this kind of M$_2$ receptor would be useful in the management of conditions, such as Alzheimer's disease, which are associated with a reduced effectiveness of cholinergic neurons. (33 ref).

353. El-Defrawy, S. R. et al. (1985). **Functional and neurochemical cortical cholinergic impairment following neurotoxic lesions of the nucleus basalis magnocellularis in the rat.** *Neurobiology of Aging,* 6(4), 325–330.
Among male Sprague-Dawley rats, the release of cortical [^{3}H]-acetylcholine (^{3}H-ACh), high-affinity choline uptake, and acetylcholinesterase was significantly reduced 7 days following injections of kainic acid (4.7 nmoles) and quinolinic acid (60, 150, and 300 nmoles) into the nucleus basalis magnocellularis. Results show that quinolinic acid, an endogenous neuroexcitant, produced a deficit of cholinergic function similar to that described in the cortical tissue of patients with senile dementia of Alzheimer's type. It is suggested that the cortical slice preparation from quinolinic acid-treated animals showing impairment of ^{3}-ACh release may be useful in assessing the action of drugs designed to improve cholinergic function. (23 ref).

354. Engström, Charlotte; Undén, Anders; Ladinsky, Herbert; Consolo, Silvana et al. (1987). **BM-5, a centrally active partial muscarinic agonist with low tremorogenic activity: In vivo and in vitro studies.** *Psychopharmacology,* 91(2), 161–167.

Investigated the effects of acute (100 ml) and 14-day administration of various doses of the centrally active oxotremorine analog, BM-5 (N-methyl-N-[1-methyl-4-pyrrolidino-2-butynyl]acetamide) (BM-5), in adult male Sprague-Dawley rats and CBA mice. Due to BM-5's regional specificity and low tremorogenic activity, it is suggested as a model compound for muscarinic agonists with therapeutic value in treating senile dementia of the Alzheimer type.

355. Fine, Alan. (1986). **Transplantation in the central nervous system.** *Scientific American,* 255(2), 52–58B.
Contends that grafts of embryonic brain tissue can be anatomically and functionally incorporated into the adult central nervous system (CNS) and suggests that this treatment can be useful in treating Parkinson's and Alzheimer's diseases in which parts of the CNS degenerate. Experimentation with rat brains has shown that grafts improved dopamine input to damaged nerve cells or improved Ss' abilities to run mazes. It is proposed that denervation supersensitivity accounts for some of the ability of embryonic neuronal transplants to reverse behavioral abnormalities in animal models of degenerative neurological diseases.

356. Fine, Alan; Pittaway, Kay; de Quidt, Marion; Czudek, Carole et al. (1987). **Maintenance of cortical somatostatin and monoamine levels in the rat does not require intact cholinergic innervation.** *Brain Research,* 406(1–2), 326–329.
Levels of somatostatin, noradrenaline, dopamine, 5-hydroxytryptamine (5-HT), and 5-hydroxyindoleacetic acid were unchanged in the neocortex of male Sprague-Dawley rats 3 or 6 mo after ibotenic acid lesion of the ipsilateral nucleus basalis that reduced cortical choline acetyltransferase levels by over 60%. These results render unlikely the possibility that non-cholinergic neurotransmitter deficits in Alzheimer's disease cortex are the consequence of cholinergic degeneration.

357. Fischer, W.; Wictorin, K.; Björklund, A.; Williams, L. R. et al. (1987). **Amelioration of cholinergic neuron atrophy and spatial memory impairment in aged rats by nerve growth factor.** *Nature,* 329(6134), 65–68.
As in Alzheimer-type dementia in humans, degenerative changes in the forebrain cholinergic system may contribute to age-related cognitive impairments in rodents. Recent studies have shown that neurotrophic protein nerve growth factor (NGF) can prevent retrograde neuronal cell death and promote behavioral recovery after damage to the septo-hippocampal connections in rats. A study is reported in which continuous intracerebral infusion of NGF over 4 wks partly reversed the cholinergic cell body atrophy and improved retention of a spatial memory task (the Morris water maze) in 24 behaviorally impaired aged rats.

358. Fisher, Abraham & Hanin, Israel. (1986). **Potential animal models for Senile Dementia of Alzheimer's Type, with emphasis on AF64A-induced cholinotoxicity.** *Annual Review of Pharmacology & Toxicology,* 26, 161–181.
Reviews the literature on ethylcholine aziridinium ion (AF64A), which has recently been proposed as a potential tool for developing an animal model for Senile Dementia of the Alzheimer's type (SDAT), a disorder in which a central cholinergic hypofunction has been implicated. The clinical, behavioral, and neuropathological features of SDAT are discussed to ascertain the relevance of AF64A-induced cholinotoxicity to the animal model of SDAT. The AF64A model is compared with other experimental models of SDAT (e.g., scopolamine- or hemicholinium-treated Ss, anoxic or hypoxic rodents, aluminum-treated Ss, aged rodents or monkeys, and excitotoxin-lesioned rats or monkeys). Overall data show that AF64A is a valuable clinical tool with which a persistent cholinergic deficiency of presynaptic origin can be induced. Implications of its apparent selectivity of action are noted.

359. Friedman, Eitan; Lerer, Barbara & Kuster, Joan. (1983). **Loss of cholinergic neurons in the rat neocortex produces deficits in passive avoidance learning.** *Pharmacology, Biochemistry & Behavior,* 19(2), 309–312.
Bilateral kainic acid lesions of the ventral globus pallidus produced a significant and selective cortical decrease in choline acetyltransferase activity in the brains of male Sprague-Dawley rats. When lesioned and control Ss were compared on performance in a step-through passive avoidance task, lesioned Ss showed a marked retention deficit 24 hrs after the initial training trial. This experimentally induced memory deficit associated with a cortical cholinergic neuronal loss resembles the deficits in senile dementia of the Alzheimer type and may provide a useful animal model for studying the disease. (33 ref).

360. Geddes, James W. et al. (1985). **Plasticity of hippocampal circuitry in Alzheimer's disease.** *Science,* 230(4730), 1179–1181.
Compared the response of the human central nervous system (CNS) to neuronal loss resulting from Alzheimer's disease (AD) with the response of male Sprague-Dawley rats to a similar neuronal loss induced by lesions of the entorhinal cortex, using 2 markers of neuronal plasticity. The similarity between the human CNS response to AD-induced denervation and the rat CNS response to lesion-induced denervation suggests that rats with lesions of the entorhinal cortex may be a model for some aspects of AD. Results indicate that the CNS is capable of a plastic response in AD. Adaptive growth responses occur along with the degenerative events. (17 ref).

361. Haigler, H. J.; Cahill, L.; Crager, M. & Charles, E. (1986). **Acetylcholine, aging and anatomy: Differential effects in the hippocampus.** *Brain Research,* 362(1), 157–160.
The response to acetylcholine (ACh) administered microiontophoretically was determined for single units in CA1 and CA3–4 areas of the hippocampi of both young (3–5 mo) and old (24–26 mo) male Fisher 344 rats. Single units in CA1 showed a greater response to ACh (20 nA) than single units in CA3–4 in young and in old Ss. However, the response to ACh in single units of young Ss was significantly greater than in single units of old Ss. It is suggested that this difference in sensitivity to ACh as a function of anatomical location as well as age has implications for the study of Alzheimer's disease. (11 ref).

362. Hallak, Marta & Giacobini, E. (1987). **A comparison of the effects of two inhibitors on brain cholinesterase.** *Neuropharmacology,* 26(6), 521–530.
Compared the effects of intramuscular, intravenous, and intraventricular doses of the cholinesterase (CHE) inhibitors physostigmine (PH) and metrifonate (ME) on brain CHE, acetylcholine (ACh), and choline in male Sprague-Dawley rats. Results suggest that ME is more likely to produce a therapeutic effect on ACh in humans than PH and that a drug that increases brain ACh with minimal effect on ACh turnover would be more suitable for treating Alzheimer's disease.

363. Hayashi, Masao & Patel, Ambrish J. (1987). **An interaction between thyroid hormone and nerve growth factor in the regulation of choline acetyltransferase activity in neuronal cultures, derived from the septal-diagonal band region of the embryonic rat brain.** *Developmental Brain Research,* 36(1), 109–120.
Established culture conditions for growing neurons from the medial frontal part of the forebrain, containing the septum and the diagonal band of Broca, of 17-day-old rat embryos in a chemically defined medium. Observations indicate that sub-

cortical cholinergic neurons, which are affected in Alzheimer's disease and in Down's syndrome, are subject to regulation by an interaction between thyroid hormone and local humoral factors such as nerve growth factor.

364. Heitkemper, Margaret M. & Marotta, S. F. (1985). **Role of diets in modifying gastrointestinal neurotransmitter enzyme activity.** *Nursing Research,* 34(1), 19–23.
Examined the effect of substrate deficiency and dietary fasting on neurotransmitter enzyme activity in the gastrointestinal tracts of 3 groups of 5 male Sprague-Dawley rats: control nontreated, choline-deficient diet for 14 days, and starvation (water only) for 3 days. The choline-deficient diet produced a decrease in adrenergic enzyme activity, and starvation decreased adrenergic enzyme activities and increased activity of the acetylcholine synthesizing enzyme in most segments of the gastrointestinal tract. Implications for treatment of Alzheimer's disease and for patients undergoing prolonged fasts are discussed. (23 ref).

365. Hurlbut, Brian J. (1987). **Basal forebrain infusion of hemicholinium in rats: Maze learning deficits and neuropathology.** *Dissertation Abstracts International,* 47(10-B), 4337.

366. Jarrard, Leonard E.; Levy, Aharon; Meyerhoff, James L. & Kant, G. Jean. (1985). **Intracerebral injections of AF64A: An animal model of Alzheimer's disease?** *Annals of the New York Academy of Sciences,* 444, 520–522.
Two experiments investigated the effects of ethylcholine aziridinium ion (AF64A) on cholinergic systems of the brain in rats. Exp I tested the effects of intracerebroventricular injections of AF64A on motivation, memory, and neurotransmitters. Exp II tested the effects of injecting AF64A into a predominantly noncholinergic brain area. Results of the 2 experiments were similar, suggesting that the influence of AF64A on memory is due to a nonspecific lesion effect rather than to a specific effect on cholinergic systems. (5 ref).

367. Kesner, Raymond P.; Adelstein, Ted & Crutcher, Keith A. (1987). **Rats with nucleus basalis magnocellularis lesions mimic mnemonic symptomatology observed in patients with dementia of the Alzheimer's type.** *Behavioral Neuroscience,* 101(4), 451–456.
College students, healthy elderly subjects, patients diagnosed with mild or moderate dementia of the Alzheimer's type, as well as rats with small or large lesions of nucleus basalis magnocellularis (NBM) were tested on an order memory task for a 6- or 8-item list of varying spatial locations. Similar patterns of order memory deficits as a function of serial order position were observed in rats with small or large NBM lesions and patients with mild or moderate dementia of the Alzheimer's type. The results provide support for the possibility that rats with NBM lesions might mimic the mnemonic symptomatology of Alzheimer's disease.

368. Kesner, Raymond P.; Crutcher, Keith A. & Measom, Michael O. (1986). **Medial septal and nucleus basalis magnocellularis lesions produce order memory deficits in rats which mimic symptomatology of Alzheimer's disease.** *Neurobiology of Aging,* 7(4), 287–295.
Male Long-Evans rats (*N* = 31) with electrolytic lesions of the medial septum or ibotenic acid lesions of the nucleus basalis magnocellularis (NBM) were tested in an order memory task for an 8-item list of varying spatial locations within an 8-arm radial maze. Results indicate that Ss with small medial septal lesions resulting in small acetylcholinesterase (AchE) depletion of dorsal hippocampal formation were impaired only for the first, but not the last choice orders of the list. Ss with large NBM lesions resulting in large AchE depletion of parietal and part of frontal cortex displayed an order memory deficit for all the choice orders of the list. The relationship between these findings and mnemonic symptomatology of Alzheimer's disease is discussed.

369. Kitt, Cheryl A. et al. (1984). **Evidence for cholinergic neurites in senile plaques.** *Science,* 226(4681), 1443–1445.
Identified cholinergic axons in the neocortices and amygdalae of 2 young (approximately 5 yrs old) and 5 old (aged 20–30 yrs) macaques (*Macaca mulatta*), using a monoclonal antibody to bovine choline acetyltransferase. Findings indicate that, in the older Ss, some cholinergic axons showed multifocal enlargements along their course. The appearance of amyloid-associated abnormal cholinergic processes was similar to that of neurites in senile plaques, suggesting that cholinergic systems give rise to some of the neurites with senile plaques. (22 ref).

370. Kordower, Jeffrey H. & Gash, Don M. (1986). **Animals and experimentation: An evaluation of animal models of Alzheimer's and Parkinson's disease.** *Integrative Psychiatry,* 4(2), 64–70.
Evaluates animal models of Alzheimer's and Parkinson's diseases, 2 classical neurologic syndromes. Animal studies have focused mainly on specific neurochemical systems involved in these disease states. The advantages and limitations of the various rodent models are examined. The need to establish valid nonhuman primate models is discussed.

371. Langston, J. William. (1986). **"Animals and experimentation: An evaluation of animal models of Alzheimer's and Parkinson's disease": Commentary.** *Integrative Psychiatry,* 4(2), 78–80.
Discusses J. H. Kordower and D. M. Gash's (1986) paper on animal models of Alzheimer's and Parkinson's disease. The use of primates as opposed to rodents in developing animal models, the creation of models of these diseases at a time in the animal life span that corresponds to the typical age of onset in humans, and future models are considered.

372. Lerer, Barbara et al. (1985). **Cortical cholinergic impairment and behavioral deficits produced by kainic acid lesions of rat magnocellular basal forebrain.** *Behavioral Neuroscience,* 99(4), 661–677.
The rat magnocellular basal forebrain (MNBF) is homologous to the human nucleus basalis of Meynert, a structure implicated in the cholinergic hypothesis of cognitive impairment in Alzheimer's disease (AD). In the present study, 18 male Sprague-Dawley rats with kainic acid lesions in the MNBF were compared with 6 unoperated controls, 10 sham-operated controls, and 6 controls injected with kainic acid in the cortical area directly above the MNBF. MNBF lesions depleted choline acetyltransferase in cortex but not in striatum or hippocampus. Cortical dopamine levels were unchanged; serotonin levels were unchanged in hippocampus and parietal cortex but decreased in frontal cortex. Compared with controls, MNBF-lesioned Ss were impaired in 24-hr retention, but not acquisition, of a passive avoidance task with escapable footshock. The groups did not differ in mean number of daily avoidances on a barpress active avoidance task, although learning was slower in MNBF-lesioned Ss. In a serial spatial discrimination reversal test, MNBF-lesioned Ss performed significantly worse than controls. This model may be useful for studying the role of the cholinergic system in memory and possibly for developing treatment strategies to alleviate the cognitive dysfunction of AD. (63 ref).

373. Levine, M. S.; Adinolfi, A. M.; Fisher, R. S.; Hull, C. D. et al. (1986). **Quantitative morphology of medium-sized caudate spiny neurons in aged cats.** *Neurobiology of Aging,* 7(4), 277–286.
Assessed some morphological alterations that occur in medium-sized spiny neurons of the caudate nucleus in 11 cats (5 1–3 yrs and 6 10+ yrs of age). All measures of dendrite length displayed statistically significant decreases of 30–40% in Ss 15 and 18 yrs of age. Results indicate that there is a sequence of

age-related changes that occurs in caudate medium-sized spiny neurons and provides a basis from which to assess functional alterations. Findings have implications for disorders of aging (e.g., Alzheimer's and Parkinson's diseases).

374. Mantione, Charles R.; Fisher, Abraham & Hanin, Israel. (1984). **Possible mechanisms involved in the presynaptic cholinotoxicity due to ethylcholine aziridinium (AF64A) in vivo.** *Life Sciences,* 35(1), 33–41.
Investigated the potential of an in vivo active cholinotoxin by administering the toxin directly into the brains of rats and mice. The neurochemical and behavioral consequences of AF64A administration were reminiscent of similar measures in patients with Alzheimer's disease. It is tentatively suggested that the AF64A-treated animal may be explored as a potential animal model of this debilitating disease state. (31 ref).

375. Morgan, David G.; May, Patrick C. & Finch, Caleb E. (1987). **Dopamine and serotonin systems in human and rodent brain: Effects of age and neurodegenerative disease.** *Journal of the American Geriatrics Society,* 35(4), 334–345.
Suggests that there are nonpathological age-related declines in the dopamine- and serotonin-containing neurotransmitter systems in human and rodent brain. In Alzheimer's disease, both pre- and postsynaptic markers of the serotonin system are reduced, including a loss of serotonin-containing raphe neurons. A hypothesis is presented to explain the typically young age-at-onset of schizophrenia and the older age-at-onset of parkinsonism, within the context of normal declines in the dopamine system occurring in the absence of neurological disorders.

376. Murphy, D. E. & Boast, C. A. (1985). **Searching for models of Alzheimer's disease: A comparison of four amnestic treatments in two behavioral tasks.** *Annals of the New York Academy of Sciences,* 444, 450–452.
Compared the effects of pentylenetetrazol (40 mg/kg, intraperitoneally), scopolamine (1.5 mg/kg, subcutaneously), ibotenic acid lesions of the nucleus basalis, and aging on the acquisition and retention of rats in an appetitive maze and in an inhibitory avoidance task. Results show that none of the 4 treatments was a viable model of the memory deficits associated with Alzheimer's disease. (7 ref).

377. Nakagawa, Yuzo; Nakamura, Shizuo; Kaśe, Yoshitoshi; Noguchi, Teruhisa et al. (1987). **Colchicine lesions in the rat hippocampus mimic the alterations of several markers in Alzheimer's disease.** *Brain Research,* 408(1–2), 57–64.
Examined the effect of colchicine-induced lesions of hippocampal cells on male Fischer rats. 12 days after infusion, pretrained colchicine-treated Ss showed a significant decrease in choice accuracy in a T-maze learning task, a local reduction in choline acetyltransferase activity, and significant losses of 55-kDa protein in the soluble fraction and 50-kDa protein in myelin and synaptosomal fractions of the hippocampi. There was a marked increase in [³H]glutamate binding in the hippocampus and cortex. Analysis revealed that the increase in glutamate binding was due to an increase in the number of glutamate receptors without significant change in their affinity. The changes caused by hippocampal infusion of colchicine resemble those seen in Alzheimer's disease, suggesting the use of colchicine-treated rats as a model for the disease.

378. Nakahiro, Masanobu et al. (1985). **Pantoyl-γ -aminobutyric acid facilitates cholinergic function in the central nervous system.** *Journal of Pharmacology & Experimental Therapeutics,* 232(2), 501–506.
In the present investigation, pantoyl-GABA (P-GABA) administered ip inhibited scopolamine- and atropine-induced locomotor activities in ICR mice. P-GABA inhibited the binding of [³H]muscimol to the brain membranes of male Sprague-Dawley rats. GABA and P-GABA enhanced K⁺

(25mM)-induced release of [³H]acetylcholine from slices of the cerebral cortex and hippocampus in a dose-dependent manner, and their effects were antagonized by bicuculline. Results suggest that P-GABA binds to GABA receptors causing enhanced cholinergic neurotransmission in the CNS. Implications for use of P-GAMA in the treatment of Alzheimer's disease and senile dementia of the Alzheimer type are discussed. (32 ref).

379. Ögren, Sven-Ove; Carlsson, S. & Bartfai, T. (1985). **Serotonergic potentiation of muscarinic agonist evoked tremor and salivation in rat and mouse.** *Psychopharmacology,* 86(3), 258–264.
Studied the oxotremorine-, arecoline- and physostigmine-induced muscarinic responses of tremor and salivation in male NMRI mice and male Sprague-Dawley rats pretreated with alaproclate, a selective 5-hydroxytryptamine (5-HT) uptake inhibitor with antidepressant properties. Results suggest a 5-HT receptor involvement in the action of alaproclate, which may exert its muscarinic potentiating effects at an as yet undefined metitepine- and danitracen-sensitive serotonergic site. Implications for the study of Huntington's chorea and Alzheimer's disease are noted. (29 ref).

380. Oreland, Lars & Gottfries, Carl-Gerhard. (1986). **Brain and brain monoamine oxidase in aging and in dementia of Alzheimer's type.** *Progress in Neuro-Psychopharmacology & Biological Psychiatry,* 10(3–5), 533–540.
Reviews studies of monoamine oxidase (MAO) activity in normal aging and Alzheimer's disease in humans and in hemitransection experiments in rats. The evidence indicates that brain MAO-B activity increases with age, the rate varying in different brain regions. Brain MAO-A activity does not change with age in humans and is decreased in rats. Brain MAO-B activity in Alzheimer's disease and senile dementia of the Alzheimer's type has been found to be higher than in age-matched controls. Increased MAO-B activity in aging is due to increased concentration of extrasynaptosomal MAO-B. Platelet MAO has also been found to increase in patients with Alzheimer's disease.

381. Patočka, J.; Bajgar, J.; Herink, J.; Skopec, F. et al. (1986). **Biochemical and morphologic changes after intracerebral administration of aziridin derivative of choline (ADCh-1) to rats.** 27th Annual Psychopharmacology Meeting (1985, Jeseník, Czechoslovakia). *Activitas Nervosa Superior,* 28(1), 46–47.
Studied the use of ADCh-1 in the design of an animal model of the cholinergic hypofunction characteristic of Alzheimer-type presenile dementia. Despite the lack of morphologic confirmation, intracerebral administration of ADCh-1 to the rat septal region biochemically modeled this presenile disorder.

382. Pepeu, Giancarlo; Casamenti, Fiorella; Pedata, Felicita; Cosi, Cristina et al. (1986). **Are the neurochemical and behavioral changes induced by lesions of the nucleus basalis in the rat a model of Alzheimer's disease?** *Progress in Neuro-Psychopharmacology & Biological Psychiatry,* 10(3–5), 541–551.
Reviews work on the neurochemical, EEG, and behavioral changes induced in the rat by lesions of the nucleus basalis. Similarities and differences between the lesions' effects and the neurochemical and clinical alterations characterizing senile dementia of Alzheimer type (SDAT) are pointed out. It is concluded that lesions of the nucleus basalis only partly mimic the complex clinical picture of SDAT. They offer, nevertheless, a useful tool for understanding the critical role of central cholinergic pathways in cognitive processes and identifying potentially useful pharmacological treatments.

383. Piercey, M. F.; Vogelsang, G. D.; Franklin, S. R. & Tang, A. H. (1987). **Reversal of scopolamine-induced amnesia and alterations in energy metabolism by the nootropic piracetam: Implications regarding identification of brain structures involved in consolidation of memory traces.** *Brain Research,* 424(1), 1–9.
Pretreatment with scopolamine prevented the acquisition of a passive avoidance task in rats. Scopolamine reduced glucose utilization in several areas of the cerebral cortex. The regional depressions in glucose metabolism observed following scopolamine treatment had some resemblance to depressions in glucose metabolism reported for Alzheimer's disease patients in positron emission tomography studies. Piracetam did not alter the energy metabolism of any of the brain regions examined; however, it completely reversed the scopolamine-induced depressions in the hippocampus. Data support the hippocampal-cholinergic theory of memory as originally formulated by B. Meyers and E. F. Domino (1964).

384. Pirch, J. H.; Corbus, M. J.; Rigdon, G. C. & Lyness, W. H. (1986). **Generation of cortical event-related slow potentials in the rat involves nucleus basalis cholinergic innervation.** *Electroencephalography & Clinical Neurophysiology,* 63(5), 464–475.
Conducted experiments with 38 male Sprague-Dawley rats to gather information regarding the role of cholinergic innervation to the cortex in the generation of event-related slow potentials. The effects of unilateral drug treatments or lesions on ipsilateral and contralateral frontal slow potential responses were examined. It was found that pharmacological depression of nucleus basalis neurons, blockade of cholinergic muscarinic receptors in the cortex, and nucleus basalis lesions that reduced cortical choline acetyltransferase activity depressed event-related slow potentials in the rat frontal cortex. The results provide evidence that cortical slow potential responses in the rat are dependent on cholinergic innervation from the nucleus basalis. These findings may be relevant to observations that patients with Alzheimer's disease have altered contingent negative variations. (French abstract) (61 ref).

385. Price, Donald L. et al. (1985). **The functional organization of the basal forebrain cholinergic system in primates and the role of this system in Alzheimer's disease.** *Annals of the New York Academy of Sciences,* 444, 287–295.
The authors discuss the anatomy and physiology of the basal forebrain cholinergic system in primates in terms of (1) the effects of aging on this system; (2) the consequences of experimental lesions of the primate basal forebrain; and (3) the changes occurring in this neuronal population in Alzheimer's disease, in aged individuals with Down's syndrome, and in certain demented patients with Parkinson's disease. (86 ref).

386. Price, Donald L.; Kitt, Cheryl A.; Struble, Robert G.; Whitehouse, Peter J. et al. (1985). **Neurobiological studies of transmitter systems in aging and in Alzheimer-type dementia.** Institute for Child Development Research Conference: Hope for a new neurology (1984, New York, New York). *Annals of the New York Academy of Sciences,* 457, 35–51.
Discusses the clinical syndrome of Alzheimer-type dementia and reviews recent advances in the area of diagnostic studies. Focus is on the nature and distribution of structural and chemical pathologies (especially those involving specific neuronal systems); the development of nonhuman primate models of aging and disease; and prospects for using these models to design and test new therapeutic approaches. Dysfunction and death of specific neuronal systems are important processes occurring in aging and in Alzheimer's and in Parkinson's disease. The availability of animal models (including aged monkeys, macaques with cholinergic deficiencies, and monkeys with nigrostriatal pathology) allows the opportunity to assess the efficacies of new pharmacotherapies, neural grafts, and trophic factors.

387. Roberts, Eugene; Bologa, Liane; Flood, James F. & Smith, Gary E. (1987). **Effects of dehydroepiandrosterone and its sulfate on brain tissue in culture and on memory in mice.** *Brain Research,* 406(1–2), 357–362.
Low concentrations of dehydroepiandrosterone (DHEA) and its sulfate (DHEAS) enhanced neuronal and glial survival and/or differentiation in dissociated cultures of 14-day mouse embryo brain. Posttrial intracisternal injection into the brains of mice undergoing active avoidance training alleviated amnesia and enhanced long-term memory. By minimizing degenerative changes in injured nerve tissue and facilitating plastic changes, DHEA and DHEAS may be of use in treatment of neurodegenerative and memory disorders in humans, including multiple sclerosis and Alzheimer's disease.

388. Salamone, John D. (1986). **Behavioural functions of nucleus basalis magnocellularis and its relationship to dementia.** *Trends in Neurosciences,* 9(6), 256–258.
Discusses the basal nucleus of Meynert's provision of a major cholinergic innervation to neocortex (consistently reduced in Alzheimer's disease) and its rat homolog—the nucleus basalis magnocellularis (NBM). Behavioral studies of NBM in rats show that the nucleus basalis is involved in the performance of tasks related to learning and memory. Lesions of this structure may provide an animal model for dementia and data on how the brain processes information and performs higher mental functions.

389. Sladek, John R.; Collier, Timothy J.; Haber, Suzanne N.; Roth, Robert H. et al. (1986). **Survival and growth of fetal catecholamine neurons transplanted into primate brain.** *Brain Research Bulletin,* 17(6), 809–818.
Examined transplants of dopamine and norepinephrine neuroblasts of the ventral mesencephalon, hypothalamus, and dorsolateral pons from fetal African green monkeys (*Cercopithecus aethiops sabaeus*) into multiple brain sites in 3 adult African green monkeys. Results indicate that the fetal catecholamine-containing neurons survived transplantation and produced extensive neuritic outgrowths, with no apparent tissue rejection. Findings provide information on nerve cell grafting as a prerequisite in the consideration of neural transplant therapy for neurological disease, especially Alzheimer's disease and Parkinsonism.

390. Sofroniew, M. V.; Isacson, O. & Björklund, A. (1986). **Cortical grafts prevent atrophy of cholinergic basal nucleus neurons induced by excitotoxic cortical damage.** *Brain Research,* 378(2), 409–415.
Damage to the neocortex of the rat was induced by the excitotoxin kainic acid, which is known to cause cell shrinkage in the part of the cholinergic basal nucleus projecting to the damaged area. Fetal cortical tissue, implanted into the neuron-depleted cortex, prevented this degenerative change. It is proposed that the basal forebrain cholinergic neurons normally receive a trophic influence from their target areas and that grafted neocortex can substitute for the loss of such trophic influence in cortex-damaged Ss. Results have implications for Alzheimer's disease.

391. Sonsalla, Patricia K. & Heikkila, Richard E. (1986). **"Animals and experimentation: An evaluation of animal models of Alzheimer's and Parkinson's disease": Commentary.** *Integrative Psychiatry,* 4(2), 70–72.
In response to J. H. Kordower and D. M. Gash's (1986) article, the present authors discuss the use of 1-methyl-4-phenyl- 1,2,3,6-tetrahydropyridine (MPTP) in creating animal models for Parkinson's disease (PD). The available information on the effects of MPTP in various experimental animals is summarized, and mechanisms involved in its neurotoxic actions are described. The impact of MPTP on basic and clinical research associated with PD is considered.

41

392. Stewart, Dwight J.; MacFabe, Derrick F. & Vanderwolf, C. H. (1984). **Cholinergic activation of the electrocorticogram: Role of the substantia innominata and effects of atropine and quinuclidinyl benzilate.** *Brain Research,* 322(2), 219–232.
Systemic injection of quinuclidinyl benzilate partially abolished low-voltage fast activity (LVFA) in the neocortex of waking Long-Evans rats, resulting in the appearance of large irregular slow waves during Type 2 behaviors (e.g., immobility, sniffing without head movement, face washing). These slow waves did not occur during Type 1 behavior (e.g., walking, head movement). Atropine sulfate produced a similar effect but was less potent. Injection of kainic acid into the substantia innominata (a) destroyed local cells that contain acetylcholinesterase (AChE) and reduced AChE staining in the ipsilateral neocortex and (b) produced large slow waves in the ipsilateral neocortex during Type 2 but not Type 1 behavior. These slow waves were abolished by pilocarpine. Data suggest that the LVFA depends on a cholinergic input to the neocortex from the substantia innominata. The relevance of these findings to Alzheimer's disease is discussed. (45 ref).

393. Stone, William S. (1986). **Circadian behaviors and memory in animal models of aging and Alzheimer's disease.** *Dissertation Abstracts International,* 47(4-B), 1778.

394. Struble, Robert G.; Price, Donald L. Jr.; Cork, Linda C. & Price, Donald L. (1985). **Senile plaques in cortex of aged normal monkeys.** *Brain Research,* 361(1–2), 267–275.
Determined the density, type, and distributions of cortical senile plaques in 15 4–31 yr old rhesus monkeys. For the 6 oldest Ss, plaque densities were highest in prefrontal and temporal cortices and lowest in occipital cortex. Neurite plaques contained many argentophilic neurites and little amyloid; mixed plaques had both neurites and amyloid; and amyloid plaques showed significant amounts of amyloid and fewer numbers of neurites. As total plaque density increased, there was a linear increase in the density of amyloid plaques, suggesting that plaques evolve from neurite, to mixed, to amyloid types. (57 ref).

395. Tomaz, Carlos & Huston, Joseph P. (1986). **Facilitation of conditioned inhibitory avoidance by post-trial peripheral injection of substance P.** *Pharmacology, Biochemistry & Behavior,* 25(2), 469–472.
Three experiments investigated the effects of the neuropeptide Substance P (SP) on performance of a conditioned inhibitory avoidance response using a single-trial inhibitory avoidance task with 290 male Wistar rats. In Exp I, SP was injected immediately after the training trial in doses of 0.5, 5, 50, 100, 250 or 500 μg/kg: The group treated with 50 μg SP/kg exhibited better avoidance than the other groups. In Exp II, the doses of SP used were 1, 50, 250 μg/kg: Only the 50 μg SP/kg treatment group showed significantly better performance. In Exp III, 50 μg/kg SP or vehicle was injected posttrial immediately or 5 hrs after the trial. Only the group in which SP was injected immediately after the training trial showed significantly better performance when tested 24 hrs later. Results are discussed in relation to the finding that patients with senile dementia of the Alzheimer type show lower cortical SP immunoreactivity than controls.

396. Troncoso, Juan C. et al. (1986). **Immunocytochemical studies of neurofilament antigens in the neurofibrillary pathology induced by aluminum.** *Brain Research,* 364(2), 295–300.
Describes an immunocytochemical analysis of spinal cord sections from aluminum-injected New Zealand rabbits. In control Ss, phosphorylated 200-kilodalton (kd) neurofilament proteins were not demonstrable in perikarya of motor neurons; in experimental Ss, perikarya and proximal axons of affected motor neurons showed striking accumulations of immunoreactivity of 1 phosphorylated epitope. It is suggested that the presence of phosphorylated 200-kd neurofilament

proteins in these regions may have important consequences for the organization of the cytoskeleton and for the transport of neurofilaments. It is noted that a similar (but not identical) pattern of accumulation has been observed in neurofibrillary tangles in Alzheimer's disease. (18 ref).

397. Wenk, Gary; Hughey, Donna; Boundy, Virginia; Kim, Anna et al. (1987). **Neurotransmitters and memory: Role of cholinergic, serotonergic, and noradrenergic systems.** *Behavioral Neuroscience,* 101(3), 325–332.
In Alzheimer's disease (AD), pathological changes are found in the basal forebrain cholinergic system (BFCS), serotonergic raphe (RA), and noradrenergic locus coeruleus (LC) systems. The present study examined the extent to which selective damage in each of these systems individually could produce an impairment of memory, one of the clinical symptoms of AD. Rats were given selective lesions by injecting ibotenic acid into the nucleus basalis magnocellularis and medial septal area (i.e., BFCS); 5,7-dihydroxytryptamine into the medial and dorsal RA; and 6-hydroxydopamine (6-OHDA) into the LC or by ip injections of (2-chloroethyl)N-ethyl-2-bromobenzylamine HCl (DSP4). Rats were tested in a delayed spatial alternation in a T-maze. BFCS lesions impaired choice accuracy with intertrial delays of 5, 30, and 60 sec. RA lesions or DSP4 injections impaired choice accuracy only when the intertrial delay was 60 sec. LC lesions (by 6-OHDA) did not impair choice accuracy at any delay. The results suggest that the pathological changes in the BFCS and RA are sufficient to produce the types of memory impairments associated with dementia, but the quantitative effects of pathology in these 2 systems are different.

398. Wenk, Gary L.; Engisch, Kathrin L.; McCall, Lisa D.; Mitchell, Susan J. et al. (1986). **[³H]ketanserin binding increases in monkey cortex following basal forebrain lesions with ibotenic acid.** *Neurochemistry International,* 9(4), 557–562.
Lesions were placed in the medial septal area, nucleus basalis, or both regions of 10 male cynomologus macaques (*Macaca fascicularis*). 10 mo later, [³H]ketanserin binding was increased in the neocortex, but not in the hippocampus, while levels of choline acetyltransferase activity decreased in the neocortex and hippocampus. Data suggest that degeneration of the basal forebrain cholinergic system may alter serotonergic function in the neocortex. Relations with the neurological changes observed in Alzheimer's disease are discussed.

399. Whishaw, Ian Q.; O'Connor, W. T. & Dunnett, S. B. (1985). **Disruption of central cholinergic systems in the rat by basal forebrain lesions of atropine: Effects on feeding, sensorimotor behaviour, locomotor activity and spatial navigation.** *Behavioural Brain Research,* 17(2), 103–115.
Conducted 2 experiments with 51 female Sprague-Dawley rats to examine Ss with ibotenic acid lesions of the nucleus basalis magnocellularis (the origin of the extrinsic cholinergic innervation of the cortex) for changes in feeding, sensorimotor behavior, nocturnal locomotor activity, and place navigation in the Morris swimming pool task, in comparison with control Ss and Ss receiving the muscarinic antagonist atropine (50 mg/kg). The lesions produced acute feeding impairments marked by weight loss and vigorous active rejection of food and water lasting 2–4 days, sensorimotor impairments in placing and orienting, and overnight hyperactivity. A similar hyperactivity was induced by atropine, lasting approximately 6 hrs following the injection. Ss with lesions or those that received atropine were similarly impaired in the acquisition of the spatial navigation task, failed to reach control levels of efficiency even once they had acquired the task, and showed small but significant retention impairments when pretrained in the absence of either treatment. Results are discussed in terms of the lesions producing a disruption of cortical cholinergic systems, with implications for the clinical disorder of senile dementia of the Alzheimer type, and in terms of

possible associated disruption to noncholinergic systems. (54 ref).

400. Wilson, Paula M. (1985). **A photographic perspective on the origins, form, course and relations of the acetylcholinesterase-containing fibres of the dorsal tegmental pathway in the rat brain.** *Brain Research Reviews,* 10(2), 85–118.
Analyses of 126 hooded rat brains suggested that the dorsal tegmental pathway (DTP) takes origin from choline acetyl-transferase (ChAT)-containing pedunculopontine and laterodorsal nuclei. Exploration of a role for the ChAT/substance P/nicotinamide-adenosine dinucleotide phosphate diaphorase DTP fibers in the failure of cholinergic mechanisms that characterize Alzheimer's disease may follow corroboration of the diagonal band/basal nucleus of Meynert afferents. (141 ref).

401. Wisniewski, Henryk M.; Sturman, John A. & Shek, Judy W. (1982). **Chronic model of neurofibrillary changes induced in mature rabbits by metallic aluminum.** *Neurobiology of Aging,* 3(1), 11–22.
A slurry of aluminum powder injected into the brains of New Zealand rabbits produced neurofibrillary changes in neurons of the spinal cord and cerebrum. This chronic animal model of neurofibrillary changes, induced in a mature nervous system, will allow better investigations of alterations in biochemistry, pathology, behavior, and cognition. Results are discussed in terms of research suggesting that neurofibrillary changes impair some cognitive functions and possible implications for senile dementia of the Alzheimer type. (11 ref).

402. Yokel, Robert A. (1983). **Repeated systemic aluminum exposure effects on classical conditioning of the rabbit.** *Neurobehavioral Toxicology & Teratology,* 5(1), 41–52.
Excessive aluminum exposure and accumulation has been implicated as the cause of 2 disorders that involve learning deficits (dialysis encephalopathy and Alzheimer's disease). To develop an animal model, 61 female New Zealand White rabbits were given 20 A1 lactate injections (0, 25, 50, 100, 200, or 400 µmole/kg, sc) over 4 wks. Dose-dependent weight reductions were observed. When the baseline frequency of nictitating membrane extension (NME) were determined, 2 wks later, differential classical conditioning of the NME was conducted. No treatment group differences were observed in frequency of baseline NME, amplitude of the response to shock, or shock threshold to produce NME, suggesting no aluminum effects on the Ss' ability to perform the response. All Ss developed the discrimination. The 2 highest dose groups acquired the CR less well than controls, as shown by a lower percent of CRs in the 2nd half of the conditioning sessions (80 and 74% of controls) and a greater latency to onset of the CR (327 and 310 msec vs 261 msec for controls). Results indicate that chronic systemic exposure of adult rabbits to A1 results in learning deficits not due to sensory or motor impairment of the learned response. (33 ref).

403. Ziegler, Dewey K. (1986). **"Animals and experimentation: An evaluation of animal models of Alzheimer's and Parkinson's disease": Commentary.** *Integrative Psychiatry,* 4(2), 73.
Discusses J. H. Kordower and D. M. Gash's (see PA, Vol 74: 30510) review of the contributions of animal research to the study of Alzheimer's and Parkinson's diseases and the problems associated with conclusions drawn from these studies. Emphasis is on the difficulty of studying these disorders in primates.

EPIDEMIOLOGY & DIAGNOSIS

404. Agbayewa, M. Oluwafemi. (1986). **EEG and CT scan in Alzheimer's disease.** *Journal of Clinical Psychiatry,* 47(4), 217–218.
Examined the results of EEGs and computerized tomographic (CT) scans performed during 1 yr on 188 dementia patients (aged 60+ yrs). Findings indicate that abnormal EEGs are a more reliable finding than CT scans and should be the technique of choice when differentiating between Alzheimer's disease and the "pseudodementias."

405. Amaducci, Luigi A.; Fratiglioni, Laura; Rocca, Walter A.; Fieschi, Cesare et al. (1986). **Risk factors for clinically diagnosed Alzheimer's disease: A case-control study of an Italian population.** *Neurology,* 36(7), 922–931.
Conducted a case-control study of 116 patients (aged 40–80 yrs) with the clinical diagnosis of Alzheimer's disease (AD) in 7 Italian centers. 116 hospital controls and 97 population controls were matched to the cases by age, sex, and region of residence. A structured questionnaire was administered to the next-of-kin of cases and controls by trained interviewers to identify possible risk factors. Genetic, viral, toxic, immunologic, medical, surgical, and personality factors were examined. Dementia among 1st- or 2nd-degree relatives and advanced age of the mother at S's birth (over 40 yrs of age) were associated with AD.

406. Arie, Tom. (1984). **Prevention of mental disorders of old age.** *Journal of the American Geriatrics Society,* 32(6), 460–465.
Discusses developments linking transmissible causes, identification of genetic markers, and more careful analysis to the prevention of dementias and other mental disorders of old age (MDOA). Dementia of the Alzheimer type, multi-infarct dementia, and depression are discussed separately. It is suggested that ways in which the personality can be influenced toward resilience is important for prevention of MDOA. (44 ref).

407. Barclay, Laurie L.; Zemcov, Alexander; Blass, John P. & Sansone, Joseph. (1986). **"Survivors-only bias in estimating survival in Alzheimer's disease and vascular dementias": Reply.** *Neurology,* 36(7), 1009–1010.
Responds to criticism by J. Habbema and D. Dippel (1986) concerning the present authors' (1985) article on survival in Alzheimer's disease. The authors maintain that their conclusion that Alzheimer's disease is associated with a higher life expectancy than the vascular dementias is justified.

408. Barclay, Laurie L.; Zemcov, Alexander; Blass, John P. & McDowell, Fletcher H. (1985). **Factors associated with duration of survival in Alzheimer's disease.** *Biological Psychiatry,* 20(1), 86–93.
Compared survival rates in different subgroups of 199 patients with dementia of the Alzheimer type (DAT) using a computerized data base, a data retrieval system, and a computer program using the actuarial method of life-table analysis. The 71 men had a shorter duration of survival than the 128 women. Ss younger than 65 yrs at onset had a decreased relative duration of survival compared with Ss over 65 at onset, suggesting a more malignant course. Ss with a longer duration of illness tended to die sooner, but this effect was not significant. Patients with high behavioral scores on a scale by J. A. Haycox (1984), indicating more severe behavioral impairment, had lower survival rates at 500 days than patients with low scores. Factors associated with decreased duration of survival in DAT include male sex, presenile onset, and increased severity of behavioral impairment. (16 ref).

409. Berg, Leonard et al. (1984). **Predictive features in mild senile dementia of the Alzheimer type.** *Neurology,* 34(5), 563–569.

43 Ss (aged 63.8–81.2 yrs) with mild senile dementia of the Alzheimer type, diagnosed and staged by clinical research criteria, were studied with clinical, psychometric, EEG, visual evoked potential, and computerized tomography (CT) measures. During the 12 mo following entry into the study, 21 Ss progressed to moderate or severe dementia, 21 remained mild, and 1 was lost to follow-up. Many of the clinical and psychometric measures of impairment were predictive of the progression to moderate or severe dementia. Electrophysiologic and CT measures were not. In a discriminant function analysis, the scores on 2 measures (the Digit Symbol subtest of the WAIS and an aphasia battery) correctly predicted the stage of dementia 1 yr later in 95% of the Ss. (21 ref).

410. Bigler, Erin D. et al. (1984). **Volumetric CAT measures and neuropsychological performance in Alzheimer's disease.** *International Journal of Neuroscience,* 24(3–4), 291–294.
Generated, by computer, the following measures from the computed axial tomography scans of 31 patients (mean age 69.8 yrs) with degenerative disorder (Alzheimer's type): brain surface area, brain volume, ventricular surface area, ventricular volume (VV), and an atrophy index (AI). Results indicate that VV and the AI measures were the most sensitive for the detection of degenerative morphological brain changes in relationship to neuropsychological impairment in the Ss. (9 ref).

411. Bondareff, William; Raval, Janak; Colletti, Patrick M. & Hauser, Douglas L. (1988). **Quantitative magnetic resonance imaging and the severity of dementia in Alzheimer's disease.** *American Journal of Psychiatry,* 145(7), 853–856.
The T_2 component of the magnetic resonance imaging (MRI) signal was measured in 11 brain loci in 6 demented elderly patients (aged 68–83 yrs) diagnosed as having probable Alzheimer's disease. T_2 values and relative amount of periventricular high-intensity foci were significantly correlated with dementia severity, indicated by the score on a dementia scale developed by G. Blessed et al (1968). Although the mean T_2 value for left hemispheric structures was more closely correlated with the dementia score, T_2 values did not differ significantly in the right and left hemispheres or in gray and white matter. Findings suggest that more severe dementia in Alzheimer's disease is associated with more water in the brain.

412. Breitner, John C. & Folstein, Marshal F. (1984). **Familial Alzheimer Dementia: A prevalent disorder with specific clinical features.** *Psychological Medicine,* 14(1), 63–80.
The early literature on Alzheimer dementia (AD) describes the clinical features of aphasia, apraxia, and agraphia as characteristic. The authors investigated the hypothesis that these features would specifically identify the familial form of AD (FAD). Since pedigree studies had suggested that FAD is an autosomal dominant genetic disorder, it was hypothesized that the 1st-degree relatives of language-disordered or apractic AD probands would show at least 50% lifetime risks of dementia. Using standardized methods, 3,500 nursing home patients (aged 50+ yrs) were screened for stringently defined AD cases and tested for agraphia. 150 cases met the clinical criteria for AD. Of a final sample of 62, 39 were unable to write. Clinical and family histories were obtained from multiple informants. 33 age-, race-, and sex-matched nondemented controls were also examined. Language disorder and apraxia were found in 78% of AD cases; they strongly predicted familial aggregation of dementia, with a 90-yr lifetime incidence among relatives exceeding 50%, or 7 times the control values. Results suggest that language disorder and apraxia specifically identify a distinct clinical entity, FAD, that is among the commonest forms of senile dementia. (45 ref).

413. Brown, Paul; Salazar, Andres M.; Gibbs, Clarence J. & Gajdusek, D. Carleton. (1982). **Alzheimer's disease and transmissible virus dementia (Creutzfeldt-Jakob disease).** *Annals of the New York Academy of Sciences,* 396, 131–143.
Creutzfeldt-Jakob disease (CJD), like Alzheimer's disease (AD), presents as a progressive mental deterioration, but from an early stage is associated with neurological abnormalities that include cerebellar, visual, pyramidal, and extrapyramidal signs. Myoclonus, with or without other movement disorders, occurs later in most CJD patients. However, similarities in symptomatology and clinical evolution make it difficult to differentiate the 2 disorders; and pathologic, genetic, and biologic comparisons between AD and CJD suggest a similar pathogenesis for AD and the spongiform virus encephalopathies. The comparison of AD and CJD depends on the results of attempts to transmit the diseases to experimental animals, which have succeeded for CJD but not for AD. (44 ref).

414. Brun, Arne & Englund, Elisabet. (1986). **Brain changes in dementia of Alzheimer's type relevant to new imaging diagnostic methods.** *Progress in Neuro-Psychopharmacology & Biological Psychiatry,* 10(3–5), 297–308.
Correlated gray and white matter changes and their topography to the results of brain imaging methods in more than 75 patients with dementia of the Alzheimer's type. Ss were investigated patho-anatomically, and findings were correlated with psychiatric and neurophysiologic follow-up studies. Some of the findings are that the degenerative gray matter process showed a regionally varying accent according to a pattern consistent and typical for the disease. This corresponded to metabolic changes on regional cerebral blood flow, positron emission tomography, and single photon emission computerized tomography and thus is considered to be of diagnostic value. This pattern was largely symmetric.

415. Carlsson, Arvid. (1986). **Searching for antemortem markers premature.** *Neurobiology of Aging,* 7(5), 400–401.
In commenting on the review by E. Hollander et al (1986), the author argues that searching for diagnostic markers of Alzheimer's disease may not be the best strategy, given the poor nosology of dementia disorders. An open-minded search for biochemical and functional changes in dementia disorders of various types is seen as more appropriate.

416. Carnes, Molly. (1984). **Diagnosis and management of dementia in the elderly.** *Physical & Occupational Therapy in Geriatrics,* 3(4), 11–24.
After pointing out that while dementia increases in prevalence with age it is not a normal part of aging, the cognitive and neurological processes of normal aging are outlined. Also discussed are issues in the diagnosis of dementia, types of dementia (Alzheimer's, multi-infarct, mixed, or other), and evaluation of patients with suspected dementia (e.g., by mental status and physical examinations, interviews, and laboratory tests for hypothyroidism, renal failure, or nutritional deficiencies). The cause of dementia, particularly of the Alzheimer type, is outlined, and suggestions for management of these patients are presented. (40 ref).

417. Chandra, V.; Philipose, V.; Bell, P. A.; Lazaroff, A. et al. (1987). **Case-control study of late onset "probable Alzheimer's disease."** *Neurology,* 37(8), 1295–1300.
Conducted a case-control study on 64 cases of probable Alzheimer's disease with late onset of illness (after age 70 yrs) and 64 controls matched by age, race, and sex. Information was obtained on birth order, lifetime medical and surgical history, personal characteristics, exposure to toxins and animals, and a family history of various illnesses. None of the variables studied, including family history of dementia, reached statistical significance. An antecedent history of head trauma with loss of consciousness, though not statistically significant, was more frequently found in cases than in controls.

418. Chui, Helena C.; Teng, Evelyn L.; Henderson, Victor W. & Moy, Arthur C. (1985). **Clinical subtypes of dementia of the Alzheimer type.** *Neurology,* 35(11), 1544–1550.
Evaluated clinical subtypes of dementia of the Alzheimer type by comparing age at onset, aphasia, family history, and motor disorder in 146 individuals (mean age 68.4 yrs) with progressive dementia. Early onset was significantly associated with more prevalent and more severe language disorder. 45% of all Ss had familial history of dementia, but relative familial risk could not be differentiated based on age at onset or aphasia. Independent of duration of illness, myoclonus and non-iatrogenic extrapyramidal disorder were associated with greater severity of dementia. (43 ref).

419. Colgan, John; Naguib, Mohsen & Levy, Raymond. (1986). **Computed tomographic density numbers: A comparative study of patients with senile dementia and normal elderly controls.** *British Journal of Psychiatry,* 149, 716–719.
Compared cranial computed tomography scans of 48 patients (mean age 77.9 yrs) with senile dementia of the Alzheimer type and 40 normal elderly volunteers (mean age 75 yrs). The demented group had significantly larger lateral ventricles than the controls, but did not differ significantly from the controls with respect to attenuation density in any of the regions studied.

420. Creasey, Helen; Schwartz, Michael A.; Frederickson, Harold; Haxby, James V. et al. (1986). **Quantitative computed tomography in dementia of the Alzheimer type.** *Neurology,* 36(12), 1563–1568.
22 men (45–84 yrs old) and 17 women (55–81 yrs old) with dementia of the Alzheimer type (DAT), including a history of progressive cognitive loss, were compared with 36 healthy controls (44–85 yrs old) for brain atrophy as measured by computed tomography (CT). DAT patients had more brain atrophy and ventricular dilatation than did controls. The male DAT patients with mild dementia had a larger mean 3rd ventricle volume, whereas male patients with severe dementia had larger lateral and 3rd ventricle volumes, more cerebrospinal fluid (CSF), and less gray matter than did controls. Correlations between several dementia scales and CT measures in the DAT patients indicated that brain atrophy and ventricular dilatation were related to the severity of dementia.

421. Cutler, Neal R. et al. (1985). **Brain metabolism as measured with positron emission tomography: Serial assessment in a patient with familial Alzheimer's disease.** *Neurology,* 35(11), 1556–1561.
Measured regional cerebral metabolic rates for glucose with positron emission tomography and ¹⁸F-fluoro-2-deoxydextroglucose on 3 occasions at 8-mo intervals, in a 57-yr-old man with Alzheimer's disease of 2.5 yrs duration and with a family history of neuropathologically confirmed Alzheimer's disease. No differences in regional cerebral metabolic rates for glucose were found between the S and 12 healthy men on the initial scan, whereas metabolism on the 2nd and 3rd scans was reduced significantly in the parietal lobes and bilaterally in some parietal lobe regions. Memory loss was demonstrable at the 1st scan, but other aspects of cognitive performance remained within normal limits: scores on the Wechsler Adult Intelligence Scale (WAIS), Boston Naming Test, and Two-Dimensional Block Construction. Results show that memory loss can precede a measurable reduction of cerebral metabolism in early Alzheimer's disease but that later reductions in parietal lobe metabolism may not be accompanied by additional measurable neuropsychological deficits. (29 ref).

422. Davis, Kenneth L. & Mohs, Richard C. (1986). **Authors' response to commentaries on Hollander *et al.,* antemortem marker paper.** *Neurobiology of Aging,* 7(5), 406–407.

Responds to series of commentary papers by L. F. Jarvik and S. S. Matsuyama, B. C. Winblad et al, E. K. Perry and R. H. Perry, E. Giacobini, M. J. de Leon and A. E. George, S. I. Rapoport et al, A. Carlsson, J. T. Hartford, and M. Roth (1986) concerning the review of antemortem markers in Alzheimer's disease by E. Hollander et al (1986).

423. de Leon, Mony J. (1980). **Computed tomography evaluations of brain–behavior relationships in senile dementia of the Alzheimer's type.** *Dissertation Abstracts International,* 41(4-B), 1308–1309.

424. de Leon, Mony J. & George, Ajax E. (1986). **Structural and functional neuroimaging in Alzheimer's disease.** *Neurobiology of Aging,* 7(5), 396–398.
In commenting on the review by E. Hollander et al (1986), the authors note that the evolution of neuroimaging technics has improved the understanding of both gross structural and physiological alterations associated with normal aging and with Alzheimer's disease (AD). The authors share the view that neuroimaging will contribute to the development of antemortem markers for AD.

425. Ebmeier, K. P.; Besson, J. A.; Crawford, J. R.; Palin, A. N. et al. (1987). **Nuclear magnetic resonance imaging and single photon emission tomography with radio-iodine labelled compounds in the diagnosis of dementia.** *Acta Psychiatrica Scandinavica,* 75(5), 549–556.
Identified white matter lesions and T¹ changes for 22 Alzheimer's patients (DAT Ss [aged 53–81 yrs]), 18 multiple infarct dementia patients (MID Ss [aged 46–88 yrs]), and 10 controls (aged 42–80 yrs). Results indicate that although nuclear magnetic resonance could not differentiate between the 2 diseases, single photon emission tomography showed parietal lesions in 19 out of 21 DAT Ss and in 4 out of 18 MID Ss.

426. Erkinjuntti, Timo; Ketonen, L.; Sulkava, R.; Vuorialho, M. et al. (1987). **CT in the differential diagnosis between Alzheimer's disease and vascular dementia.** *Acta Neurologica Scandinavica,* 75(4), 262–270.
Examined 68 Alzheimer's disease (AD) patients (aged 40–69 yrs), 79 multi-infarct dementia (MID) patients (aged 48–92 yrs), and 46 patients (aged 53–90 yrs) with probable vascular dementia (PVD), using computed tomography (CT). 88.6% of MID and 41.3% of PVD patients, compared with 1 AD patient, had at least 1 brain infarct on CT. White matter low attenuation (WMLA) also differentiated MID and PVD from AD, especially among Ss aged 75 yrs or less with low or moderate dementia. In all types, brain atrophy on CT had a positive correlation with degree of dementia. It is concluded that infarcts and WMLA on CT, but not brain atrophy, are of diagnostic value in differentiating between vascular and degenerative dementia.

427. Fisk, Albert A. & Pannill, Fitzhugh C. (1987). **Assessment and care of the community-dwelling Alzheimer's disease patient.** *Journal of the American Geriatrics Society,* 35(4), 307–311.
Conducted a 2-yr study of 159 community-dwelling Alzheimer's disease (AD) patients (average age 77 yrs). Ss were not as disabled as commonly supposed, having only a moderate reduction in cognitive function, as measured by the Mini-Mental Status Examination (MMS), and physical activities of daily living (ADLs), but were more dependent in their instrumental ADLs. 47% lived alone, and 39% had not been out of the home in the previous week, making isolation a major concern. During the study, 34% went into nursing homes. Initial mean MMS scores of these Ss was 12.4 compared to 16.6 for Ss who remained at home, but ADL mean scores were not significantly different. The management of AD patients—including medication use, daycare, education

and support for family caregivers, and nursing home placement—is discussed.

428. Gainotti, G. (1979). **Le demenze degenerative dell'eta pre-senile e senile. Aspetti clinici e problemi fisiopatologici. / Degenerative dememtia of presenile and senile ages: Clinical aspects and physiopathogenic problems.** *Archivio di Psicologia, Neurologia e Psichiatria,* 40(4), 556–585.
Alzheimer's disease is differentiated from depressive pseudodementia, multi-infarct dementia, normal hydrocephalus, and Creutzfeldt-Jacob's disease. In Alzheimer's disease, the following are noted: (a) a relationship between aging and senile dementia, (b) changes in brain aluminum distribution, (c) association with slow-virus infections, (d) the role of immunological factors, and (e) a central cholinergic deficit. (French, English, & German summaries) (62 ref).

429. Gershon, Samuel & Herman, Stephen P. (1982). **The differential diagnosis of dementia.** *Journal of the American Geriatrics Society,* 30(11, Suppl), 58–66.
While the 2 major types of dementia, Alzheimer's disease and multi-infarct dementia, are irreversible, perhaps 20% of dementias are secondary to treatable causes and are reversible. The most important of these is the pseudodementia of depression. The differential diagnosis of these disorders and other causes of dementia secondary to disease or therapy are discussed. (21 ref).

430. Giacobini, Ezio. (1986). **Brain acetylcholine: A view from cerebrospinal fluid (CSF).** *Neurobiology of Aging,* 7(5), 392–396.
Reviews the CSF studies reported in the article of E. Hollander et al (1986). In particular, conflicting results reported in the literature with regard to acetylcholine, related enzymes, and choline are discussed.

431. Gutzmann, Hans. (1984). **Frontallappensyndrome bei (prä-)senilen Demenzen vom Alzheimer-Typ: Eine korrelations-statistische Untersuchung. / Frontal lobe syndromes in senile dementia of Alzheimer type: An intercorrelative study.** *Zeitschrift für Gerontologie,* 17(3), 128–131.
Studied a group of gerontopsychiatric patients (55–84 yrs of age) with mild to severe dementia. Clinical instruments included a psychological assessment system and a battery of tests. Structural changes of the brain were detected by computerized tomography (CT). A number of correlations between clinical and morphological variables were found. The statistical analysis of most of the variables correlating with the CT determinants of the frontal lobe revealed a consistency with the classical frontal lobe syndrome. The relations of the remaining items to the symptomatology of normal-pressure hydrocephalus are discussed. (11 ref).

432. Harrell, Lindy E.; Callaway, Ross & Sekar, B. Chandra. (1987). **Magnetic resonance imaging and the diagnosis of dementia.** *Neurology,* 37(3), 540–543.
Describes 7 64–78 yr old patients with clinical, laboratory, and computed tomography evidence of primary degenerative dementia (Alzheimer's and Pick's). Results show that magnetic resonance imaging (MRI) demonstrated regions in white matter consistent with cerebral infarction. It is suggested that MRI may be a sensitive way to differentiate multi-infarct dementia and primary degenerative dementia.

433. Hartford, James T. (1986). **A review of antemortem markers of Alzheimer's disease.** *Neurobiology of Aging,* 7(5), 401–402.
Comments on the review of antemortem markers in Alzheimer's disease (AD) by E. Hollander et al (1986). It is suggested that current theories regarding the etiology of AD tend to derive from 1 of 4 possible causes: a genetically acquired autosomal dominant trait, a slow viral infection, an environmental toxin, or a systemic metabolic illness. Progress

in advancing knowledge to increased understanding of AD is hampered by the inability to reliably and consistently make an antemortem diagnosis. Current criteria are overinclusive and result in as much as a 30% error of overdiagnosis of patients later found to have another neurological disorder or no dementia.

434. Henderson, A. S. & Jorm, A. F. (1987). **Is case-ascertainment of Alzheimer's disease in field surveys practicable?** *Psychological Medicine,* 17(3), 549–555.
Examines what is presently known about reliability and validity of Alzheimer's disease (AD) at 2 stages of ascertainment: the diagnosis of dementia and the diagnosis of AD itself with the exclusion of other causes of dementia.

435. Hollander, Eric; Mohs, Richard C. & Davis, Kenneth L. (1986). **Antemortem markers of Alzheimer's disease.** *Neurobiology of Aging,* 7(5), 367–387.
Examines approaches to the development of antemortem markers of Alzheimer's disease. Among the procedures discussed are neurochemical and histopathologic studies of the cholinergic system, concentrating on cerebrospinal fluid (CSF) and blood plasma; genetic studies; imaging and electrophysiological studies; and neuroendocrine studies.

436. Hurley, Anne D. & Sovner, Robert. (1986). **Dementia, mental retardation, and Down's syndrome.** *Psychiatric Aspects of Mental Retardation Reviews,* 5(8), 39–44.
Reviews the Diagnostic and Statistical Manual of Mental Disorders (DSM-III) criteria for the diagnosis of dementia, its etiology and clinical course, and the differentiation of dementia from other causes of intellectual impairment such as depression or delirium. Behavioral and personality changes associated with dementia are described, and the deficits that characterize successive stages of Alzheimer's disease are outlined. The diagnosis and management of mentally retarded persons with dementia are discussed, and the high incidence and early onset of Alzheimer's disease in Down's syndrome patients is noted. It is contended that many cases of dementia in the mentally retarded are initially misdiagnosed as being of psychological origin; this can have tragic consequences because dementia can be caused by reversible medical illnesses. It is emphasized that dementia should be considered a possible diagnosis in any middle-aged or older retarded person who develops behavioral problems. (16 ref).

437. Jacoby, R. J. (1984). **CT-Untersuchung in der Demenz—heute und in der Zukunft. / CT in the investigation of dementia: Present and future.** *Zeitschrift für Gerontologie,* 17(3), 132–135.
The role of computerized tomography (CT) in the diagnosis of senile dementia of the Alzheimer type (SDAT) is discussed. Data show that although SDAT is closely correlated with brain atrophy (sulcal and ventricular dilatation), there is a significant overlap with the normal elderly population; that is, within the demented population, CT changes correlate only weakly with cognitive impairment. However, taken together with other clinical indices, results indicate that CT can be useful both for the assessment of SDAT and the exclusion of treatable lesions. Newer computer methods of analysis and technical improvements have promise for future clinical and research advances in this area. (14 ref).

438. Jagust, William J.; Budinger, Thomas F. & Reed, Bruce R. (1987). **The diagnosis of dementia with single photon emission computed tomography.** *Archives of Neurology,* 44(3), 258–262.
Investigated, in 9 Alzheimer's disease (AD), 2 multi-infarct dementia (MID), and 5 healthy control Ss (aged 63–79 yrs), whether single photon emission computed tomography (SPECT) measurements of regional cerebral blood flow (rCBF) would demonstrate the same temporoparietal deficits that have been seen in positron emission tomography (PET)

studies and evaluated the utility of SPECT in differentiating the Ss with varying clinical severities of AD from Ss with MID and controls. Results show that the SPECT rCBF pattern of temporoparietally diminished blood flow was similar to the pattern seen using PET with a variety of metabolic and flow tracers and allowed differentiation of AD Ss from controls and MID Ss.

439. Jarvik, Lissy F. & Matsuyama, Steven S. (1986). **Antemortem markers in Alzheimer disease: Have we looked at the forest and missed the trees?** *Neurobiology of Aging,* 7(5), 387–388.
In commenting on the review of antemortem markers for Alzheimer's disease by E. Hollander et al (1986), the authors suggest that the possible heterogeneity of the disease and analysis by group comparisons may have obscured the homogeneous subgroups of patients. Interdisciplinary collaborative investigations are needed to identify clinically and biologically meaningful subgroups.

440. Johnson, Keith A.; Davis, Kenneth R.; Buonanno, Ferdinando S.; Brady, Thomas J. et al. (1987). **Comparison of magnetic resonance and roentgen ray computed tomography in dementia.** *Archives of Neurology,* 44(10), 1075–1080.
Compared the utility of magnetic resonance imaging (MRI) and roentgen ray computed tomography (CT) in assessing 26 Alzheimer's patients (aged 59.9–79.2 yrs), 8 patients (aged 56–85.3 yrs) with vascular or mixed dementia, and 2 patients (aged 77 and 79 yrs) with Parkinson's disease with dementia. Abnormalities in subcortical white matter and hippocampus, enlargement of basal and sylvian cisterns, and ventriculomegaly were more evident on MRI than CT scans, but qualitative ratings in all other brain regions were similar. Dementia severity was correlated with periventricular white matter abnormalities on both images.

441. Johnson, Keith A.; Mueller, Stefan T.; Walshe, Thomas M.; English, Robert J. et al. (1987). **Cerebral perfusion imaging in Alzheimer's disease: Use of single photon emission computed tomography and iofetamine hydrochloride I 123.** *Archives of Neurology,* 44(2), 165–168.
Compared iofetamine hydrochloride I 123 (IMP) uptake in 15 patients (aged 58–81 yrs) with severe disease (in whom the clinical diagnosis of Alzheimer's disease was highly probable) with the uptake in 9 healthy controls (aged 56–81 yrs). In Ss with clinically diagnosed advanced Alzheimer's disease, images made with IMP and single photon emission computed tomography detected regional alterations in cortical tracer uptake, distinguishing these Ss from the controls.

442. Jorm, Anthony F. (1985). **Subtypes of Alzheimer's Dementia: A conceptual analysis and critical review.** *Psychological Medicine,* 15(3), 543–553.
Proposes criteria necessary for establishing the existence of qualitatively different subtypes of a disorder and reviews the literature on Alzheimer's dementia (AD), suggesting subtypes on the basis of either psychological or neuropathological data. It is concluded that, as yet, this research has not met the criteria for establishing qualitatively different subtypes. Studies of AD Ss have yielded evidence of quantitative variability (i.e., in severity of dementia and slope of decline); these findings appear to be related to factors of etiological significance. The possibility that this quantitative variability could provide the basis for subtyping is discussed. (3 ref).

443. Kamo, H.; McGeer, P. L.; Harrop, R.; McGeer, E. G. et al. (1987). **Positron emission tomography and histopathology in Pick's disease.** *Neurology,* 37(3), 439–445.
Reports the results of pre- and postmortem examination of a 75-yr-old man with Pick's disease and severe dementia. Results show that a sharply decreased cortical metabolic rate for glucose was obtained in specific gyri, especially in the frontal lobes, where there was extensive gliosis and neuronal loss.

More moderate decreases were found in areas with numerous Pick bodies and inflated neurons but less gliosis. The positron emission tomography pattern was sufficiently distinctive to suggest that it might be possible to distinguish Pick's from Alzheimer's disease premortem.

444. Katzman, Robert. (1986). **Alzheimer's disease.** *New England Journal of Medicine,* 314(15), 964–973.
Notes that a consensus on diagnostic criteria for Alzheimer's disease (AD) has developed and that major epidemiologic studies are now under way. The first data on age-specific incidence have been reported, and a number of risk factors has been discovered. Knowledge of the changes that occur in the brains of AD patients has advanced rapidly, including appreciation of the selectivity of the pattern of cell loss and of the anatomical distribution of the major pathological markers. The involvement of specific neurotransmitter systems, particularly the ascending cholinergic system and the somatostatin-cell system in the cerebral cortex and the hippocampus, has been delineated. Especially exciting is the beginning of the molecular characterization of the abnormal and unique fibrous proteins in the brains of AD patients.

445. Khachaturian, Zaven S. (1985). **Progress of research on Alzheimer's disease: Research opportunities for behavioral scientists.** *American Psychologist,* 40(11), 1251–1255.
Presents recommendations for research needs in the behavioral sciences to improve the diagnosis of Alzheimer's disease (AD). Among the suggestions made are longitudinal studies of individuals suffering from AD and of general aged populations; studies of environmental factors, normal aging, and other diseases producing dementia; and research on diagnostic techniques such as neuroimaging, electrophysiological studies, and psychological testing. (1 ref).

446. Khachaturian, Zaven S. (1985). **Diagnosis of Alzheimer's disease.** *Archives of Neurology,* 42(11), 1097–1105.
Describes a research workshop on Alzheimer's disease (AD), the participants of which included 37 scientists and physicians divided among 6 disciplines (neurochemistry, neuropathology, neuroradiology, neurology, neuropsychology, and psychiatry). Major themes of the workshop included longitudinal studies, diagnosis and etiology, molecular genetics, environmental factors, normal aging, and other diseases producing dementia. Diagnostic methods and markers discussed included neuroimaging, biological and chemical markers, and electrophysiological markers. Down's syndrome was proposed as a useful model of AD. The autopsy criteria for the diagnosis of AD were also outlined. (14 ref).

447. Knesevich, John W.; Toro, Felix R.; Morris, John C. & LaBarge, Emily. (1985). **Aphasia, family history, and the longitudinal course of senile dementia of the Alzheimer type.** *Psychiatry Research,* 14(3), 255–263.
Examined the role of aphasia and family history in 43 patients with clinically defined senile dementia of the Alzheimer type (SDAT) and 43 controls matched for age, sex, race, and education. Ss were administered a semistructured diagnostic interview and a battery of psychometric tests on 3 occasions over 2½ yrs. Findings demonstrate the confounding effect of aphasia on the use of narrowly based methods of staging dementia as well as on the results of psychometric testing, even with nonverbal measures. Ss who were aphasic had a more rapidly progressive course of dementia but a lower prevalence of familial cases. Risks of developing SDAT for the parents and siblings of aphasic and nonaphasic probands are discussed.

448. Kokmen, Emre; Offord, Kenneth P. & Okazaki, Haruo. (1987). **A clinical and autopsy study of dementia in Olmsted County, Minnesota, 1980–1981.** *Neurology,* 37(3), 426–430.

Studied clinical records and autopsy protocols from 350 cases in which an autopsy was done in Olmstead County, Minnesota over a 2-yr period. Results show that the overall autopsy rate was 33.6%, and autopsy rate for those aged 60 yrs or more was 29%. Preselected criteria were used for diagnosis of dementia. 32 demented and 68 nondemented Ss had complete autopsies; all were more than 60 yrs old. 23 of 32 demented patients had Alzheimer's disease. The frequency of cerebral infarcts among the nondemented Ss was significantly higher than among the demented Ss.

449. Lauter, H. (1970). **Concerning late forms of Alzheimer's disease and its relation to senile dementia.** *Psychiatria Clinica,* 3(3), 169–189.
Reports 52 cases of Alzheimer's disease with onset after age 70. The morphological differentiation from senile dementia could be made despite the high age at onset on the basis of severity of cortical atrophy and of the great density of the histological changes. The clinical picture was similar to that of a control group of 40 female patients with senile dementia who were under observation or undergoing inpatient treatment and the majority of whom showed focal symptoms in the form of aphasic, apractic, or agnostic disturbances. However, the late Alzheimer cases were in some respects clearly different from the classical forms of that illness as they are found during adulthood and the praesenium. Particularly remarkable is the fact that the clinical localizing tendency becomes weaker with increasing age. Alzheimer's disease and senile dementia are not 2 different disease entities but are merely special types within the framework of a phase-specific pathomorphosis, to which the identical disease process in different life periods is subjected. Such a unitary nosological theory is not only in accord wih the identical morphological findings; the genetic findings are also entirely in line with this concept.

450. Loewenstein, Richard J. et al. (1982). **Disturbances of sleep and cognitive functioning in patients with dementia.** *Neurobiology of Aging,* 3(4), 371–377.
Reviews the relationship of sleep, circadian rhythms, and cognitive impairment in dementia patients and collected all-night sleep EEG data for 9 relatively young and relatively unimpaired patients (aged 52–70 yrs) with presumptive Alzheimer's disease and for 8 age-matched controls. Delta sleep time and delta sleep percentage (Stages 3 and 4), but not REM sleep measures, were significantly reduced in the patients. (58 ref).

451. Mayeux, Richard; Stern, Yaakov & Spanton, Susan. (1985). **Heterogeneity in dementia of the Alzheimer type: Evidence of subgroups.** *Neurology,* 35(4), 453–461.
Reviewed records of 121 consecutive patients (mean age 68.6 yrs) with dementia of the Alzheimer type (DAT). Ss with myoclonus or extrapyramidal signs had greater intellectual decline and functional impairment in daily activities. Assessment measures included the Mini-Mental State Examination, Brief Psychiatric Rating Scale, Columbia University Parkinson's Disease Rating Scale, and family history data. Among patients studied over 4 yrs, there were 4 groups: benign—little to no progression; myoclonic—severe intellectual decline and frequent mutism after younger onset; extrapyramidal—severe intellectual and functional decline and frequent psychotic symptoms; and typical—a gradual progression of intellectual and functional decline but without other distinguishing features. Except for the group with myoclonus, no subgroup was segregated by age at onset or other demographic variables. Results suggest that DAT is heterogeneous and that certain clinical manifestations (e.g., motor abilities) may be useful in predicting outcome. (42 ref).

452. McGeer, P. L.; Kamo, H.; Harrop, R.; McGeer, E. G. et al. (1986). **Comparison of PET, MRI, and CT with pathology in a proven case of Alzheimer's disease.** *Neurology,* 36(12), 1569–1574.
Positron emission tomography (PET) with flurodeoxyglucose (FDG), magnetic resonance imaging (MRI), and computed tomography (CT) were carried out in a male patient with Alzheimer's disease 16 mo before he died at age 83 yrs. At autopsy, the gross appearance of the brain correlated with MRI and CT, which showed some regional atrophy. These were much less revealing than PET, which correlated with microscopic findings of neuronal loss and proliferation of glia. In areas of severe metabolic impairment, there was a profound loss of neurons, extensive gliosis, and a diminished appearance of plaques. It is concluded that PET-FDG is a better measure of the severity of Alzheimer's disease than MRI or CT, because it reflects the degree of neuronal pathology.

453. McGeer, Patrick L.; McGeer, Edith G.; Kamo, Hisaki & Wong, Kathy. (1986). **Positron emission tomography and the possible origins of cytopathology in Alzheimer's disease.** *Progress in Neuro-Psychopharmacology & Biological Psychiatry,* 10(3–5), 501–518.
Reviews the results and provides some new data obtained with the techniques of positron emission tomography (PET), immunohistochemistry, and electron microscopy in the study of Alzheimer's disease (AD). PET studies show that the local cerebral metabolic rate for glucose declines in the cerebral cortex in AD. Evidence is presented for the possible presence of viral particles of the double-stranded DNA type in AD brain tissue.

454. Meyer, John S.; Rogers, Robert L. & Mortel, Karl F. (1986). **"Cerebral blood flow in dementia": Reply from the authors.** *Neurology,* 36(11), 1542–1543.
Responds to M. D. O'Brien's (1986) discussion of the present authors' (R. L. Rogers et al, 1986) findings concerning decreases in cerebral blood flow (CBF) and vascular dementia. The present authors note that CBF declined about 2 yrs before the onset of symptoms in all of their risk-factored volunteers who developed multi-infarct dementia. The present authors agree that there may be a bias in the Hachinski index but note that their diagnoses were also based on other criteria.

455. Mindham, R. H.; Steele, Cynthia; Folstein, Marshal F. & Lucas, Jane. (1985). **A comparison of the frequency of major affective disorder in Huntington's disease and Alzheimer's disease.** *Journal of Neurology, Neurosurgery & Psychiatry,* 48(11), 1172–1174.
Compared 27 patients (mean age 70.5 yrs) with Alzheimer's disease with 27 patients (mean age 63.8 yrs) with Huntington's disease for psychiatric morbidity prior to the onset of dementia. The Huntington's disease group showed twice the incidence of major affective disorder. This finding suggests a specific relationship between Huntington's disease and major affective disorder rather than the latter being a nonspecific prodromal feature of dementia. (6 ref).

456. Miniszek, N. A. (1983). **Development of Alzheimer disease in Down syndrome individuals.** *American Journal of Mental Deficiency,* 87(4), 377–385.
Autopsies have indicated that people with Down's syndrome (DS) who live longer than 40 yrs develop the brain pathology of Alzheimer's disease. Because of their initially low levels of mental functioning, DS persons' clinical symptoms frequently go undetected until the disease is advanced and deterioration severe. Study of this doubly inflicted population is critical to development of appropriate assessment methods and to the study of the role of genetics in aging. A preliminary investigation of the Adaptive Behavior Scale (ABS) as a potential diagnostic tool is presented. An examination of the records of

6 DS patients (aged 53–65) and 6 age-, sex-, and IQ-matched non-DS patients confirmed the regression of older DS persons. In an examination of ABS protocols (C. J. Fogelman, 1975), the ABS clearly differentiated the regressed from the well-functioning DS Ss, offering promise as a practical assessment device. (25 ref).

457. Mohs, Richard C.; Breitner, John C.; Silverman, Jeremy M. & Davis, Kenneth L. (1987). **Alzheimer's disease: Morbid risk among first-degree relatives approximates 50% by 90 years of age.** *Archives of General Psychiatry,* 44(5), 405–408.
Investigated the familial aggregation of Alzheimer's disease (AD) in relatives of probands by the family history method. Informed consent was obtained from responsible relatives of 50 biologically unrelated patients (aged 51–85 yrs) with AD and 45 matched controls (aged 46–85 yrs). 34 (13.9%) of 244 AD proband relatives over 45 yrs old and 9 (4.3%) of 211 comparable control relatives had evidence of cognitive impairment. 23 proband relatives (67.6% of those with dementia) and 4 control relatives were eventually judged to have probable AD. A cumulative morbid risk of 45.9% among relatives of AD probands by 86 yrs of age is indicated. The possibility of genetic causes for AD is suggested.

458. Mölsä, Pekka K.; Marttila, R. J. & Rinne, U. K. (1986). **Survival and cause of death in Alzheimer's disease and multi-infarct dementia.** *Acta Neurologica Scandinavica,* 74(2), 103–107.
Studied the survival rate and causes of death in 218 patients with Alzheimer's disease (AD) and 115 patients with multi-infarct dementia (MID). The survival prognosis was found to be less favorable in MID than AD. The dementia disorder was the underlying cause of death in 68% of the AD patients vs 38% of the MID patients. 33% of the MID patients died of an acute cerebrovascular accident vs only 9% of the AD patients.

459. Neary, D.; Snowden, J. S.; Shields, R. A.; Burjan, A. W. et al. (1987). **Single photon emission tomography using ^{99m}Tc-HM-PAO in the investigation of dementia.** *Journal of Neurology, Neurosurgery & Psychiatry,* 50(9), 1101–1109.
Carried out single photon emission tomographic imaging of the brain using ^{99m}Tc-hexamethyl propyleneamine oxime (^{99m}Tc HM-PAO) in 41 patients with a clinical diagnosis of Alzheimer's disease, non-Alzheimer frontal-lobe dementia, and progressive supranuclear palsy. Independent assessment of reductions in uptake revealed posterior hemisphere abnormalities in the majority of the Alzheimer group, and selective anterior hemisphere abnormalities in both other groups. Findings are consistent with observed patterns of mental impairment. Results suggest that the imaging technique has potential value in the differential diagnosis of primary cerebral atrophy.

460. Nee, Linda E. (1985). **Studying the family.** Special Issue: Alzheimer's disease. *Geriatric Nursing,* 6(3), 154–156.
Discusses the relationship between family history and the incidence of Alzheimer's disease (AZD). Findings of a study involving 12 women and 4 men who were admitted to the National Institutes of Health in 1983–1984 show that 25% had not had periods of psychosocial dysfunction prior to AZD, 56% had marked dysfunction in the family of origin, 68% had marked dysfunction in the marital family, and 25% had a 1st-degree relative with AZD. 75% of the total group had experienced unusual stress in the family of origin. The role of genetically determined stress factors and inherited genes for AZD is discussed, and a Canadian family with 8 generations of AZD is described. (8 ref).

461. Ninos, Mary & Makohon, Rennie. (1985). **Functional assessment of the patient.** Special Issue: Alzheimer's disease. *Geriatric Nursing,* 6(3), 139–142.

Discusses the need for functional assessment (FA) of patients with Alzheimer's disease (AZD) to identify areas in which independence and control can be maintained, contributing to the patient's self-esteem and helping to conserve family resources. A comprehensive FA of the person with AZD requires the skills of the social worker, occupational therapist, and neuropsychologist, along with those of the nurse and physician. Nurses, by virtue of the quality and quantity of time spent with patients, are best able to begin the FA and coordinate the care plans. The nursing assessment examines function in 3 domains—the physical, psychosocial, and cognitive—within the context of the environment. Areas of assessment within each of these domains are presented and discussed. It is concluded that it is important to differentiate AZD patients' functional ability—how they manage their environment—from their performance on neuropsychological tests. The nursing assessment of patient functioning distinguishes between the two. Simultaneously, it provides a framework for integrating practice with research and applying progress to patient care. (11 ref).

462. O'Brien, M. D. (1986). **Cerebral blood flow in dementia.** *Neurology,* 36(11), 1542.
Comments on the report by R. L. Rogers et al (1986) of a decrease in cerebral blood flow (CBF) before there was clinical evidence of vascular dementia but that CBF was relatively preserved in patients with Alzheimer's disease and fell only with advancing dementia. The present author notes that he first postulated this difference in 1970. The present author also notes that the Hachinski index is useful but contains a bias that must increase with age.

463. Perry, E. K. & Perry, R. H. (1986). **CNS cholinergic markers and Alzheimer's disease.** *Neurobiology of Aging,* 7(5), 390–391.
Markers of central nervous system (CNS) cholinergic activity are not yet established despite their potential value in the diagnosis of Alzheimer's disease. As the review by E. Hollander et al (1986) suggests, it is shown that blood or cerebrospinal fluid (CSF) parameters have not yet proved useful in this respect, although the prospects for probing the brain directly are much more hopeful. Among other issues, some of the problems and possibilities concerning cholinergic receptor probes are considered in relation to the status of cholinergic muscarinic and nicotinic receptors in Alzheimer's disease.

464. Rapoport, Stanley I.; Atack, John R.; May, Conrad & Grady, Cheryl L. (1986). **Commentary on antemortem markers of Alzheimer's disease.** *Neurobiology of Aging,* 7(5), 398–400.
In a comment on the review of antemortem markers of Alzheimer's disease by E. Hollander et al (1986), the authors show that longitudinal studies of lateral ventricular volume using quantitative computer-assisted tomography, combined with studies of cerebral metabolism and of cognitive dysfunction using positron emission tomography and neuropsychological tests, constitute a battery of markers that describe Alzheimer's disease in relation to severity.

465. Reisberg, Barry; Ferris, Steven H. & Franssen, Emile. (1985). **An ordinal functional assessment tool for Alzheimer's-type dementia.** *Hospital & Community Psychiatry,* 36(6), 593–595.
Presents an instrument that characterizes aspects of Alzheimer's patients' daily functioning in terms of 16 functional assessment stages, ranging from normality to the most severe dementia. The instrument can help clinicians to determine rapidly whether the nature of the dementing process is consistent with uncomplicated senile dementia of the Alzheimer type and to differentiate various complications of Alzheimer's disease from the natural progression of the illness. (7 ref).

466. Rosenstock, Harvey A. (1970). **Alzheimer's presenile dementia: A review of 11 clinically diagnosed cases.** *Diseases of the Nervous System,* 31(12), 826–829.
Reviews the early course of 11 patients wih clinically diagnosed Alzheimer's disease. Principal findings indicate that (a) Alzheimer's presenile dementia is distinguishable clinically from other idiopathic dementias of the presenium. (b) There is a predictable course of early amnesia, disorientation, confusion, apraxia, and impaired perceptual organization. (c) Depression and other psychiatric symptoms are not uncommon in the early stages of the illness. (d) EEG changes occur early and include diffuse slowing and loss of the dominant alpha rhythm. The pneumoencephalogram may reveal generalized cortical atrophy and/or ventricular dilatation. (e) The early occurrence of confabulation, focal neurological deficits, incontinence, muscular atrophy, and convulsions would suggest a disorder other than Alzheimer's disease.

467. Roth, Martin. (1986). **"Antemortem markers of Alzheimer's disease": A commentary.** *Neurobiology of Aging,* 7(5), 402–405.
Argues that E. Hollander et al (1986) have performed a valuable service in their comprehensive review of the literature of antemortem markers in Alzheimer's disease. The discovery of objective and reliable indices in vivo of an illness of obscure causation constitutes a forward step in scientific progress toward its accurate diagnosis and discovery of its etiology. When markers that have a satisfactory correlation with clinical diagnosis on the one hand and postmortem findings on the other have been developed, an acceleration of progress almost invariably follows.

468. Schoenberg, Bruce S.; Anderson, Dallas W. & Haerer, Armin F. (1985). **Severe dementia: Prevalence and clinical features in a biracial US population.** *Archives of Neurology,* 42(8), 740–743.
In a Mississippi county containing 49.1% Black and 50.1% White residents, 80 of 23,842 residents were identified with severe dementia (i.e., requiring constant supervision). Although no striking differences were found between groups in incidence, age-adjusted prevalence rates were higher for Blacks and for females. Prevalence is a function of both incidence and survival. In a screening of 5,489 40–64 yr old residents, 3 Ss were identified with severe dementia, 1 of whom had primary chronic progressive dementia. (10 ref).

469. Serby, Michael; Chou, James C. & Franssen, Emile H. (1987). **Dementia in an American-Chinese nursing home population.** *American Journal of Psychiatry,* 144(6), 811–812.
Of 58 demented residents (aged 59–100 yrs) in an American-Chinese nursing home, 44 (75.9%) had multi-infarct dementia, 7 (12.1%) had possible Alzheimer's disease, 4 (6.9%) had other dementias, and 3 (5.2%) had unknown disorders. It is conluded that Alzheimer's disease was relatively less prevalent than in US nursing homes overall.

470. Shibayama, Hiroto; Kasahara, Y. & Kobayashi, H. (1986). **Prevalence of dementia in a Japanese elderly population.** *Acta Psychiatrica Scandinavica,* 74(2), 144–151.
Conducted a psychiatric epidemiological study of 3,106 community residents (aged 65+ yrs) selected from the whole Aichi Prefecture of Japan. The prevalence of dementia was estimated to be 5.8% (moderate and severe, 2.2%; mild, 3.6%) of the aged population in the community. Cerebrovascular dementia or multi-infarct dementia was found in 2.8%, senile dementia of the Alzheimer type in 2.4%, and dementia due to other causes in 0.6%.

471. Stern, Matthew B.; Gur, Ruben C.; Saykin, Andrew J. & Hurtig, Howard I. (1986). **Dementia of Parkinson's disease and Alzheimer's disease: Is there a difference?** *Journal of the American Geriatrics Society,* 34(6), 475–478.

Reviews similarities and differences in the pathophysiology of dementias associated with Parkinson's disease (PD) and Alzheimer's disease (AD). The clinical characteristics of dementia in PD and the effects of antiparkinsonian medications on cognition are discussed. It is concluded that PD and AD may coexist in some patients, but a more coherent synthesis of the available evidence favors a unique chemical disequilibrium in the dementia of PD that will ultimately differentiate its clinical pathophysiology and treatment from AD.

472. Sulkava, Raimo. (1982). **Alzheimer's disease and senile dementia of Alzheimer type: A comparative study.** *Acta Neurologica Scandinavica,* 65(6), 636–650.
Investigated clinical and neuropsychological findings, EEG, and blood and cerebrospinal fluid parameters in 36 patients with Alzheimer's disease (AD) and 35 patients with senile dementia of Alzheimer type (SDAT). Both groups were unable to take care of themselves and showed other symptoms such as disorientation, hallucinations, and aggressiveness. There were more women among senile Ss and more familial cases among presenile Ss. The average duration of the symptoms was longer in presenile Ss than in senile. Extrapyramidal signs were found in over 60% of all Ss. Four presenile and 2 senile Ss had epileptic seizures. A positive correlation was found between the EEG abnormality and the severity of dementia in AD but not in SDAT. It is concluded that it is artificial to separate AD and SDAT at the age of 65 yrs because they compose a single clinical entity. (27 ref).

473. Treves, Therese et al. (1986). **Present dementia in Israel.** *Archives of Neurology,* 43(1), 26–29.
Conducted a nationwide epidemiologic study in Israel of presenile dementia of the Alzheimer type (PDAT) with onset through age 60 yrs. When national neurologic disease register and clinical records of all patients discharged from hospitals from 1974–1983 with a diagnosis suggestive of dementia were reviewed, data show 71 Jewish Ss with onset of PDAT during this period. Age of onset was 43–60 yrs, and the median survival rate was 8.1 yrs, with slightly longer survival if onset occurred before age 55 yrs. The incidence of PDAT was found to be significantly higher in those born in Europe or the US than in those born in Asia or Africa. Findings are consistent with the hypothesis that the disease in European- and American-born Jews reflects a single nosologic entity. (14 ref).

474. Veroff, Amy E.; Pearlson, Godfrey D. & Ahn, Hyo S. (1982). **CT scan and neuropsychological correlates of Alzheimer's disease and Huntington's disease.** *Brain & Cognition,* 1(2), 177–184.
Cortical and subcortical dementia syndromes differ in areas of primary neuropathology and clinical characteristics. Conventional computerized tomography (CT) scan interpretation, visual inspection of pictures, has not been useful in studying dementia. Recent studies of the digitally stored CT attenuation values have found systematic variations with normal aging and aphasia subtypes. In the present study of numerical CT scan information, 4 Alzheimer's disease and 2 Huntington's disease patients (aged 55–65 yrs) were administered the WAIS and Wechsler Memory Scale. Findings indicate a double dissociation of frontal- and temporal-lobe density values, and a significant correlation between left temporal-lobe density and verbal-ability measures in the Alzheimer's disease patients. Results indicate that Alzheimer's and Huntington's disease can be differentiated by analysis of numerical CT scan density information. (15 ref).

475. Wagner, Henry N. (1985). **Probing the chemistry of the mind.** *New England Journal of Medicine,* 312(1), 44–46.
Discusses the use of positron-emission tomography (PET) and simple radiation detectors to examine the localization, concentration, and chemical forms of peptides arising in or having effects on the CNS. Specific uses of PET scans include

assessment of regional cerebral blood flow in Alzheimer's patients, examination of the mechanisms of antidepressant and neuroleptic treatments, and the classification of neuropsychiatric disorders. Overall, PET represents a new way to examine the chemistry of the mind. (9 ref).

476. Whall, Ann. (1985). **Alzheimer's disease and depression.** *Journal of Gerontological Nursing,* 11(3), 33.
Notes that the diagnosis of Alzheimer's disease is a diagnosis of exclusion that may overlook depression as the cause of disorder. It is noted that depression is a common reversible condition with symptoms similar to AD; Ss in the early stages of AD are also depressed. Differential diagnosis is important to the appropriate treatment of both disorders.

477. White, Roberta F. (1987). **Differential diagnosis of probable Alzheimer's disease and solvent encephalopathy in older workers.** *Clinical Neuropsychologist,* 1(2), 153–160.
Presents 4 case histories to illustrate the differential diagnosis of the effects of exposure to industrial solvents vs Alzheimer's disease and discusses research findings with regard to assessing cognitive problems in older workers. Issues discussed include the prevalence of such problems, patterns of neuropsychological dysfunction, and proposed principles of diagnosis. These principles concern the assessment of IQ, language, retrograde memory, attention and visuospatial skills, and progression of cognitive decline.

478. Wilson, Robert S. et al. (1982). **Computed tomography in dementia.** *Neurology,* 32(9), 1054–1057.
Examined computerized tomographies (CTs) of patients with senile dementia of the Alzheimer type and of age-matched normal controls. Cerebral atrophy measures were available on 42 patients and 38 controls (mean age 69 yrs), and density measures were available for 19 patients (mean age 71.7 yrs) and 33 controls (mean age 67.9 yrs). Cerebral atrophy was associated with advancing age and the presence, but not the degree, of dementia. CT density numbers in 14 separate brain regions were not related to age or to the presence or degree of dementia. Findings fail to support other reports of decreased CT density in dementia and suggest that the role of CT scan in the evaluation of dementia is limited to ruling out mass lesions. (17 ref).

479. Winblad, Bengt; Fowler, Christopher J. & Marcusson, Jan. (1986). **Critique of antemortem markers of Alzheimer's disease.** *Neurobiology of Aging,* 7(5), 388–389.
Suggests that the review of antemortem markers for Alzheimer's disease (AD) by E. Hollander et al (1986) is somewhat overbiased toward the cholinergic hypothesis of AD. Some data of relevance to the article, without being an alternative viewpoint per se, are presented.

480. Yerby, M. S. et al. (1985). **A new method of measuring brain atrophy: The effect of aging in its application for diagnosing dementia.** *Neurology,* 35(9), 1316–1320.
Describes a method of measuring cerebral atrophy that uses computerized tomography to determine a ratio of brain parenchyma to ventricular and subarachnoid space. In 117 patients (aged 54–94 yrs) referred for evaluation of cognitive dysfunction, the method's ability to differentiate persons with senile dementia of the Alzheimer's type from those suffering from pseudodementia was found to be confounded by age and of limited utility. (29 ref).

Clinical Aspects

481. Agbayewa, M. Oluwafemi. (1986). **Earlier psychiatric morbidity in patients with Alzheimer's disease.** *Journal of the American Geriatrics Society,* 34(8), 561–564.
The medical charts of 188 Alzheimer patients (average age 79.5 yrs) and a comparison group of 80 nondemented patients matched for age and sex were retrospectively reviewed for history of psychiatric morbidity. Results show that the Alzheimer Ss were more likely to have had a psychiatric illness earlier in life, with unipolar depression and paranoid disorder being the 2 most frequent psychiatric disorders. Possible explanations for these findings are discussed, including underreporting, facility bias, functional psychiatric features as prodromal states of Alzheimer's disease, and vulnerability to psychiatric morbidity in persons who go on to develop Alzheimer's disease.

482. Boyle, Sylvia A. (1987). **The clinical manifestations of Alzheimer's disease in a Down's syndrome population.** *Dissertation Abstracts International,* 48(5-B), 1527.

483. Brednev, A. G. (1967). **On the differentio-diagnostic significance of clinical features in the early stage of Pick's disease and Alzheimer's disease.** *Zhurnal Nevropatologii i Psikhiatrii,* 67(4), 549–554.
Based on 24 cases of Pick's disease (PD) and 22 of Alzheimer's disease (AD), a medical analysis of the 2 pathologies is presented, accompanied by accounts of behavioral and mental disorders characterizing them. The initial period of AD is almost twice that of PD. The clinical picture of PD is more complex and polymorphous because of the greater variability of local atrophies. The frontal lobes are drawn into the atrophic process the earliest and the most often, making the pseudoparalytic syndrome and lack of spontaneity the major signs of PD. However, in primarily temporal and parieto-temporal atrophic localization, speech-motor hyperactiviity is observed, while in frontal-temporal atrophy lack of motor spontaneity may be combined wih speech hyperactivity. In these cases differentiation between PD and AD is the most difficult. In the initial period of AD, speech-motor activity is usually heightened, in correspondence with the predominance of disorders in the temporo-parietal divisions of the cortex in this disease. Better preservation of the formal and higher ethico-moral functions in AD may be explained by the lesser damage of the frontal lobes. Dementia in PD from the very beginning exhibits a cruder character, leading to earlier hospitalization.

484. Campbell-Taylor I. (1985). **Dimensions of clinical judgment in the diagnosis of Alzheimer's disease.** *Dissertation Abstracts International,* 45(8-B), 2524.

485. Dalton, Arthur J. & Crapper-McLachlan, Donald R. (1986). **Clinical expression of Alzheimer's disease in Down's syndrome.** *Psychiatric Clinics of North America,* 9(4), 659–670.
Suggests that the presence of trisomy 21 in Down's syndrome (DS) may be a risk factor predisposing to the development of Alzheimer's disease (AD). Neuropathologic studies conducted over more than 50 yrs have consistently documented the similarities of the lesions found in DS with those found in the brains of patients of normal karyotypes with AD. Some conflicting clinical observations of dementia are reviewed, and some major problems associated with clinical investigations are identified. A case of DS with confirmed AD at autopsy illustrates the power of the longitudinal approach in delineating the natural course of dementia in DS.

486. Duara, Ranjan; Grady, Cheryl L.; Haxby, James V.; Sundaram, M. et al. (1986). **Positron emission tomography in Alzheimer's disease.** *Neurology,* 36(7), 879–887.
Studied 21 patients (mean age range 63–65 yrs) with dementia of the Alzheimer's type (DAT) and 29 healthy age-matched male controls (mean age 63 yrs) using positron emission tomography (PET) and [18F]-2-fluoro-2-deoxydextroglucose to measure regional cerebral glucose consumption in the resting state. Reductions in ratio measures of relative metabolism in some parietal, temporal, and frontal regions were found in mild, moderate, and severe DAT groups. A significant increase in right–left metabolic asymmetry, particularly in parietal regions, also was seen in mild and mod-

erate groups. Only in the severely demented Ss was the absolute cerebral metabolic rate reduced significantly from control values. It is concluded that PET is useful in quantifying regional cerebral dysfunction in DAT, even in the early stages of the disease.

487. El-Sobky, Adel; Darwish, A. K. & El-Shazly, M. (1985). **Serial dexamethasone suppression test (DST) in depression and senile dementia of the Alzheimer type (SDAT).** *Psychiatric Hospital,* 16(4), 187–191.
Administered the DST serially over an 18 mo period to 61 adults (aged 18–89 yrs) with SDAT or endogenous depression. Findings indicate that the DST had an overall sensitivity of 70% in depressive Ss. Test results were gradually normalized in depressives who responded to treatment and remained positive in depressives who were resistant to treatment. DST sensitivity in depressives was decreased in Ss aged over 65 yrs. DST sensitivity in the SDAT Ss was 22.8%. DST profiles in this group were unrelated to the clinical picture and were characterized by decreased basal cortisol levels, greater suppression than in depressed Ss, and more positive DST results in the morning than in the afternoon.

488. Erkinjuntti, Timo. (1987). **Differential diagnosis between Alzheimer's disease and vascular dementia: Evaluation of common clinical methods.** *Acta Neurologica Scandinavica,* 76(6), 433–442.
193 consecutively admitted adult demented patients were examined to evaluate the role of common clinical methods in the differential diagnosis between Alzheimer's disease (AD) and vascular dementia (VD). Ss fulfilling criteria for VD were divided into multi-infarct dementia (MID) and probable vascular dementia (PVD). Absence of cardio- and cerebrovascular diseases, corticospinal tract signs, and gait disorders differentiated AD from MID and PVD. 88.6% of the MID Ss and 41.3% with PVD had brain infarct on computerized tomography. Ischemic scores seemed to be useful in the differential diagnosis between AD and VD.

489. Erkinjuntti, Timo; Ketonen, Leena; Sulkava, Raimo; Sipponen, Jorma et al. (1987). **Do white matter changes on MRI and CT differentiate vascular dementia from Alzheimer's disease?** *Journal of Neurology, Neurosurgery & Psychiatry,* 50(1), 37–42.
Magnetic resonance imaging (MRI) showed white matter changes in all 29 patients (mean age 68.7 yrs) with vascular dementia and in 8 out of 22 patients (mean age 64 yrs) with Alzheimer's disease. The corresponding figures for computed tomography (CT) were 26 and 1, respectively. White matter changes are suggested to be a useful diagnostic aid in the differential diagnosis between vascular dementia and Alzheimer's disease.

490. Filinson, Rachel. (1984). **Diagnosis of senile dementia Alzheimer's type: The state of the art.** *Clinical Gerontologist,* 2(4), 3–23.
Contends, on the basis of a review of the medical literature, that there are inadequacies in diagnostic practices with regard to senile dementia Alzheimer's type (SDAT) and that there is differential emphasis on the type of error typically made in diagnosis–overdiagnosis. The precision of diagnosis of SDAT is undermined by a lack of consistency in naming and classification of this type of disorder; although DSM-III standards have been developed, they are not widely applied. The majority of empirical work on misdiagnosis stresses the overdiagnosis of SDAT in cases where dementialike symptoms have been produced by functional disorders or overmedication. These findings can only apply to those who have been referred for evaluation; little attention has been paid to those seeking but not referred for diagnostic evaluation or to factors that might impede referral for diagnosis. It is suggested that attempts to identify and perfect diagnostic methods falter

unless there is a postmortem autopsy to confirm the presence and severity of the disease. (3½ ref).

491. Gauthier, Serge. (1985). **Practical guidelines for the antemortem diagnosis of senile dementia of the Alzheimer type.** Eighth Annual Meeting of the Canadian College of Neuropsychopharmacology: Perspectives in Canadian neuropsychopharmacology (1985, London, Canada). *Progress in Neuro-Psychopharmacology & Biological Psychiatry,* 9(5–6), 491–495.
Suggests that senile dementia of the Alzheimer type (SDAT) is the most common type of dementia in the elderly but is difficult to diagnose antemortem. Clinical assessment gives an 80% degree of accuracy of diagnosis. Now that specific therapy for SDAT is possible, diagnosis has to be more definite. Assessment of SDAT includes clinical history, physical examination, and imaging techniques such as computerized tomography and magnetic resonance imaging. Positron emission tomography using ^{18}F-2-deoxyglucose is currently the best imaging technique for diagnosing SDAT in vivo. A cortical biopsy with histology and assay of choline acetyltransferase is required to give a diagnosis of definite SDAT. (14 ref).

492. Gauthier, Serge; Robitaille, Yves; Quirion, Remi & Leblanc, Richard. (1986). **Antemortem laboratory diagnosis of Alzheimer's disease.** *Progress in Neuro-Psychopharmacology & Biological Psychiatry,* 10(3–5), 391–403.
Reviews the literature concerning and describes the authors' own experience with diagnostic laboratory procedures for Alzheimer's disease. Procedures covered involve conventional studies, including routine laboratory work-up and EEG; cerebrospinal fluid (CSF) analysis; imaging techniques, including computed tomography, nuclear magnetic resonance, and positron emission tomography; and cortical biopsy, including surgical technique, histological analysis, and biochemical analysis.

493. Gustafson, Lars & Nilsson, Lennart. (1982). **Differential diagnosis of presenile dementia on clinical grounds.** *Acta Psychiatrica Scandinavica,* 65(3), 194–209.
57 patients (mean age 57.6 yrs) were studied for differential diagnosis among dementias. Three rating scales were used for identification of Alzheimer's disease (AD), Pick's disease (PD), and multi-infarct dementia (MID). Their validity was tested against verified diagnoses in 28 Ss. The rating scale of ischemic score consisting of 13 items such as abrupt onset, stepwise progression, fluctuating course, history of strokes, and neurological symptoms and signs, identifies patients with MID. This can also be achieved by the 2 rating scales for diagnosis of AD and PD, which in turn can be used for the differentiation between these 2 dementias. The rating scale for diagnosis of AD contains clinical features such as early spatial disorientation, apraxia, aphasia, agnosia, logoclonia, and increased muscular tension. The rating scale for PD contains such clinical features as early loss of insight, early signs of disinhibition, echolalia, mutism, and amimia. Results show that the differentiation between the major types of presenile dementia can be achieved by a systematic rating of the clinical features. (51 ref).

494. Hamill, Robert W. & Buell, Stephen J. (1982). **Dementia: Clinical and basic science aspects.** *Journal of the American Geriatrics Society,* 30(12), 781–787.
Reexamines the following basic tenets regarding alterations of higher intellectual function in the elderly: gait and posture, cranial nerves, motor system, sensory systems, reflexes, differential diagnosis, and Alzheimer's disease. (32 ref).

495. Hauser, W. Allen; Morris, Marcia L.; Heston, Leonard L. & Anderson, V. Elving. (1986). **Seizures and myoclonus in patients with Alzheimer's disease.** *Neurology,* 36(9), 1226–1230.

Reviewed 8 patients with dementia and autopsy findings of Alzheimer's disease (AD) to identify patients with seizures or myoclonus after onset of dementia. Group mean ages at time of dementia onset ranged from 69.1 to 73.5 yrs. Eight had seizures, and 8 others had myoclonus. The incidence of seizures was 10 times more than expected in a reference population. Seizures occurred in any stage of AD, but myoclonus was often a late manifestation. Both seizures and myoclonus are manifestations of AD and may be seen at any time in the course of the illness.

496. Hendricks, Robert D. (1985). **Psychological assessment as an aid in the differentiation of Senile Dementia of the Alzheimer's Type (SDAT) and depressive pseudodementia.** *Dissertation Abstracts International,* 45(12-B, Pt 1), 3941–3942.

497. Heyman, A.; Wilkinson, W. E.; Hurwitz, B. J.; Helms, M. J. et al. (1987). **Early-onset Alzheimer's disease: Clinical predictors of institutionalization and death.** *Neurology,* 37(6), 980–984.
Made follow-up observations of 92 White patients (aged 51.3–74.6 yrs) with early-onset Alzheimer's disease to determine the demographic, clinical, and neuropsychological factors predictive of institutionalization or death. The cumulative mortality rate 5 yrs after entry into the study was 23.9%, compared with an expected rate of 9.5%. The 5-yr cumulative rate of admission to nursing homes was 62.8%. The language ability of the Ss on entry to the study, their scores on a brief screening test of cognitive function, and their overall ratings of clinical dementia were predictors of subsequent institutional care and death. The age of the Ss had a significant modifying effect on these predictive factors, resulting in a greater risk of institutionalization and death in younger Ss with severe cognitive impairment as compared with older Ss with the same degree of dysfunction.

498. Huff, F. Jacob; Boller, Francois; Lucchelli, Federica; Querriera, Richard et al. (1987). **The neurologic examination in patients with probable Alzheimer's disease.** *Archives of Neurology,* 44(9), 929–932.
Analyzed the neurological examination findings on 95 Alzheimer's disease (AD) patients (aged 65.7 yrs) and 81 healthy controls (aged 61.9 yrs) to determine which neurologic abnormalities are useful for differentiating AD from controls. Factors other than mental status that were useful in the clinical diagnosis of AD were (in order of decreasing odds ratio) the presence of release signs, olfactory deficit, impaired stereognosis or graphesthesia, gait disorder, tremor, and abnormalities on cerebellar testing. These abnormalities are discussed in terms of pathological AD effects on underlying central nervous system (CNS) structures.

499. Jenike, Michael A. & Albert, Marilyn S. (1984). **The dexamethasone suppression test in patients with presenile and senile dementia of the Alzheimer's type.** *Journal of the American Geriatrics Society,* 32(6), 441–444.
Performed the dexamethasone suppression test (DST) on 18 patients, aged 55–79 yrs, with presenile and senile dementia of the Alzheimer's type. Objective cognitive testing showed that 13 Ss were mildly to moderately impaired, and 5 were moderately to severely impaired. The Hamilton Rating Scale for Depression yielded normal results in all Ss. DST results were abnormal in only 1 of the mildly impaired Ss but in 4 of the 5 moderately impaired Ss. Data suggest that the DST may be a useful clinical tool in mildly impaired patients with Alzheimer's disease but is likely to be confounded by disease in moderately to severely impaired patients. (16 ref).

500. Kłoszewska, Iwona & Bogucki, Andrzej. (1985). **Diagnostyka kliniczna pierwotnie zwyrodnieniowych zespołów otępiennych. / Clinical diagnosis of primary degenerative dementia syndromes.** *Psychiatria Polska,* 19(3), 219–225.

Discusses clinical, computerized tomographic, EEG, and positron emission tomographic diagnosis of primary degenerative dementia syndromes (e.g., Huntington's chorea, Alzheimer's disease, Parkinsonism). The diagnostic criteria of Diagnostic and Statistical Manual of Mental Disorders (DSM-III) and the Dementia Study Group of Washington University are discussed.

501. Kolata, Gina. (1986). **Genetic screening raises questions for employers and insurers.** *Science,* 232(4748), 317–319.
Discusses ethical dilemmas surrounding the potential development of tests for genetically related disorders such as Alzheimer's disease. A survey of persons at risk for Huntington's chorea is outlined that showed that most Ss wished to be tested. The potential for discrimination in employment and insurance coverage is considered with reference to the current situations of persons with epilepsy or at high risk for acquired immune deficiency syndrome.

502. Kral, V. A. (1982). **Depressive Pseudodemenz und Senile Demenz vom Alzheimer-Typ: Ein Pilot-Studie. / Depressive pseudodementia and Alzheimer's disease: A pilot study.** *Nervenarzt,* 53(5), 284–286.
Examined the etiology, symptomatology, and prognosis of depressive pseudodementia in elderly patients and compared them with those of elderly patients with senile dementia of Alzheimer's type. The case histories of 22 depressive pseudodementia patients, ages 62–78 yrs, who had been treated for 4–18 yrs, were analyzed. The absence of organic abnormalities in the brain and the restoration of intellectual function with treatment were found to differentiate the syndrome of depressive pseudodementia from that of senile dementia of Alzheimer's type. All 22 depressive pseudodementia patients responded favorably to a combination of antidepressants, neuroleptics, and psychotherapy, although the incidence of recidivism was great. 20 of the patients eventually manifested the typical symptoms of the progressive senile dementia of Alzheimer's type. (10 ref).

503. Kulczycki, Jerzy & Jedrzejczak, Tomasz. (1984). **Kliniczne und zisternographische Differentialdiagnose zwischen präseniler Demenz und Hakim-Syndrom. / Differential diagnosis of presenile dementia and Hakim-Syndrome on the basis of clinical and the radionuclide cisternography examinations.** *Psychiatrie, Neurologie und medizinische Psychologie,* 36(11), 674–677.
Compared 27 patients with Hakim syndrome and 11 with Alzheimer's disease on clinical and "radionuclide cisternography" examination data. In all cases, dementia was a stable symptom. Ss with Hakim syndrome had an early gait disturbance, ataxia, and epileptic seizures. Aphasia, apraxia, and psychotic disorders were found only in Alzheimer's Ss. Radionuclide cisternography showed ventricular retention and absence of parasagital accumulation only in Ss with Hakim syndrome. (English & Russian abstracts) (11 ref).

504. London, Eric; de Leon, Mony J.; George, Ajax E.; Englund, Elisabet et al. (1986). **Periventricular lucencies in the CT scans of aged and demented patients.** *Biological Psychiatry,* 21(10), 960–962.
Examined the contribution of computed tomography (CT) to the differential diagnosis between Alzheimer's disease (AD) and multi-infarct dementia (MID) in 314 patients. Findings indicate that white matter periventricular lucencies do not substantially help in making the differential diagnosis between AD and MID, although they are more frequent in vascular dementias.

505. Luxenberg, J. S.; May, C.; Haxby, James V.; Grady, C. et al. (1987). **Cerebral metabolism, anatomy, and cognition in monozygotic twins discordant for dementia of the Alzheimer type.** *Journal of Neurology, Neurosurgery & Psychiatry,* 50(3), 333–340.

Studied a pair of 59-yr-old male monozygotic twins—1 of whom was diagnosed as having dementia of the Alzheimer type (DAT)—using positron emission tomography (PET), quantitative analysis of cerebral computed tomography (CT), magnetic resonance imaging (MRI), and neuropsychological testing. Findings show that PET scanning, quantitative CT scanning, MRI scanning, and neuropsychological tests distinguish the changes of DAT in a pair of identical twins apparently discordant for this malady. Unlike many past studies, the cerebral anatomical and metabolic normality of the asymptomatic twin was documented.

506. McLean, Steve. (1987). **Assessing dementia: I. Difficulties, definitions and differential diagnosis.** *Australian & New Zealand Journal of Psychiatry,* 21(2), 142–174.
Discusses the syndromal and etiological diagnosis of dementia by outlining current clinical definitions, considering differential diagnosis, and reviewing characteristics of common dementing disorders. The past emphasis on a search for treatable causes, the reliance on laboratory investigations, and the concept of subcortical dementia are questioned. Aspects of evaluation that are stressed include brief objective cognitive testing, knowledge of normal age-related cognitive changes, flexible criteria for Alzheimer's disease, and comprehensive individualized evaluation of the person.

507. Merskey, Harold et al. (1985). **Correlative studies in Alzheimer's disease.** Eighth Annual Meeting of the Canadian College of Neuropsychopharmacology: Perspectives in Canadian neuro-psychopharmacology (1985, London, Canada). *Progress in Neuro-Psychopharmacology & Biological Psychiatry,* 9(5–6), 509–514.
Describes an approach for establishing and maintaining a correlative study of Alzheimer's disease (AD) and reports on findings by the University of Western Ontario Dementia Study Group (consisting of medical faculty members), based on work done since 1977. Ss were 325 dementia patients (mean age 74 yrs) and 160 control patients (mean age 71 yrs) who served in the study up to January 1985. Autopsies were performed on 98 experimental Ss and 7 control Ss who had died. Results reveal that the accuracy of the antemortem diagnosis of dementia was low if one demanded complete precision in the clinical specification of what would be found at autopsy. There was difficulty in obtaining a sensitive measure of intellectual function in the advanced state of AD. One psychological test developed specially for the study was the Extended Scale for Dementia, which was found to have satisfactory psychometric properties. Findings support the definition of AD as a hippocampal dementia. Typical and atypical forms of AD are discussed. (20 ref).

508. Mitsuyama, Tashio. (1974). **Clinicopathological study of Alzheimer's disease: Report on six cases.** *Kyushu Neuro-psychiatry,* 20(1), 48–61.
Reports 6 cases of the presenile onset of Alzheimer's disease with dementia. The 5 males and 1 female (36–52 yrs old at the time of death) had had the disease for periods from 2 yrs 6 mo to 14 yrs. Clinically, the disease was divided into 3 distinct stages. Psychological examinations revealed severe impairment of mental functions, and all Ss showed abnormal EEG patterns. All the autopsies showed acute bronchopneumonia, marked emaciation, pleural adhesion and atrophy of the internal organs, and generalized cerebral atrophy with focal accentuation on frontal, parietal, and temporal lobes. Microscopic examinations also revealed the effects of the disease on the cerebral cortices. The evidence indicates that Alzheimer's disease is a distinct clinicopathological entity that should be distinguished from senile dementia and from other types of presenile dementia. (English summary) (52 ref).

509. Miyama, Yoshio. (1986). **Dementia: From the standpoint of pathology, Alzheimer's disease and vascular dementia.** *Kyushu Neuro-psychiatry,* 32(1), 20–28.

Discusses diagnostic discrimination between vascular dementia and Alzheimer's. In both cases, reduction in the weight and volume of the brain and an increase in the size of the ventricle and of the sulci are common gross changes in the diseased brain. The loss of neurons, deposition of lipofuscin age pigment, loss of dendritic spines, amygloid changes, senile (neuritic) plaques and the formation of neurofibrillary tangles are the major microscopic changes in the brain. These changes, commonly observed in the brains of Alzheimer's disease patients, are also observed in the brains of older persons with no sign of senile dementia. Results of pathological studies show that the brain with Alzheimer's disease had deposition of lipofuscin age pigment in the limbic neocortex (cingulate, pyriform cortex), amygdala, limbic thalamic nuclei, and mammillary body.

510. Molchanova, E. K.; Sudareva, L. O.; Selezneva, N. D. & Voskresenskaya, N. I. (1986). **Some characteristics of initial manifestations of Alzheimer's disease.** *Zhurnal Nevropatologii i Psikhiatrii,* 86(9), 1371–1375.
Conducted a retrospective study of the characteristics of the initial state of Alzheimer's disease (AD) in 46 adult patients. The psychopathological structure during the initial stage of AD, the Ss' age at disease onset, and the duration of the initial period were studied. (English abstract).

511. Mölsä, P. K.; Paljärvi, L.; Rinne, U. K. & Säkö, E. (1984). **Accuracy of clinical diagnosis in dementia.** 25th Scandinavian Congress of Neurology: Dementia and degenerative cerebral disorders (1984, Bergen, Norway). *Acta Neurologica Scandinavica,* 69(98), 232–233.
58 patients with clinical diagnoses of senile dementia Alzheimer type (SDAT), multi-infarct dementia, or a combination of neuronal degeneration of the Alzheimer type and multiple infarcts (called "combined dementia"; CD) came to autopsy, 1979–1982. Specimens were taken from the right half of the brain, and neurofibrillary tangles and neuritic plaques were quantified for neuropathological diagnoses. Results show that accurate clinical diagnosis of CD was the least reliable; these Ss were frequently found to be diagnosed as belonging in the SDAT group, presumably on the basis of primary neuronal degeneration of the Alzheimer type. (4 ref).

512. Mölsä, Pekka K. et al. (1985). **Validity of clinical diagnosis in dementia: A prospective clinicopathological study.** *Journal of Neurology, Neurosurgery & Psychiatry,* 48(11), 1085–1090.
Examined the accuracy of a clinical diagnosis of dementia in 58 patients by conducting a neuropathological investigation of each S after death. Ss were aged 59–95 yrs at time of death. Dementia was diagnosed before death if there was a primarily occurring progressive deterioration of memory and other cognitive functions. After death, Alzheimer's disease was diagnosed if there were senile plaques and neurofibrillary tangles in the neocortex. Alzheimer's disease and multi-infarct dementia were recognized with sensitivities and specificities exceeding 70%, whereas combined dementia as a separate group was relatively unreliably diagnosed. The value of Hachinski's Ischaemic Score (V. C. Hachinski et al, 1975) in differentiating between Alzheimer's disease and vascular dementias was demonstrated. Its performance was to some extent improved by assigning new weights to the items. In a logistic regression model, fluctuating course, nocturnal confusion, and focal neurological symptoms emerged as features with the best discriminating value and helped to diagnose correctly 89% of the Alzheimer and 71% of the vascular dementia patients. (20 ref).

513. Oelenberg, W.; Verspohl, F.; Menne, R. & Kutzner, M. (1987). **Congophilic angiopathy with cerebrospinal symptoms.** *European Archives of Psychiatry & Neurological Sciences,* 236(5), 281–287.

Presents the case of a patient who developed symptoms of spinal motor neuron affection 20 yrs prior to his death at the age of 79. In the course of the disease, dementia and spasticity of the legs occurred. Autopsy revealed amyloid angiopathy of the brain and cervical spinal cord, corresponding with clinical symptomatology. It is suggested that this represents a distinct disease entity, different from a variant course of Alzheimer's disease.

514. Owens, David; Dawson, James C. & Losin, Sheldon (1971). **Alzheimer's disease in Down's syndrome.** *American Journal of Mental Deficiency,* 75(5), 606–612.
Although neuropathologists describe Alzheimer's changes in the brains of all victims of Down's syndrome over 35 yrs of age, only 3 cases of clinical dementia in such individuals are described in the literature. In order to establish clinical correlates of Alzheimer's disease, psychiatric and neurologic findings obtained from a middle-aged group were compared to those of Down's syndrome patients in their early 20's. The older group exhibited significantly greater incidence of abnormality in object identification, snout reflex, Babinski sign, and palmomental sign. Both groups displayed mild hypertonia rather than hypotonia, and face–hand test was abnormal in 75% of Ss tested. While dementia is uncommon, subtle neurological changes reflect neuropathological findings present in aging sufferers of Down's syndrome.

515. Poppe, Wilhelm; Läuter, Hennig & Uchanekowna-Tibilowna, Alda. (1985). **Über den Wahrscheinlichkeitscharakter der klinischen Diagnosen Morbus Pick und Morbus Alzheimer. / On the probabilistic character of the clinical diagnoses Morbus Pick and Morbus Alzheimer.** *Psychiatrie, Neurologie und medizinische Psychologie,* 37(9), 518–528.
Analyzed 15 cases of Alzheimer's disease (AD) and 16 cases of Pick's disease (PD) to identify and compare psychopathological characteristics of these 2 degenerative diseases. While there was considerable overlap in the clinical characteristics of PD and AD, the 2 diseases clearly differed in terms of the developmental phases of dementia and of personality changes. (English & Russian abstracts).

516. Prelipceanu, D. (1985). **Sindrom psihoorganic alcoolic cronic acutizat heterotoxic. / Acute heterotoxic, chronic alcoholic psychoorganic syndrome.** *Neurologie, Psihiatrie, Neurochirurgie,* 30(1), 65–69.
Describes a case of chronic alcoholic psychoorganic syndrome that presented problems of differential diagnosis (Korsakoff-like syndrome, true Korsakoff's syndrome, idiopathic dementia, or brain tumor). When the etiological circumstances leading to the development of the clinical picture were determined, it was concluded that a partial, Alzheimer-like condition with dementia was caused by accidental carbon monoxide poisoning of a patient previously intoxicated with alcohol. (English & Russian abstracts).

517. Price, Donald L.; Whitehouse, Peter J. & Struble, Robert G. (1985). **Alzheimer's disease.** *Annual Review of Medicine,* 36, 349–356.
Discusses clinical features involved in the diagnosis of Alzheimer's disease (AD) and resulting brain abnormalities, pathogenetic factors, and therapies. AD usually presents with loss of memory, but language disorders, praxis, and perceptual distortions may be apparent in early stages and almost invariably appear in later stages. In evaluating a patient with cognitive abnormalities, it is essential to exclude treatable causes of dementia and other degenerative diseases (e.g., Huntington's disease). (60 ref).

518. Reding, Michael J. et al. (1984). **Follow up of patients referred to a dementia service.** *Journal of the American Geriatrics Society,* 32(4), 265–268.
In view of previously reported high error rates in diagnoses of dementia, 85 elderly patients referred to a rehabilitation ser-

vice for evaluation were followed for up to 4 yrs in an investigation of the validity of Ss' diagnoses. Each S was examined by a neurologist, psychiatrist, and internist; administered a series of neurological tests; and evaluated by a social worker. Medical records were reviewed, and each S was discussed by staff in conference. Follow-up evaluation was conducted by telephone or by a repeat clinical visit. Results indicate that progressive dementia occurred in 55 of the 56 Ss in whose cases it was predicted by the service, and 3-yr mortality rates were 83% for multi-infarct dementia, 57% for mixed vascular plus Alzheimer dementia, and 37% for Alzheimer's disease. Differences in death rates among the different diagnostic groups supported the validity of the clinical distinctions drawn. Results suggest that a subspecialty clinic can accurately identify progressive intellectual impairment in the elderly and that patients who have depression complicating organic brain disease are at risk for progressive intellectual impairment, even if not demented when initially examined. (19 ref).

519. Roberts, Gareth W.; Lofthouse, R.; Brown, R.; Crow, T. J. et al. (1986). **Prion-protein immunoreactivity in human transmissible dementias.** *New England Journal of Medicine,* 315(19), 1231–1233.
Reports the use of immunocytochemical methods to detect the presence of prion proteins in archival material from humans, making it a useful aid for diagnosis of Alzheimer's disease. The presence of prion-protein immunoreactivity within cerebral amyloid plaques helped to differentiate the transmissible prion dementias from Alzheimer's disease, thus extending the results of Western blots. Results are consistent with the hypothesis that scrapie or Creutzfeldt-Jakob disease prions do not cause Alzheimer's disease.

520. Sabin, Thomas D. (1987). **AIDS: The new "great imitator."** *Journal of the American Geriatrics Society,* 35(5), 467–468.
Describes how the neurological symptoms of acquired immune deficiency syndrome (AIDS) dementia can be misdiagnosed as Alzheimer's disease, especially in patients over 50 yrs of age. It is suggested that geriatricians should include AIDS in the differential diagnosis of dementia myelopathy and peripheral neuropathy.

521. Sandman, Per-Olof; Adolfsson, Rolf; Nygren, Charlotte; Hallmans, Göran et al. (1987). **Nutritional status and dietary intake in institutionalized patients with Alzheimer's disease and multiinfarct dementia.** *Journal of the American Geriatrics Society,* 35(1), 31–38.
Studied nutritional status, dietary intake, weight change, and mortality in 44 severely demented, institutionalized patients (mean age 76 yrs). Dietary intake was recorded during 5 days in 2 periods, 5 wks apart, using a weighing method. Nutritional status was assessed by anthropometric measurements and determination of circulating proteins. Energy and/or protein malnutrition was found in 50% of Ss. A comparison of Ss with or without malnutrition showed no differences in dietary intake, diagnoses, age, length of hospital stay, or duration of illness. However, malnourished Ss had had 4 times as many infectious periods treated by antibiotics as Ss with no malnutrition. 39 Ss lost weight during their hospital stay. Results suggest that malnutrition and weight loss are common findings among institutionalized, severely demented patients.

522. Shefer, V. F. (1985). **Multiinfarction dementia.** *Zhurnal Nevropatologii i Psikhiatrii,* 85(7), 976–979.
Studied 255 cases of dementia of advanced age. The clinical diagnosis was vascular dementia in 142 cases. The anatomical diagnosis was senile dementia or Alzheimer's disease in 55 cases and multiinfarction dementia (MD) in 40 cases. MD

was combined with senile dementia and Alzheimer's disease in 11 of these 40 cases. The pure form of MD constituted 11% of the 255 cases and the mixed form, 18%. (English abstract).

523. Shuttleworth, Edwin C.; Huber, Steven J. & Paulson, George W. (1987). **Depression in patients with dementia of Alzheimer type.** *Journal of the National Medical Association,* 79(7), 733–736.
Examined the severity of depression in 22 patients with dementia of Alzheimer type (DAT) by means of the Self-Rating Depression Scale and the Mini-Mental State Examination. Data indicate that the magnitude of depression did not differ as a function of disease severity. The use of appropriate antidepressant therapy is encouraged at any stage of disease in patients with DAT.

524. Small, Gary W. (1985). **Revised Ischemic Score for diagnosing multi-infarct dementia.** *Journal of Clinical Psychiatry,* 46(12), 514–517.
Discusses shortcomings of the Ischemic Score (IS), a favored clinical and research tool developed by V. C. Hachinski et al (1975) for use in differentiating Alzheimer-type from multi-infarct dementia, that interfere with standardization. To address these difficulties, the IS was revised by the present author to include anchoring statements to maximize interrater reliability, a multipoint subscale to allow for assessment of severity, and a confidence subscale to account for varied sources of data. A copy of the revised IS with Severity and Confidence subscales is appended. (13 ref).

525. Small, Gary W. & Matsuyama, Steven S. (1986). **HLA-A2 as a possible marker for early-onset Alzheimer disease in men.** *Neurobiology of Aging,* 7(3), 211–214.
Performed human lymphocyte antigen (HLA) typing on 36 patients (15 males, 21 females) with clinically diagnosed Alzheimer disease and 25 cognitively intact controls (10 males, 15 females). Antigen A2 was present in all 10 men (100%) with early-onset ($<$ 60 yrs) dementia, a frequency significantly higher than the 30% frequency found in the cognitively intact men of a comparable age. This increased A2 frequency was also significantly greater than the frequencies for all other patient subgroups, including late-onset men, early-onset women, and late-onset women. Findings suggest that HLA-A2 positive men may comprise a subgroup with increased susceptibility to early-onset disease.

526. Stern, Y.; Mayeux, R.; Sano, M.; Hauser, W. A. et al. (1987). **Predictors of disease course in patients with probable Alzheimer's disease.** *Neurology,* 37(10), 1649–1653.
Evaluated the ability of myoclonus, extrapyramidal signs, or psychosis, noted at an Alzheimer's disease patient's 1st visit, to predict 1 of 2 specific clinical endpoints: (1) impairment of intellect or (2) functional impairment in ability to perform activities of daily living. 65 patients (mean age at onset 63.8 yrs) were followed either until they reached the endpoints or to the end of the study period. Survivorship curves were drawn to predict the distribution of time to onset of an endpoint in Ss with and without the clinical signs. Time to reach the cognitive endpoint was shorter for Ss with extrapyramidal signs or psychosis compared with those without these signs and symptoms. These clinical signs did not predict the functional endpoint. It is concluded that extrapyramidal signs and psychosis may be useful predictors of intellectual decline in Alzheimer's disease.

527. Sunderland, Trey et al. (1985). **TRH stimulation test in dementia of the Alzheimer type and elderly controls.** *Psychiatry Research,* 16(4), 269–275.
Administered the thyrotropin-releasing hormone (TRH) stimulation test, previously used as a possible biological marker of depression, to 15 patients (aged 42–77 yrs) with dementia of the Alzheimer type (DAT) and 10 healthy controls (aged 48–72 yrs). Results show that 7 of 15 of the DAT Ss but none of the controls showed a blunted response with maximal changes of thyroid-stimulating hormone from baseline of $\leq$ 7 µIU/ml following injection of 500 µg of TRH. The degree of blunting did not correlate with concurrent depression ratings. (44 ref).

528. Thase, Michael E.; Liss, L.; Smeltzer, D. & Maloon, J. (1982). **Clinical evaluation of dementia in Down's syndrome: A preliminary report.** *Journal of Mental Deficiency Research,* 26(4), 239–244.
Surveyed the clinical signs and symptoms of dementia in 40 25–64 yr old institutionalized patients with Trisomy-G Down's syndrome (DS) and 40 institutionalized controls matched for age, sex, IQ, and length of hospitalization. Findings show that DS Ss had significantly greater impairment on measures of orientation, attention span, digit-span recall, visual memory, and object identification and praxis, and they were more likely to have pathological released reflexes than controls. Neuropsychiatric status tended to worsen with advancing age in DS Ss but not in controls. 45% of DS Ss aged 45 or older had a full syndrome of dementia, compared to only 5% of controls. Results support the association of dementia Alzheimer type with DS. (28 ref).

529. Tobiasch, Victor & Chrostek, M. (1981). **Die sogenannte Präsklerose (beginnende zerebrale Insuffizienz). / The so-called presclerosis (the beginning of cerebral insufficiency).** *Zeitschrift für Gerontologie,* 14(2), 129–144.
Enumerates the symptoms of 400 patients, of which the most common were (a) disturbances of memory and concentration; (b) nervousness, inward restlessness, and increased irritability; and (c) fatigue and decreased performance. Previously, if these symptoms appeared in older persons they were considered an expression of neuronal degeneration. In middle age the same syndrome was considered a sign of premature arteriosclerosis. Recently it has been shown that these symptoms are due to a degenerative process of Alzheimer's type. In many cases it is difficult to decide which kind of changes are occurring. Cues for differential diagnosis and treatment of cases seen in general practice are presented. (93 ref).

530. Wade, John P.; Mirsen, Thomas R.; Hachinski, Vladimir C.; Fisman, Michael et al. (1987). **The clinical diagnosis of Alzheimer's disease.** *Archives of Neurology,* 44(1), 24–29.
Assessed the reliability of clinical diagnosis of dementia of the Alzheimer type (DAT) in 65 47–92 yr old patients when compared with subsequent autopsies. The neurologic history was standardized; all Ss underwent standardized psychometry, EEG, and computerized tomography scanning; and an ischemic score was obtained. The diagnosis of DAT alone was made clinically in 33 of the 38 patients with morphologically proven DAT without significant evidence of other disease, so the sensitivity of diagnosis was 87%. Findings show that DAT can be diagnosed with some confidence in elderly patients with moderate to severe disease.

531. Wagner, Ortrud; Oesterreich, Klaus & Hoyer, Siegfried. (1985). **Validity of the ischemic score in degenerative and vascular dementia and depression in old age.** International Workshop: Psychiatry in aging and dementia (1984, Montecatini-Terme, Italy). *Archives of Gerontology & Geriatrics,* 4(4), 333–345.
36 male and 45 female patients (average age 66 yrs) suffering from Alzheimer type dementia (DAT) or vascular type dementia (DVT) and from depression in old age were evaluated using physical, psychiatric, psychometric, neurological, neurophysiological, and computerized tomography (CT) scan examinations. It is concluded that the combination of Ischemic Score (V. C. Hachinski et al, 1975) and EEG was most valid in differentiating DAT from DVT. Additional cranial CT scans and the psychological testing of attention and memory confirmed the diagnosis of dementia and differentiated dementia from depression in old age. (16 ref).

532. Weiler, Philip G.; Mungas, Dan & Pomerantz, Sandy. (1988). **AIDS as a cause of dementia in the elderly.** *Journal of the American Geriatrics Society,* 36(2), 139–141.
Reports on a 63-yr-old White male patient who presented with a diagnosis of Alzheimer's disease (AD) and was later found to have the acquired immune deficiency syndrome (AIDS). It has been recognized that AIDS can present initially as dementia without other neurological or clinical manifestations. In addition, human immunodeficiency virus contaminated blood transfusions in the elderly seem to be underreported. Because of these findings, dementia in the elderly may be misdiagnosed as AD or other causes of senile dementia.

Cognitive/Neuropsychological & Behavioral Aspects

533. Albert, Marilyn S. (1984). **Assessment of cognitive function in the elderly.** *Psychosomatics,* 25(4), 310–317.
Contends that neuropsychological testing of the 5 basic areas of mental function (attention, language, memory, visuospatial ability, and conceptualization) can be used to help differentiate the effects of normal aging, delirium, depression, and dementing disorders, and in developing appropriate treatment or management plans. Types of tests are outlined that can be used to examine each of these functional areas in relative isolation from one another so that a profile of spared and impaired functions can be developed. A detailed examination of the manner in which impairments affect the individual can be used to guide patient care and to identify areas of preserved function that can be used to circumvent areas of dysfunction. The meaning of test results is discussed with particular reference to Alzheimer's disease. (17 ref).

534. Appell, Julian; Kertesz, Andrew & Fisman, Michael. (1982). **A study of language functioning in Alzheimer patients.** *Brain & Language,* 17(1), 73–91.
Reviews the literature on language functioning in Alzheimer's disease and reports the performance of 25 Alzheimer patients, all of whom were aphasic to some degree, on the Western Aphasia Battery. As a group, Ss differed from normals on all language variables and from stroke patients in terms of higher fluency and lower comprehension. Spontaneous speech showed high incidence of circumlocutions and semantic jargon but no phonemic paraphasias or target approximations. Syllabic perseverations, shouting, inappropriate laughter, and mutism were late-appearing features. Transcortical sensory and Wernicke's aphasias were frequent, but Broca's and transcortical motor aphasias were notably absent. Extent of language impairment correlated with current length of hospitalization but not age. Reading, writing, and performance scores except praxis were lower than oral language scores. Findings are discussed in relation to previous results, methodology, and language organization in the brain. (28 ref).

535. Arlien-Søborg, Peter. (1984). **Chronic toxic encephalopathy in house-painters.** *Acta Neurologica Scandinavica,* 69(Suppl 99), 105–113.
Evaluated behavioral and cognitive functioning in 70 24–63 yr old housepainters consecutively referred to a hospital neurological department for suspected chronic solvent intoxication or presenile dementia of an unknown origin. Ss' most common complaint was impaired learning and memory. Data from the administration of tests measuring immediate verbal memory span, verbal learning and memory, visual-spatial learning and memory, visual construction praxis, concept formation, and vigilance and psychomotor speed indicate that the symptoms were caused at least partly by the solvents' reduction of cerebral oxidative metabolism and blood flow. Symptoms may become permanent with continued solvent exposure. Alzheimer's disease and solvent-induced encephalopathy seem to have different etiologies. (27 ref).

536. Baddeley, Alan; Logie, R.; Bressi, S.; Sala, S. Della et al. (1986). **Dementia and working memory.** Special Issue: Human memory. *Quarterly Journal of Experimental Psychology: Human Experimental Psychology,* 38(4-A), 603–618.
Explored the hypothesis that patients suffering from dementia of the Alzheimer type (DAT) are particularly impaired in the functioning of the central executive component of working memory and that this will be reflected in the capacity of patients to perform simultaneously 2 concurrent tasks. 28 DAT patients (mean age 64.9 yrs), 28 age-matched controls (mean age 64 yrs), and 20 young controls (mean age 24.3 yrs) attempted to combine performance on a tracking task with each of 3 concurrent tasks: articulatory suppression, simple reaction time (RT) to a tone, and auditory digit span. When digit span or concurrent RT were combined with tracking, the deterioration in performance shown by the DAT Ss was particularly marked.

537. Barclay, Laurie L.; Zemcov, Alexander; Blass, John P. & Sansone, Joseph. (1985). **Survival in Alzheimer's disease and vascular dementias.** *Neurology,* 35(6), 834–840.
Followed 199 patients (mean age 73.3 yrs) with Alzheimer-type dementia (ATD), 69 (mean age 75.9 yrs) with multi-infarct dementia (MID), and 43 (mean age 76.9 yrs) with mixed dementia (MIX) over a 5-yr period. All 3 diagnostic categories had comparable progression of behavioral and cognitive impairment and need for home care or institutionalization at follow-up. 50% survival from diagnosis was 2.6 yrs for MID, 2.5 yrs for MIX, and 3.4 yrs for ATD. 50% survivals from onset were longer than previous reports suggested (8.1 yrs for ATD, 6.7 for MID, and 6.2 for MIX). (22 ref).

538. Bayles, Kathryn A. et al. (1985). **Verbal perseveration of dementia patients.** *Brain & Language,* 25(1), 102–116.
Examined patterns of perseveration and frequency of carrier phrases in the verbal descriptive discourse of 65 dementia patients controlled for etiology (i.e., mild or moderate dementia associated with senile dementia of the Alzheimer's type or Huntington's disease) and severity (e.g., normal, mildly impaired, moderately impaired, severe). Ss were asked to describe 4 common environmental objects (button, nail, envelope, and marble). Results show that dementia Ss perseverated significantly more frequently than did 30 normal controls and that severity of dementia was more strongly associated than etiology with increased perseveration. Frequency of carrier phrases did not distinguish the descriptive discourse of dementia Ss from normals. Discontinuous perseveration was more common than continuous perseveration, and perseveration of ideas after an intervening response was the perseverate most typical of dementia Ss. Findings are discussed in terms of prominent theories of the cause of perseveration. (20 ref).

539. Bayles, Kathryn A. & Tomoeda, Cheryl K. (1983). **Confrontation naming impairment in dementia.** *Brain & Language,* 19(1), 98–114.
Investigated the effects of dementia etiology and severity on the confrontation naming ability of 29 Ss with Alzheimer's, 11 Ss with Huntington's, and 13 Ss with Parkinson's diseases as well as 8 Ss with multi-infarct dementia. Ss were elderly, and 33 elderly normal Ss served as controls. Ss were asked to name a set of 20 colored pictures. Although naming impairment has been reported as a consequence of dementing illness, confrontation naming was not found to be significantly impaired in mildly involved Ss. Further, although moderate Huntington's and Parkinson's Ss made more naming errors than normals, only moderate Alzheimer's disease Ss were significantly different. Regardless of etiology, most misnamings were semantically related or semantically and visually related to the stimulus. Results challenge the theory that misnamings by dementia patients result primarily from misperception. Data support the theory that naming errors are due primarily to linguistic-cognitive impairment. (16 ref).

540. Beattie, Margot T. (1987). **Attention theory applied to the assessment of attention deficits in Alzheimer's patients.** *Dissertation Abstracts International,* 48(5-B), 1507.

541. Becker, James T.; Boller, François; Saxton, Judith & McGonigle-Gibson, Karen L. (1987). **Normal rates of forgetting of verbal and non-verbal material in Alzheimer's Disease.** *Cortex,* 23(1), 59–72.
Compared rates of forgetting in 62 patients (mean age 67.4 yrs) with Alzheimer's disease (AD) and in 64 normal elderly controls (mean age 62.7 yrs). Ss were tested for immediate and delayed recall of a short verbal passage and a modified Rey complex figure. Results suggest that although AD Ss recalled less than controls, they did not forget at a faster rate during the 30 min retention interval, supporting the finding that these memory-impaired patients do not have an abnormal rate of forgetting. Data suggest that poor initial encoding of the stimuli may have been the cause of the AD patients' impaired recall.

542. Berg, Gary; Edwards, Dorothy F.; Danzinger, Warren L. & Berg, Leonard. (1987). **Longitudinal change in three brief assessments of SDAT.** *Journal of the American Geriatrics Society,* 35(3), 205–212.
Analyzed the ability of 3 brief measures to predict the course of senile dementia of the Alzheimer's type (SDAT), using 43 patients (aged 64–81 yrs) with SDAT and 57 healthy controls (aged 64–82 yrs) studied over a 30-mo period. Measures used were the Blessed Dementia Scale, the Short Portable Mental Status Questionnaire, and the Face-Hand Test. Ss were also rated on a clinical dementia rating scale based on a lengthy clinical interview. Results indicate that (1) control scores did not change over time on any of the measures; (2) when classified according to severity of SDAT, different patterns of performance emerged over time for each measure; and (3) it was difficult to accurately predict progression of SDAT from the 3 scores.

543. Bigler, Erin D.; Hubler, Donn W.; Cullum, C. Munro & Trukheimer, Eric. (1985). **Intellectual and memory impairment in dementia: Computerized axial tomography volume correlations.** *Journal of Nervous & Mental Disease,* 173(6), 347–352.
Examined the relationship between intellectual performance on the WAIS and memory functioning on the Wechsler Memory Scale (WMS) in 42 patients (mean age 67.9 yrs) with Alzheimer's disease. Ventricular volume estimates and an index of cerebral atrophy were obtained from computerized axial tomography scans of Ss and were used to examine the correlation between morphological brain change and performance on the WAIS and the WMS. Despite ventricular volumes in excess of 60% larger than normal, no significant correlations were found between ventricular size and WAIS or WMS performance. The index of pericerebral atrophy did correlate negatively with various WAIS measures, particularly Performance IQ, and some aspects of WMS performance. Results suggest that in Alzheimer's disease, pericerebral atrophy measures, but not ventricular dilation, correlate with intellectual decline and certain aspects of memory impairment. (22 ref).

544. Blackburn, I. M. & Tyrer, G. M. (1985). **The value of Luria's Neuropsychological Investigation for the assessment of cognitive dysfunction in Alzheimer-type dementia.** *British Journal of Clinical Psychology,* 24(3), 171–179.
Assessed the cognitive functioning of 15 Alzheimer-type dementia patients (aged 54–67 yrs), 13 alcoholic Korsakoff's syndrome patients (aged 49–72 yrs), and 29 normal controls (aged 51–78 yrs) using items from a revised version of the Luria-Nebraska Neuropsychological Battery (LNNB). An attempt was made to validate the LNNB with this population for use with sophisticated physiological measures of the syndromes. Results indicate that the LNNB was a sensitive as-

sessment of the 3 neuropsychological disorders. The measure was able to distinguish differences within the Alzheimer-type dementia group and among the 3 patient groups. The validity and usefulness of the LNNB for the assessment of Alzheimer-type dementia patients are discussed. (20 ref).

545. Blanken, Gerhard; Dittmann, Jürgen; Haas, J.-Christian & Wallesch, Claus-W. (1987). **Spontaneous speech in senile dementia and aphasia: Implications for a neurolinguistic model of language production.** *Cognition,* 27(3), 247–274.
Analyzed spontaneous speech production in semistandardized interviews conducted with 10 patients suffering from moderate senile dementia of the Alzheimer type, 5 Wernicke's aphasics, and 5 elderly controls without brain damage. Both patient groups showed a reduction of sentence length and a relatively selectively diminished use of nouns. Patient groups exhibited different patterns of pathological behavior on the discourse level of responding to the interviewer's questions. Results are interpreted within a proposed neurolinguistic language production model. It is argued that the formulation process may be preserved in demented patients but is disturbed in aphasia. (French abstract).

546. Boaz, Timothy L. (1987). **Speed of scanning in primary memory in patients with dementia of the Alzheimer type.** *Dissertation Abstracts International,* 48(2-B), 558.

547. Botwinick, Jack; Storandt, Martha & Berg, Leonard. (1986). **A longitudinal, behavioral study of senile dementia of the Alzheimer type.** *Archives of Neurology,* 43(11), 1124–1127.
Compared the performance of 18 Ss (aged 64–80 yrs) with mild senile dementia of the Alzheimer type (SDAT) with that of 30 healthy Ss (aged 64–81 yrs) of similar socioeconomic status (SES) on 16 behavioral tests administered 4 times over a period of 4 yrs. Normal Ss showed little decline in performance over the 4-yr period. SDAT Ss showed progressive decline on all tests. The largest percentage declines were seen with the logical memory subtest of the Wechsler Memory Scale, the Digit Symbol subscale of the Wechsler Adult Intelligence Scale (WAIS), and the Trailmaking test (S. G. Armitage, 1946). The smallest decline was seen with the Digit Span Forward subtest of the Wechsler Memory Scale. Some SDAT Ss declined more than others over the 4-yr period.

548. Bowles, Nancy L.; Obler, Loraine K. & Albert, Martin L. (1987). **Naming errors in healthy aging and dementia of the Alzheimer type.** *Cortex,* 23(3), 519–524.
Analyzed naming errors for 39 30–39 yr old and 40 70–79 yr old Ss and 10 47–71 yr old patients diagnosed with senile dementia of the Alzheimer type (SDAT). Three types of errors were identified that varied in relatedness to the target word: near synonyms, semantically related naming errors, and unrelated naming errors. Older adults made relatively more related errors than did younger adults. SDAT patients were distinguished by the number of unrelated responses given. SDAT patients who scored within the normal range were also identified by the high number of response attempts relative to the number of initial errors. It is suggested that error patterns on naming tasks may serve as clinical markers to distinguish healthy older persons with mild naming disorders from patients with SDAT.

549. Branconnier, Roland J.; Cole, Jonathan O.; Spera, Karen F. & DeVitt, Donald R. (1982). **Recall and recognition as diagnostic indices of Malignant Memory Loss in Senile Dementia: A Bayesian analysis.** *Experimental Aging Research,* 8(3–4), 189–193.
Evaluated the discriminative validity and relative predictive values of recall and recognition as diagnostic screening tests for the malignant memory loss of senile dementia of the Alzheimer type (SDAT). 36 patients (mean age 71.13) with mild to moderate SDAT and 40 normal controls (mean age 68.85 yrs) served as Ss. It is concluded that while both recall

58

and recognition have discriminative validity under experimental conditions, a recognition test is the preferred diagnostic instrument when screening for the malignant memory loss of SDAT. (30 ref).

550. Breen, Alan R. et al. (1984). **Cognitive performance and functional competence in coexisting dementia and depression.** *Journal of the American Geriatrics Society,* 32(2), 132–137.
Examined the impact of depression on the intelligence, memory, and functional competence of 35 elderly community residents (aged 57–88 yrs) with senile dementia of the Alzheimer's type. Outpatients with either dementia (n = 21) or dementia coexisting with depression (n = 14) were given the WAIS, Wechsler Memory Scale (WMS), and Dementia Rating Scale. No significant group differences were found for the Verbal and Performance IQ subscales of the WAIS, or the WMS memory quotient. Ss with coexisting dementia and depression earned significantly lower full-scale IQ scores than Ss with only dementia. Analysis of WAIS and WMS subtest scores and profiles revealed no difference between the 2 groups. Significant associations were found among the various cognitive measures and functional competence in both groups, but the patterns of these relationships differed. Intellectual measures accounted for the greatest proportion of functional competence variance in Ss with dementia, whereas memory measures accounted for the greatest proportion of variance in the Ss with coexisting dementia and depression. The overlap between test scores and subtest profiles indicated that the WAIS and WMS were not effective for the clinical differentiation of depressed and nondepressed Alzheimer's patients. It is suggested that future research assess intellectual abilities and functional competence in examining the impact of depression or dementia. (29 ref).

551. Brinkman, Samuel D. & Braun, Paul. (1984). **Classification of dementia patients by a WAIS profile related to central cholinergic deficiencies.** *Journal of Clinical Neuropsychology,* 6(4), 393–400.
Scored WAIS protocols according to the formula reported by P. A. Fuld (1984), using 62 37–86 yr old Ss classified as having Alzheimer-type dementia (AD) or multi-infarct dementia (MID) on the basis of clinical criteria. Results show that the profile correctly classified 13 of 23 AD Ss and 37 of 39 MID Ss. Although the formula is similar to Wechsler's deterioration quotient, the latter produced a greater number of false positives. The profile was not biased by age, sex, or severity of impairments. It is suggested that the neuropsychological investigation of AD that emphasizes the deficiencies of cholinergic neurotransmission may be a fruitful avenue for further investigation. (17 ref).

552. Brinkman, Samuel D.; Largen, John W.; Gerganoff, Stefan & Pomara, Nunzio. (1983). **Russell's Revised Wechsler Memory Scale in the evaluation of dementia.** *Journal of Clinical Psychology,* 39(6), 989–993.
Administered the revised Wechsler Memory Scale (WMS-R) to 31 elderly normal Ss (mean age 69 yrs) and 25 patients (mean age 66 yrs) with suspected Alzheimer's disease matched for age and education. The patient group performed significantly less well than the control group on all WMS-R subtests. Impairments were found in both semantic and figural memory in the patient group. Results are discussed with respect to the clinical utility of the WMS-R as a memory screening procedure. (16 ref).

553. Brody, Elaine M.; Kleban, Morton H.; Moss, Miriam S. & Kleban, Ferne. (1984). **Predictors of falls among institutionalized women with Alzheimer's disease.** *Journal of the American Geriatrics Society,* 32(12), 877–882.
49 69–94 yr old women with senile dementia of the Alzheimer type were studied longitudinally and evaluated annually on 21 variables of physical, social, emotional, self-care,

and cognitive functioning. A substudy of falls that Ss experienced used data from 2 such annual evaluations. Clinical ratings by the interdisciplinary team estimated (1) the Ss' changes in function during the preceding year and (2) the current levels of the Ss' functioning. Separate regressions for each of the 2 yrs returned identical significant patterns indicating that ratings of physical vigor were significantly related to number of falls. Those Ss who had been among the most vigorous in the group but who had shown significant declines in the preceding year were the most vulnerable to falls; Ss who had been rated as the least vigorous but whose levels of vigor had been stable during the year tended to have fewer falls. There were corresponding significant declines in emotional and cognitive scales. At the 1st evaluation, declines in individual activities and high levels of depression correlated independently with falls, apart from physical vigor. At the 2nd evaluation, Ss who tended to fall the most were those who showed the least decline in their social relationships. (19 ref).

554. Brouwers, Pim et al. (1984). **Differential perceptual-spatial impairment in Huntington's and Alzheimer's dementias.** *Archives of Neurology,* 41(10), 1073–1076.
Examined the visuoperceptual and constructive abilities of patients with Alzheimer's disease (AD) or Huntington's disease (HD). 10 patients (aged 27–55 yrs) with a diagnosis of HD, 14 patients (aged 50–68 yrs) with suspected AD, and 25 age-matched normal adults served as Ss. Ss were given standardized road-map direction, complex figure, mosaic comparison, and stylus maze tests; the tasks assessed directional sense with reference to personal space, visual discrimination, and constructional skills. Performance of Ss with AD was found to be significantly impaired on tasks involving extrapersonal perception and construction but not on the test of personal space. Visuoconstructive performance by Ss with HD was not significantly impaired, while salient deficits were apparent when manipulation of personal space was required. These differential patterns of defects may have been aligned with neuropathologic changes in different cortical and subcortical structures, respectively, in Ss with AD and HD. (17 ref).

555. Bucht, Gösta & Adolfsson, R. (1983). **The Comprehensive Psychopathological Rating Scale in patients with dementia of Alzheimer type and multiinfarct dementia.** *Acta Psychiatrica Scandinavica,* 68(4), 263–270.
Interviewed 18 patients (mean age 63.6 yrs) diagnosed as having Alzheimer's disease (AD) and 20 patients (mean age 71.8 yrs) diagnosed as having multi-infarct dementia (MID), using a subscale of the Comprehensive Psychopathological Rating Scale (CPRS). This subscale consisted of items measuring psychopathological symptoms commonly seen in dementia patients. The primary purpose was to evaluate whether a difference in psychopathology between AD and MID could be observed during a semistructured psychiatric interview using the CPRS. In both groups, the duration of illness was similar and the dementia mild to moderate. All Ss were subjected to somatic, psychiatric, laboratory, neurophysiologic, and neuroradiologic examinations to obtain the correct clinical diagnoses. Results show that Ss with AD had a more variable psychopathology than Ss with MID. Ss with MID were rated lower on all items, especially those concerning verbal and personal contact. (23 ref).

556. Budzenski, Carol A. (1986). **An analysis of memory dysfunction in senile dementia of the Alzheimer's type, multi-infarct dementia, and pseudodementia.** *Dissertation Abstracts International,* 47(4-B), 1713.

557. Burch, Earl A. & Andrews, Susan R. (1987). **Comparison of two cognitive rating scales on medically ill patients.** *International Journal of Psychiatry in Medicine,* 17(2), 193–200.

Tested the applicability of the cognitive portion of W. G. Rosen and colleagues' (1984) Alzheimer's disease assessment scale (ADAS-COG) as a screening instrument on a psychiatric consultation service. The ADAS-COG compared favorably with the Mini-Mental State Examination, but it appeared to be less influenced by educational level. The advantages and disadvantages of using each of these tests on a psychiatric consultation service are discussed.

558. Buschke, Herman. (1984). **Cued recall in amnesia.** *Journal of Clinical Neuropsychology,* 6(4), 433–440.
Used a search procedure to control processing during learning with 10 53–73 yr old normal Ss and 7 36–67 yr old patients (4 Ss with Alzheimer's disease or senile dementia of the Alzheimer's type and 3 Ss with amnesia due to other etiologies). Results show apparently normal cued recall by some amnesic Ss with impaired free-recall learning. It is suggested that their ability to encode and retrieve may be relatively intact when they are induced to carry out effective processing during learning. When processing is controlled during learning, cued recall may be useful for neuropsychological evaluation of residual learning and memory capacity. (20 ref.)

559. Butters, Nelson et al. (1983). **The effect of verbal mediators on the pictorial memory of brain-damaged patients.** *Neuropsychologia,* 21(4), 307–323.
14 patients (mean age 44.9 yrs) with Huntington's disease (HD), 11 patients (mean age 53.5 yrs) with alcoholic Korsakoff's syndrome (AKS), 11 patients (mean age 64.5 yrs) with Alzheimer's disease (AD), 10 patients (mean age 53.1 yrs) with right-hemisphere lesions (RHL), and 11 "young" (mean age 44 yrs) and 11 "old" (mean age 64.4 yrs) controls were administered the Make a Picture Story Test. In this test, they attempted to associate specific human and animal figures with particular scenic backgrounds. Under 1 condition, no explicit verbal cues were provided to help Ss associate the figures with the scenes; in a 2nd condition, stories linking the figures to the background scenes were read to Ss during the study period. Although all 4 groups were impaired in picture-context recognition under the "no-story" condition, the groups differed significantly in their ability to use the stories to improve pictorial memory. HD and RHL Ss' picture recognition showed significant improvement when stories were provided; AKS and AD Ss failed to use verbal material in a productive manner. The groups also differed in their tendency to make intrusion (perseverative) errors on the picture-context recognition task. These differences may be related to the combination of language, cognitive, and motivational deficits associated with each disease. (French & German abstracts) (63 ref.)

560. Butters, Nelson; Granholm, Eric; Salmon, David P.; Grant, Igor et al. (1987). **Episodic and semantic memory: A comparison of amnesic and demented patients.** *Journal of Clinical & Experimental Neuropsychology,* 9(5), 479–497.
Episodic and semantic memory tasks were administered to 13 Alzheimer's disease (AD), 12 Huntington's disease (HD), and 9 alcoholic Korsakoff (AK) patients matched for overall severity of dementia. Mean age range of Ss and controls was 45.08–68.39 yrs. Although all patient groups were severely and equally impaired on memory for passages, only the AD and AK patients emitted numerous intrusion errors. On both fluency tasks, the HD and AK patients demonstrated severe and moderate deficits, respectively, whereas the mild AD patients were impaired only on the category fluency task. AD and AK patients made more perseverative errors than did the HD patients on letter fluency. Findings suggest that AD and HD patients' impairments on episodic and semantic memory tasks reflect different underlying processes.

561. Caltagirone, C.; Benedetti, N.; Nocentini, U. & Gainotti, G. (1985). **Demenza e pseudo-demenza depressiva: diagnosi differenziale su base neuropsicologica. / Dementia and depressive pseudo-dementia: Diagnosis on a neuropsychological basis.** *Archivio di Psicologia, Neurologia e Psichiatria,* 46(2), 216–233.
Examined the diagnostic value of a neuropsychological battery—the Mental Deterioration Battery—to differentiate the dementia syndrome from depressive pseudo-dementia with 29 Ss with depressive pseudo-dementia, 32 Ss with initial stages of Alzheimer's disease, and 53 control Ss. The average test scores for a single test varied considerably, but when placed in relation to results on overall examination, accurate diagnoses resulted in 90% of the controls. The maximum discriminating threshold for diagnosis was quantified from test results, but social, familial, and other variables should be considered in the clinical situation. It is concluded that neuropsychological methodology can minimize diagnostic risk in differentiating dementia, despite symptomatic overlap, if individual tests are placed in the context of complete battery performance. (English abstract) (36 ref.)

562. Caltagirone, C.; Masullo, C.; Benedetti, N. & Nocentini, U. (1985). **Profilo di compromissione neuropsicologica in pazienti affectti da Morbo di Parkinson. / Dementia in Parkinson's Disease: A neuropsychological study.** *Schweizer Archiv für Neurologie, Neurochirurgie und Psychiatrie,* 136(3), 7–23.
Conducted a neuropsychological study of cognitive impairment in 57 Ss with idiopathic Parkinson's disease (PD) and 32 Ss with Alzheimer's disease (AD). Two different subgroups of PD patients (those with and without dementia) were identifiable, regardless of mean age, age of onset, and duration of treatment. Type of treatment seemed to play a specific role in the appearance of dementia in PD in that anticholinergics were assumed almost exclusively by demented PD patients. Cognitive impairment was consistently more evident in AD Ss than in PD Ss with dementia; in addition, demented PD Ss showed a pattern of impairment similar to that exhibited by patients affected by frontal lobe lesions. This result supports neuroanatomical and neurochemical data on the involvement of the whole dopaminergic system in PD and the role played by the ventromedial tegmental area projecting to the frontal cortex. It is concluded that a specific pattern of cognitive impairment in PD well-differentiated from demented patients of different etiology, suggests beneficial effects on PD patients of dopaminergic agonists, which may stimulate the prefrontal region that is probably involved in the cognitive impairment of PD patients. (37 ref.)

563. Cantone, G.; Orsini, A.; Grossi, D. & de Michele, G. (1978). **Verbal and spatial memory span in dementia: An experimental study of 185 subjects.** *Acta Neurologica,* 33(2), 175–183.
90 controls were compared with 95 patients with dementia of varied etiology, including Huntington's chorea, multi-infarct dementia, simple cerebral atrophy, Alzheimer's disease, senile dementia, and Pick's disease, on verbal span (VS) measured by the Wechsler digit span and on spatial span (SS) measured by Corsini's block-tapping test. None of the controls had a VS or SS less than 4, but 35% of the patients had a VS less than 4 and 60% had an SS less than four. The VS:SS ratio was significantly poorer only in patients with Alzheimer's disease. It is concluded (a) that damage in Alzheimer's disease is less symmetrical than other forms of dementia with preference for space functions and that this may be because Alzheimer's patients are not seen until the disease is advanced and (b) that further research is necessary on the slowly developing dementias to determine if the VS:SS ratio shows similar discrepancies in the terminal phases of the disease. (12 ref.)

564. Celsis, Pierre; Agniel, Alain; Puel, Michèle; Rascol, André et al. (1987). **Focal cerebral hypoperfusion and selective cognitive deficit in dementia of the Alzheimer type.** *Journal of Neurology, Neurosurgery & Psychiatry,* 50(12), 1602–1612.
Investigated regional cerebral blood flow using single photon emission computed tomography and xenon-133 intravenous injection in 6 57–75 yr olds with dementia of the Alzheimer type (DAT) with atypical focal clinical presentation, and in 20 age-matched healthy controls. DAT Ss had a progressive and preponderant cognitive deficit and a focal hypoperfusion that correlated with neuropsychological findings; the average flow did not significantly differ from that of controls. It is suggested that the assessment of concordant hemodynamic and neuropsychological focal abnormalities could be useful in the diagnosis of atypical cases of DAT.

565. Cole, Martin G. & Dastoor, Dolly P. (1987). **A new hierarchic approach to the measurement of dementia.** *Psychosomatics,* 28(6), 298–304.
Describes a hierarchic dementia scale, a new instrument for assessing cognitive impairment. The scale is based on Piagetian concepts, neuropsychological findings, and the hierarchic nature of decline in mental function. Performance of 20 specific functions such as orienting reflexes and comprehension can be rapidly pinpointed over a wide range of impairment. Scale reliability and validity, tested in 50 demented patients, was high. Study with the scale of the course of Alzheimer's disease in 13 patients defined a variety of patterns in their mental decline.

566. Corwin, June; Serby, Michael; Conrad, Patricia & Rotrosen, John. (1985). **Olfactory recognition deficit in Alzheimer's and Parkinsonian dementias.** *IRCS Medical Science: Psychology & Psychiatry,* 13(3–4), 260.
Seven groups of patients—11 with Alzheimer's disease (AD), 5 with Parkinson's disease ([PD] 4 of whom were demented), 12 demented alcoholics, 10 nondemented alcoholics, 19 young controls, 15 middle-aged controls, and 20 elderly controls—were evaluated with the Guild Memory Test and a cognitive interview and were tested on a 2-alternative forced-choice olfactory test. Results indicate that Ss with AD and PD performed worse on the olfactory recognition task than all other groups, even when age and degree of dementia were factored out. (6 ref).

567. Coyne, Andrew C.; Liss, Leopold & Geckler, Cheri. (1984). **The relationship between cognitive status and visual information processing.** *Journal of Gerontology,* 39(6), 711–717.
Examined susceptibility to visual masking in 16 Ss (mean age 60.8 yrs) displaying evidence of Alzheimer's disease and in 21 cognitively intact Ss (mean age 64.6 yrs). Results indicate that the cognitively impaired group was more susceptible to the perceptual interference of a visual mask than was the cognitively intact group. In addition, the impaired group was particularly susceptible to masking by a visual pattern (which had similar figural characteristics to target stimuli) as compared to masking by random noise (which had figural characteristics unrelated to the target). Susceptibility to masking was found to be negatively correlated with performance on the WAIS—R Information subtest and with rated level of cognitive functioning. It is concluded that this pattern of results represents an acceleration of changes in perceptual processing typically associated with normal human aging. (14 ref).

568. Cummings, Jeffrey L. (1987). **Dementia syndromes: Neurobehavioral and neuropsychiatric features.** *Journal of Clinical Psychiatry,* 48(5, Suppl), 3–8.
Reviews the neurobehavioral and neuropsychiatric characteristics of dementia syndromes and the principles to be applied for accurate clinical diagnosis. Syndromes considered include those related to degenerative disorders such as Alzheimer's disease, stroke-related dementia, myelinoclastic disorders such as multiple sclerosis, traumatic conditions, hydrocephalus, inflammatory conditions, toxic conditions associated with substance abuse or medications, and psychiatric disorders such as depression. It is emphasized that etiologic classification depends on a combination of historical, clinical, radiologic, and EEG considerations.

569. Cummings, Jeffrey L. & Benson, D. Frank. (1986). **Dementia of the Alzheimer type: An inventory of diagnostic clinical features.** *Journal of the American Geriatrics Society,* 34(1), 12–19.
Describes the development of an inventory presenting characteristics useful in the clinical identification of dementia of the Alzheimer type (DAT). The inventory includes aphasia, amnesia, abnormal cognition and visuospatial skills, inappropriate lack of concern, and normal motor functions. In a retrospective study of 50 consecutive dementia patients, the DAT inventory correctly identified 100% of DAT Ss and 94% of non-DAT cases. It is concluded that use of positive criteria can aid in the identification of DAT and can facilitate recognition of treatable illnesses masquerading as DAT. (71 ref).

570. Cummings, Jeffrey L.; Benson, Frank; Hill, Mary A. & Read, Stephen. (1985). **Aphasia in dementia of the Alzheimer type.** *Neurology,* 35(3), 394–397.
Speech and language assessment in 30 patients (mean age 71.34 yrs) with dementia of the Alzheimer type and in 70 normal controls (mean age 42.4 yrs) who were spouses or family members of the patient revealed that all Alzheimer patients were aphasic. The language disorder resembled transcortical sensory aphasia. Increasing language impairment correlated with increasing severity of dementia. Aphasia was present regardless of the age of onset or family history of dementia. It is suggested that aphasia is an important diagnostic criterion of Alzheimer-type dementia. (22 ref).

571. Cummings, Jeffrey L.; Houlihan, John P. & Hill, Mary A. (1986). **The pattern of reading deterioration in dementia of the Alzheimer type: Observations and implications.** *Brain & Language,* 29(2), 315–323.
13 61–82 yr olds with dementia of the Alzheimer type (DAT) were tested for their ability to read aloud and to read with comprehension. Measures included the Mini-Mental State Examination, Boston Diagnostic Aphasia Examination, and Western Aphasia Battery. Reading aloud was preserved in all but the most severely impaired Ss and was relatively independent of intellectual deterioration. Reading comprehension declined progressively with increasing dementia severity and correlated well with quantitative mental status assessments. Results suggest that the pattern of reading deterioration may aid in the clinical identification of DAT, that the disturbance of reading comprehension is a linguistic deficit rather than a product of visual–perceptual disturbances, and that the alexia is more consistent with an instrumental loss than a de-developmental model of dementia. (27 ref).

572. Cummings, Jeffrey L.; Miller, Bruce; Hill, Mary A. & Neshkes, Robert. (1987). **Neuropsychiatric aspects of multi-infarct dementia and dementia of the Alzheimer type.** *Archives of Neurology,* 44(4), 389–393.
Investigated the association between certain features (i.e., delusions, depression, hallucinations) and dementia severity, as well as the interrelationship of the behavioral changes in 30 patients (aged 62–78 yrs) with dementia of the Alzheimer type (DAT) and 15 patients (aged 60–86 yrs) with multi-infarct dementia (MID). The frequency of delusion in DAT and MID differed little. Hallucinations occurred more frequently in MID than in DAT. Depression was more common in MID than in DAT.

61

573. Cushman, Laura A. & Caine, Eric D. (1987). **A controlled study of processing of semantic and syntactic information in Alzheimer's Disease.** *Archives of Clinical Neuropsychology,* 2(3), 283–292.
Investigated the ability of 13 mildly and moderately impaired Alzheimer's disease (AD) patients and 17 age- and education-matched elderly controls to process syntactic and semantic information. Ss identified and corrected sentential errors and completed a homophone-spelling task. Results indicate that AD Ss were equivalent to controls in their ability to detect various types of sentential errors. AD Ss were impaired in their ability to correct both types of errors, although performance was superior for syntactically based corrections. The homophone-spelling task did not reveal a significant differential sensitivity of AD Ss and controls to syntactic vs semantic information. Possible mechanisms underlying variations in the language-related performance of AD Ss are noted.

574. Dalton, A. J.; Crapper, D. R. & Schlotterer, G. R. (1974). **Alzheimer's disease in Down's syndrome: Visual retention deficits.** *Cortex,* 10(4), 366–377.
Attempted to document changes in memory associated with Alzheimer's disease in Down's syndrome and to develop procedures for detecting the onset of this process. 40 hospitalized adult Ss participated in a study employing delayed-matching-to-sample performance as a measure of short term visual retention. Aging patients with Down's syndrome made significantly more errors than 2 control groups of younger patients with Down's syndrome and 2 control groups of retarded patients, matched for age, without Down's anomaly. Results indicate that the early signs of Alzheimer's disease can be detected in aging patients with an underlying primary amentia of Down's syndrome. It is suggested (a) that the early course of the disease may be the same both in individuals of normal intellect who develop Alzheimer's disease and in persons with Down's syndrome, all of whom can be expected to develop the disease in later life, and (b) that the underlying brain mechanisms controlling higher functions such as memory may be similarly altered in both types of patients.

575. Dastoor, Dolly P. & Cole, Martin G. (1986). **The course of Alzheimer's disease: An uncontrolled longitudinal study.** *Journal of Clinical & Experimental Gerontology,* 7(4), 289–299.
Conducted an uncontrolled, longitudinal study over 48 mo to assess the course of dementia in 13 patients (aged 47–88 yrs) with a diagnosis of Alzheimer's disease or primary degenerative dementia. Ss were evaluated every 12 mo using a newly developed hierarchic dementia scale that rates the severity of dementia. With one exception, Ss' scores declined consistently over time, but considerable interindividual variation occurred in patterns of decline of the different subscale functions. Patterns of decline varied in both early- and late-onset groups but were more rapid in the younger group. It is suggested that it may be necessary to reconsider the common conception that Alzheimer's disease is a homogeneous condition that follows a uniform course. (13 ref).

576. Davis, Paul E. & Mumford, Susan J. (1984). **Cued recall and the nature of the memory disorder in dementia.** *British Journal of Psychiatry,* 144, 383–386.
Investigated the retrieval deficit hypothesis of forgetting in senile dementia, using a cued recall technique. Ss were 18 patients (mean age 76.9 yrs) with Alzheimer's disease and 18 age-matched, cognitively unimpaired Ss. Memory for lists of words was tested with either no cues given at the time of recall, or alternatively by cueing the S either with the word's 1st letter or its semantic category. Both types of cues significantly improved the recall of controls, whereas only the letter cue led to an improvement in recall among Ss with dementia. Results do not support a retrieval deficit explanation of forgetting in dementia but instead suggest the possibility of a processing deficit at the acquisition stage. (19 ref).

577. Degrell, István et al. (1985). **Dementias, psychological tests, and neurotransmitters.** International Workshop: Psychiatry in aging and dementia (1984, Montecatini-Terme, Italy). *Archives of Gerontology & Geriatrics,* 4(4), 365–371.
Investigated the intelligence, dementia, verbal (VQ), and performance (PQ) quotients of MAWI (Hungarian standardized version of the Wechsler Adult Intelligence Scale [WAIS]) data for 23 patients (mean age range 51.9–68.8 yrs) suffering from multi-infarct, primary degenerative, and alcoholic dementia (MID, PDD, AlcD). In a 2nd series of investigations, homovanillic acid (HVA) and 5-hydroxyindoleacetic acid (5-HIAA) were measured in lumbar cerebrospinal fluid (CSF) from 23 patients (mean age range 59.4–77.5 yrs) with presenile dementia, senile dementia of Alzheimer's type, and MID. They were compared to 16 neurotic controls (mean age 29 yrs) and to each other. Results show that AlcD could be differentiated from other types of dementia mainly by the values of VQ and PQ, the Hewson Index 5, and by objective profile analysis. MID could hardly be differentiated from PDD, but the objective profile analysis helped. No decrease was found in the concentrations of HVA and 5-HIAA in lumbar CSF of demented patients compared to controls, but there was an elevation in 5-HIAA concentration. (7 ref).

578. de Leon, Mony J.; Potegal, M. & Gurland, B. (1984). **Wandering and parietal signs in senile dementia of Alzheimer's type.** *Neuropsychobiology,* 11(3), 155–157.
21 70–92 yr old nursing home patients with senile dementia of Alzheimer's type (SDAT) were administered a mental status questionnaire and 7 tests of demonstrated usefulness in detecting parietal dysfunctions. Hospital staff were interviewed to determine the occurrence in Ss of wandering and of navigation problems. Data revealed that 5 of the Ss were wanderers, and their parietal test scores, but not their mental status scores, were significantly lower than the other Ss. It appears that wandering in SDAT patients may be associated with parietal lobe signs and that this association is not solely the consequence of a generalized intellectual breakdown. This behavioral result is consistent with the physiological evidence that in some patients SDAT may have a predilection for a more severe involvement of parietal lobe. Thus, wandering in an SDAT patient may be a readily distinguishable sign that he/she belongs to a parietal lobe-impaired subgroup. (21 ref).

579. Direnfeld, Lorne K.; Albert, Martin L.; Volicer, Ladislav; Langlais, Philip J. et al. (1984). **Parkinson's disease: The possible relationship of laterality to dementia and neurochemical findings.** *Archives of Neurology,* 41(9), 935–941.
Studied the relationship of disease laterality to neuropsychological and neurochemical features in patients with idiopathic Parkinson's disease (PD). 10 PD Ss, 10 Ss with Alzheimer's type senile dementia, and 12 normal controls underwent neuropsychological testing; and cerebrospinal fluid (CSF) levels of homovanillic acid (HVA), 3,4-dihydroxyphenylacetic acid, 3-methoxy-4-hydroxyphenylglycol, 5-hydroxyindoleacetic acid, serotonin, and acetylcholinesterase (AChE) were measured. PD Ss were classified in terms of greater disease involvement in the left (Group L) or the right side of the body (Group R). Group L Ss showed greater neuropsychological impairments than did Group R Ss, and also had significantly higher CSF levels of HVA and AChE. These findings of neuropsychological and neurochemical differences between groups L and R suggest functional or anatomic asymmetries of dopaminergic systems in the central nervous system (CNS). (83 ref).

580. Doty, Richard L.; Reyes, Patricio F. & Gregor, Thomas P. (1987). **Presence of both odor identification and detection deficits in Alzheimer's disease.** *Brain Research Bulletin,* 18(5), 597–600.

Administered the University of Pennsylvania Smell Identification Test and a forced-choice phenyl ethyl alcohol odor-detection threshold test to 25 patients diagnosed as having mild to moderately severe Alzheimer's disease. Compared to 25 age-, gender-, and race-matched normal controls, Ss evidenced consistent and marked decrements on both types of olfactory tests. Findings indicate that both odor identification and odor detection problems are present in dementia of the Alzheimer's type.

581. Doyle, Glen C.; Dunn, Susan I.; Thadani, Indra & Lenihan, Patricia. (1986). **Investigating tools to aid in restorative care for Alzheimer's patients.** *Journal of Gerontological Nursing,* 12(9), 19–24.
Describes a method of functional assessment for use with Alzheimer's patients in a skilled nursing facility. The method involved the use of P. Rameizl's (1983) CADET self-care assessment scale and L. Libow's (1981) FROMAJE. 25 patients (aged 67–91 yrs) in an Alzheimer's unit were administered both scales, and results suggest that both are useful for providing assessments of abilities and deficits in Alzheimer's patients.

582. Drevets, Wayne C. & Rubin, Eugene H. (1987). **Erotomania and senile dementia of Alzheimer type.** *British Journal of Psychiatry,* 151, 400–402.
Presents a case of erotomania in a 75-yr-old female with senile dementia of Alzheimer type (SDAT) that demonstrates the presence of an elaborately systematized delusion in SDAT.

583. El-Awar, Munir; Becker, James T.; Hammond, Katherine M.; Nebes, Robert D. et al. (1987). **Learning deficit in Parkinson's disease: Comparison with Alzheimer's disease and normal aging.** *Archives of Neurology,* 44(2), 180–184.
Examined whether the learning performance of 12 Parkinson's disease (PD) patients (mean age 67.6 yrs) differed from that of 12 controls (mean age 66.2 yrs) and 10 Alzheimer's disease (AD) patients (mean age 66.8 yrs) and explored the extent of variability of PD performance. Results indicate that performance of the PD Ss was impaired in the initial acquisition of the paired associates, but their retention of the associations over time was normal. Further analysis indicated that the PD Ss actually consisted of 2 subgroups. One did not differ from controls in its learning abilities; the other showed a learning pattern that in many respects did not differ from that of the AD Ss.

584. Emery, Olga B. (1985). **Language and aging.** *Experimental Aging Research,* 11(1), 3–60.
Investigated linguistic patterning in the aged. Linguistic patterning was used as an indicator of synthetic mental activity in 20 normal elderly adults (aged 75+ yrs), 20 elderly adults (aged 75+ yrs) with senile dementia Alzheimer's type (SDAT), and 20 normal pre-middle-aged adults (aged 30–42 yrs). Significant differences in linguistic patterning were analyzed to determine if a shift occurs between pre-middle-age and old-age and, if so, what the structural components of such a shift are. Linguistic data were gathered in the form of recorded utterances; Ss also completed measures of memory and thought. Results show significant differences between the normal elderly sample and the pre-middle-aged sample on tests of cognitive function of language, memory, and thought, with a direct relationship between performance deficits and increased age. A sequence of deficits was found in the normal elderly group, such that the syntactic forms mastered latest in development, and concomitantly the most complex, were the forms that showed the quickest and/or greatest processing deficits. The performance of the SDAT elderly was quantitatively and qualitatively inferior to that of the normal elderly. It is concluded that SDAT is a process that involves a de-differentiation and de-socialization in which there occurs a separation of thought from language. Data point to a particular patterning of linguistic deficits that cannot be accounted for by existing models of aphasia. (256 ref).

585. Emery, Olga B. (1986). **Linguistic cues in the differential diagnosis of Alzheimer's disease.** *Clinical Gerontologist,* 6(1), 59–61.
Contends that linguistic cues are among the first to appear in the progressive degeneration of higher-order cortical processes in Alzheimer's disease and that the patterning of linguistic deterioration follows an orderly predictable progression. It is argued that language deteriorates in the reverse order of language development. Linguistic cues for determination of Alzheimer's disease are discussed.

586. Emery, Olga B. & Emery, Paul E. (1983). **Language in senile dementia of the Alzheimer type.** *Psychiatric Journal of the University of Ottawa,* 8(4), 169–178.
Investigated the language patterning, as a higher order cortical activity, in 20 71–91 yr olds with senile dementia of the Alzheimer type (SDAT), 20 75–93 yr old normal Ss, and 20 normal pre-middle-aged Ss who served as a performance baseline. Ss' responses to 13 instruments and individual interviews were analyzed linguistically. Results show that in SDAT Ss, there was a direct relationship between linguistic deficits and linguistic complexity, with a concomitant inverse relation between linguistic deterioration and sequence of language development. (60 ref).

587. Erker, Gerard J. (1987). **A comparative neuropsychological study of dementia of the Alzheimer type and multi-infarct dementia.** *Dissertation Abstracts International,* 47(8-B), 3517.

588. Erkinjuntti, Timo; Laaksonen, R.; Sulkava, Raimo; Syrjäläinen, R. et al. (1986). **Neuropsychological differentiation between normal aging, Alzheimer's disease and vascular dementia.** *Acta Neurologica Scandinavica,* 74(5), 393–403.
Studied a random sample of 182 elderly (aged 50+ yrs) community residents in Finland and 211 demented patients using A. L. Christensen's (1975) neuropsychological battery based on A. R. Luria's (1970) methods. A steady but selective cognitive impairment was observed with increasing age in normal healthy Ss, with mnestic, conceptual, and arithmetic functions most sensitive to the effects of aging. Age-related changes could be clearly differentiated from the changes found in patients with mild degrees of dementia. The battery also differentiated patients with mild, moderate, and severe dementia from each other on the basis of their social competence.

589. Feher, Edward; Largen, John W.; Barr, Deborah L. & Smith, Robert C. (1984). **Relationships between cerebral atrophy imaged by CT scanning and neuropsychological test results in Alzheimer's disease.** *International Journal of Neuroscience,* 24(3–4), 315–317.
Studied the computed axial tomography (CAT) scans of 35 patients (mean age 66.4 yrs) with Alzheimer's disease (AD) and 17 normal controls (mean age 64.1 yrs). Several measures of atrophy were taken, and the Ss were administered a neuropsychological test battery. The 2 groups differed significantly on all atrophy measures. However, few of the correlations between atrophy measures and neuropsychological test results were significant, arguing against simple brain–behavior relationships between CAT scan atrophy and neurobehavioral consequences of AD. (6 ref).

590. Field, Robert I. (1987). **Neuropsychological deficits in solvent encephalopathy and Alzheimer's Disease.** *Dissertation Abstracts International,* 48(4-B), 1150–1151.

591. Fillenbaum, Gerda G.; Heyman, Albert; Wilkinson, William E. & Haynes, Carol S. (1987). **Comparison of two sceening tests in Alzheimer's disease: The correlation and reliability of the Mini-Mental State Examination and the Modified Blessed Test.** *Archives of Neurology,* 44(9), 924–927.
Assessed the reliability and correlation of the Mini-Mental State Examination (MMSE) and the Blessed Orientation-Memory-Concentration Test (BOMC), using 36 Alzheimer's patients (mean age 65 yrs). 24 Ss judged to have less severe cognitive impairments were reassessed after 1 mo. Findings indicate that among Ss with disease onset before age 70 yrs, MMSE and BOMC scores are highly correlated and reliable. Factor analysis indicated that both tests measure conceptually comparable aspects of cognitive functioning (e.g., educational components, recent memory). It is suggested that the BOMC is preferable to the MMSE because of administrative advantages.

592. Filley, Christopher M. & Heaton, Robert K. (1987). **"Neuropsychological features of early and late-onset Alzheimer's disease": In reply.** *Archives of Neurology,* 44(8), 797–798.
Replies to comments by E. Koss and R. P. Friedland (1987) on an article by the present authors (1986), in which patients with onset of Alzheimer's disease before age 65 yrs were found to have more language impairment than patients with later onset.

593. Filley, Christopher M.; Kelley, John & Heaton, Robert K. (1986). **Neuropsychologic features of early- and late-onset Alzheimer's disease.** *Archives of Neurology,* 43(6), 574–576.
Studied neuropsychologic measures of brain function in 15 men and 8 women with early-onset and 9 men and 9 women with late-onset Alzheimer's disease. The performance of the 2 groups was compared on measures of overall function and left and right hemisphere function. Memory impairment, language ability, and spatial relations were assessed. By gross measures of IQ it appeared that left hemisphere function was more affected in younger Ss. Memory impairment was severe in both groups. Language was more severely impaired in the early-onset group. Spatial relations testing revealed a significantly higher error rate for the late-onset group, suggesting selective right hemisphere involvement in these Ss. It appears that left hemisphere vulnerability exists for younger Ss with Alzheimer's disease. Results do not clarify the question of whether early-onset and late-onset Alzheimer's disease are 2 distinct disorders.

594. Filley, Christopher M.; Kobayashi, Joyce & Heaton, Robert K. (1987). **Wechsler intelligence scale profiles, the cholinergic system, and Alzheimer's disease.** *Journal of Clinical & Experimental Neuropsychology,* 9(2), 180–186.
Evaluated 41 patients (mean age 65.68 yrs) with putative Alzheimer's disease (AD) to determine the diagnostic utility of a profile of Wechsler Adult Intelligence Scale (WAIS) subtests that has been proposed by P. A. Fuld (1984) to identify cholinergic dysfunction. Specificity of the formula was evaluated using Wechsler results of 42 older normals (mean age 63.95 yrs) and 30 patients (mean age 58.33 yrs) who were being evaluated for dementia but who did not have AD. One of the 42 normals and 5 of the patient controls showed a positive Wechsler profile. Data indicate that because of the Fuld formula's low sensitivity, a negative Wechsler profile cannot be used to help rule out AD. Although specificity of the formula is high, the diagnostic value of a positive Wechsler profile is modest even under the most favorable AD base rate conditions.

595. Flicker, Charles; Ferris, Steven H.; Crook, Thomas; Bartus, Raymond T. et al. (1986). **Cognitive decline in advanced age: Future directions for the psychometric differentiation of normal and pathological age changes in cognitive function.** *Developmental Neuropsychology,* 2(4), 309–322.

Reviews the research on cognitive losses associated with normal aging and with the early stages of senile dementia of the Alzheimer type in order to identify the changes in cognitive function that are age-dependent, dementia-dependent, neither, or both. A table is presented comparing clinical status with relative decline in sensorimotor processing, recent memory, concept formation, visuospatial praxis, attention, immediate memory, syntax and phonology, naming, remote memory, visual acuity, and visuoperceptual abilities. The authors conclude that more peripherally mediated skills are sensitive to aging, whereas the more central, long-established cognitive structures are sensitive to dementia.

596. Flicker, Charles; Ferris, Steven H.; Crook, Thomas & Bartus, Raymond T. (1987). **A visual recognition memory test for the assessment of cognitive function in aging and dementia.** *Experimental Aging Research,* 13(3), 127–132.
17 18–30 yr old nondemented Ss, 23 nondemented elderly adults, and 51 elderly patients with senile dementia of the Alzheimer type (SDAT) were administered a computerized visual recognition memory (VRM) task, which elicited significant differences in performance between the 3 groups of Ss. In a discriminant analysis, the VRM test scores correctly classified 72.6% of the aged and early SDAT Ss. Thus, the task appears to be useful for the assessment of treatment effects on age-related cognitive dysfunction.

597. Flicker, Charles; Ferris, Steven H.; Crook, Thomas; Reisberg, Barry et al. (1988). **Equivalent spatial-rotation deficits in normal aging and Alzheimer's disease.** *Journal of Clinical & Experimental Neuropsychology,* 10(4), 387–399.
Two tests of spatial-rotation ability were administered to 17 young normals (aged 18–30 yrs), 23 aged normals (aged 62–83 yrs), and 51 patients (aged 56–86 yrs) with diagnoses of Alzheimer's disease (28 with early dementia and 23 with advanced dementia). A computerized version of the Boston Naming Test assessed the Ss' capacity for mental rotation. On the Standardized Road-Map Test, spatial-rotation ability was assessed. Performance on both tasks was progressively worse in the young normal, aged normal, early dementia, and advanced dementia groups. Both tasks demonstrated a clear spatial-rotation deficit in the elderly. Although the spatial-rotation effect was superimposed on deficits in naming and left-right orientation in the demented Ss, the magnitude of the rotation effect did not significantly differ in the aged normal vs the early dementia group on either task.

598. Flicker, Charles; Ferris, Steven H.; Crook, Thomas & Bartus, Raymond T. (1986). **The effects of aging and dementia on concept formation as measured on an object-sorting task.** *Developmental Neuropsychology,* 2(1), 65–72.
Investigated abstract problem-solving abilities in elderly normals and in patients with senile dementia of the Alzheimer type (SDAT). A pair of tasks was administered to 17 young normals (ages 18–30 yrs), 22 aged normals (ages 62–83 yrs), and 51 patients (ages 56–86 yrs) with SDAT. 25 household items were simultaneously displayed on a video monitor screen. Ss were required to select a subgroup of 8 of the 25 items. Aged normals were unimpaired on this task, whereas early dementia Ss were modestly impaired, and advanced dementia Ss were markedly impaired. On the concept-formation task, the selection principle defining the subgroup of 8 items was deduced by the S. All groups performed significantly more poorly on the concept-formation than on the control task. The increase in errors was greatest in early dementia patients, less in aged normals, and least in young normals and advanced dementia patients. The performance of the severely demented Ss on the concept-formation task approached floor levels.

599. Flicker, Charles; Ferris, Steven H.; Crook, Thomas & Bartus, Raymond T. (1987). **Implications of memory and language dysfunction in the naming deficit of senile dementia.** *Brain & Language,* 31(2), 187–200.
In 2 experiments, 23 18–30 yr old normals, 51 62–83 yr old normals, and 90 56–86 yr olds with either mild-to-moderate or severe senile dementia of the Alzheimer type (SDAT) were administered tests of language function and remote memory. On all tests, elderly normals exhibited a mild, nonsignificant performance decrement relative to the young normals. Advanced SDAT Ss were markedly impaired on all of the tests. Early dementia Ss were most impaired, relative to aged normals, on tests of object naming, category instance fluency, and remote memory. Results are consistent with the notion that the language dysfunction in eary SDAT is due to a deficit in semantic memory function in which general, categorical information remains available whereas information about specific attributes becomes less accessible.

600. Folstein, Marshal F. & Whitehouse, Peter J. (1983). **Cognitive impairment of Alzheimer Disease.** *Neurobehavioral Toxicology & Teratology,* 5(6), 631–634.
Proposes that the clinical signs of Alzheimer's disease can be quantified and correlated with neuropathological evidence of the disease. These clinical signs, which include amnesia, aphasia, and apraxia, can be screened by using instruments such as the Mini-Mental State Examination. Each of these cognitive functions can be quantified using specific tests. However, further research is needed to develop normative data for more detailed psychological assessment tests of specific cognitive deficits. (44 ref).

601. Freedman, Morris & Oscar-Berman, Marlene. (1986). **Selective delayed response deficits in Parkinson's and Alzheimer's disease.** *Archives of Neurology,* 43(9), 886–890.
Performance on tests of delayed alternation (DA) and delayed response (DR) for 15 Ss (mean age 72.3 yrs) with idiopathic Parkinson's disease (PD) and dementia was compared with that of 14 Ss (mean age 68 yrs) with Alzheimer's disease (AD), 22 normal controls (mean age 64.7 yrs), and 13 Ss (mean age 62.3 yrs) with PD without dementia. In AD Ss, DA and DR were both significantly impaired, whereas in PD Ss with dementia significant deficits occurred only on DR. It is suggested that the pattern of deficits on these tasks can provide clues about the anatomic and neurobehavioral mechanisms of the cognitive dysfunction in PD and AD.

602. Freedman, Morris & Oscar-Berman, Marlene. (1987). **Tactile discrimination learning deficits in Alzheimer's and Parkinson's diseases.** *Archives of Neurology,* 44(4), 394–398.
Administered tactile learning tasks to 11 patients with Alzheimer's disease (AD [mean age 68.2 yrs]), 13 patients with idiopathic Parkinson's disease (PD [mean age 72.4 yrs]), 13 patients with PD without dementia (mean age 62.3 yrs), and 22 normal controls (mean age 64.7 yrs). The tasks consisted of a tactile original learning (TOL) and a tactile reversal learning (TRL) component. TOL was severely impaired in AD Ss compared to demented PD Ss. AD and demented PD Ss were significantly impaired on TRL.

603. Fulbright, Richard L. (1986). **Neuropsychological correlates of Alzheimer's disease.** *Dissertation Abstracts International,* 46(8-B), 2805.

604. Fuld, Paula A. (1984). **Test profile of cholinergic dysfunction and of Alzheimer-type dementia.** *Journal of Clinical Neuropsychology,* 6(4), 380–392.
Studied the effect of cholinergic deficiency on intellectual changes found in dementia Alzheimer-type (DAT) in 3 studies using 19 19–25 yr old normal Ss to whom scopolamine (1 mg, sc), an anticholinergic, had been administered 1 hr before testing with the WAIS and 77 36–83 yr old Ss referred for neurological examination (and WAIS administration) for de-

mentia. Results show that 10 normal Ss showed that the expected profile was associated with cholinergic neurotransmitter dysfunction: A ([Information + Vocabulary] ÷ 2) > B ([Similarities + Digit Span] ÷ 2) > C ([Digit Symbol + Block Design] ÷ 2) ≤ D (Object Assembly), A > D. The same subtest profile was found in 44% of Ss with DAT and was 96% specific to this disorder. It is suggested that the association of this profile with drug-induced cholinergic deficiency indicates that cholinergic deficiency of DAT might be responsible for intellectual changes seen in the disease. (35 ref).

605. Gandolfo, Carlo; Vecchia, R.; Moretti, C.; Brusa, G. et al. (1986). **WAIS testing in degenerative and multi-infarct dementia.** *Acta Neurologica,* 8(1), 45–50.
Performed a psychometric study using the Wechsler Adult Intelligence Scale (WAIS) on 65 patients (mean age 65.6 yrs) with senile dementia of the Alzheimer type (SDAT) and 21 patients (mean age 61.8 yrs) with multi-infarct dementia (MID). The WAIS did not differentiate between SDAT and MID but proved to be sufficiently sensitive for evaluating the degree of dementia in SDAT Ss. (Italian abstract) (20 ref).

606. Gewirth, Letitia R.; Shindler, Andrea G. & Hier, Daniel B. (1984). **Altered patterns of word associations in dementia and aphasia.** *Brain & Language,* 21(2), 307–317.
Studied the word associations of 38 demented, 17 aphasic, and 22 normal Ss; each group's mean age was 45.3+ yrs. Responses from a word association test indicate that both normal and brain-injured Ss made judgments about the grammatical class of the word stimulus. Certain stimulus words elicited paradigmatic responses, whereas other words elicited syntagmatic responses. The mechanism producing syntagmatic responses seemed relatively resistant to deterioration in dementia or aphasia. However, in dementia the mechanism that generated paradigmatic responses became progressively less efficient (possibly due to a loss of semantic markers) so that more random responses emerged. Anomic aphasics showed a pattern of word associations similar to that of Ss with mild dementia. Broca's aphasics retained enough self-monitoring mechanisms so that few idiosyncratic and perseverative responses were made while more null responses occurred. Wernicke's aphasics showed a marked shift away from a paradigmatic word association strategy, possibly due to an inability to access semantic markers or a true loss of these markers. (26 ref).

607. Gorissen, J.-P. (1986). **Een differentiële beschrijving van de SDAT-patiënt met twee gedragsobservatieschalen: de BOP en de GOS-G. / A differential description of the SDAT-patient with the BOP and the GOS-S.** *Tijdschrift voor Gerontologie en Geriatrie,* 17(1), 17–24.
Studied the ability of the Dutch version of the Stockton Geriatric Rating Scale (BOP) and an adaptation of the Dutch version (GOS-S) to differentiate between Alzheimer-type senile dementia (ATSD) and other psychoorganic symptoms in elderly patients. Ss were 15 55–88 yr olds with ATSD and 16 48–85 yr olds with multi-infarct dementia, Korsakoff dementia, epilepsy and dementia, organic psychosyndrome, frontal syndrome, schizophrenia, or posttraumatic stress disorder. Total, subscale, and item scores were compared. (English abstract).

608. Gottlieb, Gary L.; Gur, Raquel E. & Gur, Ruben C. (1988). **Reliability of psychiatric scales in patients with dementia of the Alzheimer type.** *American Journal of Psychiatry,* 145(7), 857–860.
For 43 patients (aged 55–88 yrs) with probable Alzheimer's disease who were screened for psychiatric disorders, the interrater reliability of the Global Deterioration Scale, Brief Psychiatric Rating Scale, and Hamilton Rating Scale for Depression was high (intraclass correlation, 0.82–0.998). As expected, the prevalence of psychiatric symptoms in this sample was low. The score on the Self-Rating Depression Scale correlated

with the score on the rater-administered Hamilton Depression scale in Ss whose Alzheimer's disease was of low severity ($n = 24$) but not high severity ($n = 19$).

609. Grady, Cheryl L.; Haxby, James V.; Horwitz, B.; Berg, G. et al. (1987). **Neuropsychological and cerebral metabolic function in early vs late onset dementia of the Alzheimer type.** *Neuropsychologia,* 25(5), 807–816.
Examined cerebral metabolism and cognitive performance in 34 early and late onset dementia of the Alzheimer type (DAT) patients (aged 45–81 yrs) who had equivalent duration and severity of illness. Regional cerebral metabolic rates for glucose were measured in the resting state by positron emission tomography using [18F]2-fluoro-2-deoxy-dextro glucose. A cross-sectional analysis showed no significant differences between the 2 groups in performance on neuropsychological tests, but the early onset Ss showed significantly more parietal metabolic dysfunction. Analysis showed no significant differences between early and late onset Ss in rate of cognitive decline. Results do not support the hypothesis of different subgroups in DAT based on age at onset or suggest a faster rate of cognitive decline in younger patients.

610. Grimes, Alison M. et al. (1985). **Central auditory function in Alzheimer's disease.** *Neurology,* 35(3), 352–358.
Studied the relationship between cerebral atrophy, brain glucose metabolism, and auditory dysfunction, using computerized and positron emission tomography scan data. 38 43–76 yr old patients with Alzheimer's disease (AD) and 25 50–74 yr old normal adults were tested. Results show that the central auditory (dichotic) function of Ss with AD was significantly impaired when compared with the control group. Significant relationships were observed between dichotic scores and IQ, cortical atrophy in the temporal lobes, and cerebral glucose metabolism in the left temporal lobe. Comparing atrophy and glucose metabolism in the temporal lobes, contralateral ear effects in dichotic performance and an interaction of asymmetry of atrophy with dichotic performance were observed that were consistent with previous models of dichotic listening in other forms of temporal lobe pathology. (36 ref).

611. Grossi, D.; Orsini, A. & Ridente, G. (1977). **Preliminary remarks about a neuropsychological study of organic dementia.** *Acta Neurologica,* 32(5), 682–696.
28 patients, 35–65 yrs old, with organic dementia were examined, mainly comparing 15 patients having Huntington's chorea (HC) with 7 having Alzheimer's or Pick's disease (AP) on (a) copying geometric designs, (b) copying crosses, (c) WAIS digit span, and (d) spatial memory span according to Corsi's block tapping test. The AP group performed much worse on copying designs and crosses than the HC group; the HC group improved cross reproduction on a 2nd trial, but the AP group did not. Spatial memory span relative to verbal memory or digit span was maintained in HC but deteriorated in AP. For the HC group, errors were mostly inversion or elision of blocks tapped, whereas simplification (maintenance of the geometric design formed by the taps but disregard for the sequence of taps) occurred in the AP group. The following hypotheses are offered to explain the data: (a) Spatial memory disturbances in syndromes of dementia are tied to temporal factors of memory. (b) Deterioration of cortical functions in HC is slow and symmetrical for all functions. (c) Deterioration in AP selectively affects spatial perception independent of the localization of the atrophic process. (English summary) (9 ref).

612. Grossi, D. & Orsini, A. (1978). **The Visual Crosses Test in dementia: An experimental study of 110 subjects.** *Acta Neurologica,* 33(2), 170–174.
35 controls were compared with 75 patients with dementia of varied etiology on the Visual Crosses Test, which requires the reproduction of the spatial arrangement of 8 crosses. Results show that (a) the dementia groups, composed of Huntington's chorea, multi-infarct dementia, simple cerebral atrophy, Alzheimer's disease, senile dementia, and Pick's disease, had significantly fewer correct reproductions than the controls, and (b) the Alzheimer patients did not have any correct reproductions and were not able to improve their spatial reproduction on a 2nd trial. It is concluded that disorders of spatial arrangement are not specific to Alzheimer's disease, but that because of the rapid development of the disease patients do not come under observation until the spatial disorder is advanced. (Italian summary) (2 ref).

613. Hagberg, Bo. (1983). **Cognitive impairment and test taking attitudes in organic dementia: A comparison between diffuse pre- and postcentral lesions.** *Psychological Research Bulletin, Lund U.,* 23(2), 10 p.
Studied 12 patients (mean age 58 yrs) with Alzheimer's disease or diffuse cortical atrophy (fronto-temporal accentuation) once each year for 1–6 yrs using psychometric and psychiatric methods. All Ss had homogeneous-type lesions and a degree of cognitive impairment. Six of the Ss had mainly diffuse precentral lesions, and the other 6 had mainly diffuse postcentral lesions. Results show that in the precentrals, there was an inverted verbal/performance discrepancy, and significantly more frequent signs of behavior deviations were found in the test situation than found with the postcentrals. It is argued that potentially intact intellectual functions are disturbed not primarily due to cognitive reduction per se, but rather because of general behavior disintegration. (26 ref).

614. Harris, S. J. & Dowson, J. H. (1982). **Recall of a 10-word list in the assessment of dementia in the elderly.** *British Journal of Psychiatry,* 141, 524–527.
49 residents of homes for the elderly with a history of impaired memory compatible with senile Alzheimer dementia were assessed by a paired-associate learning test (PALT) and a 10-word-list recall test. The latter discriminated between groups categorized according to severity of cognitive impairment by the PALT. The word recall test may be suitable for the assessment of memory and for the evaluation of change in clinical trials of treatments for dementia. (9 ref).

615. Harrold, Rose M. (1987). **Object naming in Alzheimer's Disease: What is the cognitive deficit?** *Dissertation Abstracts International,* 48(1-B), 290.

616. Hart, Robert P.; Kwentus, Joseph A.; Hamer, Robert M. & Taylor, John R. (1987). **Selective reminding procedure in depression and dementia.** *Psychology & Aging,* 2(2), 111–115.
Patients with mild dementia of the Alzheimer's type (DAT), patients with major depression, and normal elderly control Ss were administered a verbal learning task using the selective reminding procedure. Depressed patients were impaired on total recall and the proportion of items retained from one trial to the next without reminding and did not benefit from imagery in retaining items over consecutive trials. The DAT patients were impaired on all measures derived from the test, including storage and recognition memory. With the exception of the ability to benefit from imagery, all of the measures distinguished depressed and mild DAT patients. These findings are consistent with deficient encoding in DAT and performance deficits as a function of effortful cognitive processing in depression.

617. Hart, Robert P.; Kwentus, Joseph A.; Wade, James B. & Hamer, Robert M. (1987). **Digit symbol performance in mild dementia and depression.** *Journal of Consulting & Clinical Psychology,* 55(2), 236–238.
Patients with mild dementia of the Alzheimer's type (DAT), patients with major depression, and normal control Ss completed the Wechsler Adult Intelligence Scale (WAIS) Digit Symbol test and a measure of incidental memory for the digit-symbol pairs. Mild DAT and depressed patients had equiv-

alent deficits in psychomotor speed, but DAT patients recalled fewer digit-symbol items. Although the standard administration of the Digit Symbol test has limited utility in differential diagnosis, the addition of a brief measure of incidental memory may be clinically useful as part of the battery of neuropsychological tests used to distinguish early dementia from depression.

618. Hart, Robert P.; Kwentus, Joseph A.; Taylor, John R. & Harkins, Stephen W. (1987). **Rate of forgetting in dementia and depression.** *Journal of Consulting & Clinical Psychology,* 55(1), 101–105.
Patients with mild dementia of the Alzheimer's type (DAT), patients with major depression, and normal control subjects were examined for rate of forgetting line drawings of common objects after the groups had been equated for acquisition by the variation of stimulus exposure time. Depressed and DAT patients demonstrated learning impairments, but only the DAT group showed rapid forgetting in the first 10 min after learning to criterion. This finding suggests that some form of deficient consolidation contributes to memory loss in DAT but not in depression and implicates the disruption of different psychobiological mechanisms in these disorders. The rate of forgetting paradigm may be clinically useful for distinguishing patients with early DAT from elderly depressed patients with memory deficits. (53 ref).

619. Hart, S. A.; Smith, C. M. & Swash, M. (1985). **Recognition memory in Alzheimer's disease.** *Neurobiology of Aging,* 6(4), 287–292.
Two experiments examined recognition memory for several types of stimulus material in 15 Alzheimer's disease patients (mean age 68 yrs) and in 12 normal elderly controls (mean age 72 yrs). Although performance deficits were demonstrated for verbal and abstract stimuli (geometric shapes and histology slides), memory for faces was relatively intact in the patient group. Patients made more false positive responses than controls, but this could not be accounted for by a general disinhibition of responding. The possibility that a contextual processing deficit may explain the pattern of false positive responding is discussed in relation to previous findings of drug studies in Alzheimer's disease. (33 ref).

620. Hart, Siobhan; Smith, Christine M. & Swash, Michael. (1986). **Intrusion errors in Alzheimer's disease.** *British Journal of Clinical Psychology,* 25(2), 149–150.
Used the Object Learning test of the Kendrick Battery for the Detection of Dementia in the Elderly to study the incidence of intrusion errors in 20 patients (mean age 66.3 yrs) with Alzheimer's disease (AD) and 15 controls (mean age 69.5 yrs) without neurological or psychiatric disability. Although such errors constituted a higher proportion of the responses made by patients than by controls, suggestions that patients with AD show a propensity for prior-list intrusion errors were not supported. (12 ref).

621. Hart, Siobhan; Smith, Christine M. & Swash, Michael. (1988). **Word fluency in patients with early dementia of Alzheimer type.** *British Journal of Clinical Psychology,* 27(2), 115–124.
Assessed the relative fluency with which 15 older adults with Alzheimer-type dementia (DAT) retrieved words with specified 1st letters and belonging to semantically defined categories. Ss with DAT were always less fluent than controls, but, like the 12 normal elderly Ss, patients were more efficient in accessing words belonging to semantic categories. Deficits in retrieving words with specified 1st letters were greater than those predicted on the basis of verbal intellectual ability. No differences in word fluency were detected in presenile and senile patients. Data support the conclusion that word fluency may prove useful in the detection of early dementia.

622. Hart, Siobhan; Smith, Christine M. & Swash, Michael. (1986). **Assessing intellectual deterioration.** *British Journal of Clinical Psychology,* 25(2), 119–124.
20 patients (mean age 66.3 yrs) with Alzheimer-type dementia were assessed on the Wechsler Adult Intelligence Scale (WAIS), the Schonell Graded Word Reading Test, and the National Adult Reading Test (NART). 15 normal control Ss (mean age 69.5 yrs) were administered the WAIS and the NART. The regression equations of H. E. Nelson and P. McKenna (1975) and the tables of Nelson (1982) were used to estimate premorbid Full Scale IQ on the basis of WAIS Vocabulary subtest score and performance on each of the reading tests. The data were analyzed to assess the relative utility of these methods and of WAIS Verbal–Performance IQ discrepancy in the assessment of intellectual deterioration. Findings suggest that performance on the NART was the best indicator of premorbid level of functioning in terms of the size of predicted–obtained discrepancies. (19 ref).

623. Hartman, Marilyn D. (1988). **A cognitive-neuropsychological study of semantic representation in Dementia of the Alzheimer Type.** *Dissertation Abstracts International,* 48(9-B), 2781–2782.

624. Haxby, James V. & Rapoport, Stanley I. (1985). **Asymmetry of brain metabolism and cognitive function.** *Geriatric Nursing,* 6(4), 200–203.
Studied the functional significance of regional cerebral metabolism in Alzheimer's disease (AD) in 10 right-handed AD patients (mean age 64.4 yrs) and in 10 control Ss (mean age 62.4 yrs). The following neuropsychological tests were administered: the Mattis Dementia Scale, the Wechsler Adult Intelligence Scale (WAIS), and 2 delayed memory tests from the Wechsler Memory Scale. Ss also took a test of comprehension of syntactic relations in single, orally presented sentences, and a test of the ability to copy geometric figures of varying complexity. In AD Ss, the indices of neuropsychological asymmetry were correlated significantly with metabolic asymmetry in the cerebral hemispheres and in the frontal and parietal lobe cortices. Asymmetry of syntax comprehension and drawing also correlated with occipital metabolic asymmetry. Lower left hemisphere regional metabolism of glucose was associated with worse language function, and vice versa. It is concluded that because no relation between metabolic rate and neuropsychological deficits was obtained in control Ss, the relation in early AD clearly is caused by the underlying developing disease process. (38 ref).

625. Hewitt, K. E.; Carter, G. & Jancar, J. (1985). **Ageing in Down's syndrome.** *British Journal of Psychiatry,* 147, 58–62.
Hypothesized that Down's syndrome patients nearing the end of their lifespan would show gross cognitive and behavioral deterioration characteristic of dementia of Alzheimer's type in the normal population. 23 50–61 yr old hospitalized patients with Down's syndrome were administered the Stanford-Binet Intelligence Scale and were engaged in a structured interview. Findings show that psychological testing indicated that significant intellectual deterioration, which was unrelated to chronological age, sex, length of hospitalization, or earlier mental age, had occurred in 9 Ss. Clinically, there was no evidence in any S of active physical illness, focal neurological signs, or dementia, but significant associations were found between intellectual deterioration and decreased visual acuity, hearing loss, and macrocytosis. (23 ref).

626. Hier, Daniel B.; Hagenlocker, Karen & Shindler, Andrea G. (1985). **Language disintegration in dementia: Effects of etiology and severity.** *Brain & Language,* 25(1), 117–133.
Compared the speech characteristics on a standardized picture description task of 26 Ss (mean age 73.6 yrs) with presumed senile dementia of the Alzheimer type (SDAT) and

13 Ss (mean age 64.4 yrs) with stroke-related dementia (SRD) to those of 15 normal Ss (aged 60+ yrs). Data show that, compared to normal Ss, dementia Ss used fewer total words, fewer unique words, fewer prepositional phrases, fewer subordinate clauses, and more incomplete sentence fragments. Lexical deficits were more severe than syntactic ones, indicating that lexicon is more vulnerable to disruption in dementia than syntax. Greater dementia severity among SDAT Ss was associated with marked difficulties in accessing the mental lexicon. Greater dementia severity in SRD Ss was associated with laconic speech that was syntactically less complex. The speech characteristics of mild SDAT Ss showed similarities to those of anomic or semantic aphasia, whereas the speech of the more advanced SDAT Ss showed similarities to Wernicke's or transcortical sensory aphasia. The speech of Ss with more severe SRD showed some similarities to Broca's aphasia. The most important nonlinguistic deficit in both dementia groups was a failure to make relevant observations during the picture description task. Perseverations were present in the speech of both groups, whereas aposiopesis, logorrhea, and palilalia were more typical of the SDAT Ss and laconic speech more characteristic of the SRD Ss. (31 ref).

627. Houlihan, John P.; Abrahams, Joel P.; LaRue, Asenath A. & Jarvik, Lissy F. (1985). **Qualitative differences in vocabulary performance of Alzheimer versus depressed patients.** *Developmental Neuropsychology,* 1(2), 139–144.
Compared qualitative differences in the language abilities of 7 Alzheimer's disease, 7 depressed, and 7 normal elderly Ss (mean age 74 yrs). A previously developed qualitative scoring system for the Wechsler Adult Intelligence Scale (WAIS) Vocabulary subtest was used. Alzheimer Ss were found to give poor explanations as definitions more frequently than did the depressed and normal Ss who did not differ from one another. Also, the Alzheimer Ss tended to give superior synonyms as definitions less frequently than did the other 2 groups. Findings are consistent with a clinical descriptive model of Alzheimer's disease, which includes language deficits as part of the disorder. It is suggested that this language pattern has clinical application to the detection of early language changes in Alzheimer's disease.

628. Huber, Steven J.; Shuttleworth, Edwin C.; Paulsen, George W.; Bellchambers, Maree J. et al. (1986). **Cortical vs subcortical dementia: Neuropsychological differences.** *Archives of Neurology,* 43(4), 392–394.
Examined the possible distinction between cortical and subcortical dementia by using a neuropsychological test battery specifically designed to evaluate proposed differences among 14 Ss (mean age 65.3 yrs) with dementia of the Alzheimer type (DAT), 38 Ss (mean age 64.9 yrs) with idiopathic Parkinson's disease, and 20 normal controls (mean age 61.7 yrs). The test battery included quantitative measures of overall mental function, memory, language, apraxia, attention, and visuospatial skills, and a scale for depression. Results suggest that there are qualitative and quantitative differences in the dementia syndromes, consistent with the cortical-subcortical hypothesis.

629. Huff, F. Jacob; Becker, J. T.; Belle, S. H.; Nebes, R. D. et al. (1987). **Cognitive deficits and clinical diagnosis of Alzheimer's disease.** *Neurology,* 37(7), 1119–1124.
Used cognitive deficits detected by neuropsychological testing (NT) to evaluate clinical diagnosis of Alzheimer's disease (AD). There were 79 AD Ss (mean age 67.4 yrs) and 86 controls (mean age 62.6 yrs). Deficits were defined with respect to performance of controls according to procedural guidelines set by a NINCDS-ADRDA Work Group that was under the auspices of the US Department of Health and Human Services. The most frequent deficits were in recent memory and lexical-semantic language abilities. Clinical diagnosis of AD was compared with diagnosis based on a criterion of 2 or more cognitive deficits both on initial NT

and on testing repeated a year later in some Ss. Initial clinical diagnosis identified 96% of cases who met the criterion when first tested and 100% of those with multiple deficits at follow-up. Specificity with respect to the criterion was 86% on initial testing and 89% at follow-up. Findings support the validity of clinical diagnosis of AD using the NINCDS-ADRDA criteria.

630. Huff, F. Jacob; Corkin, Suzanne & Growdon, John H. (1986). **Semantic impairment and anomia in Alzheimer's disease.** *Brain & Language,* 28(2), 235–249.
Investigated impairment in naming visually presented objects in 2 experiments, using a total of 23 patients (mean age 65.3 yrs) with Alzheimer's disease (AD) and 18 healthy controls (mean age 62 yrs). Impaired object naming correlated with difficulty in listing the names of objects from a specified semantic category and with erroneous selection of words semantically related to the correct names for objects in a name recognition test. Results suggest that patients with AD had a semantic impairment characterized by inability to distinguish among objects that are members of the same semantic category and that this impairment was associated with difficulty in producing the names for objects. Semantic impairment was present in Ss with normal ability to discriminate visually presented shapes, indicating that the semantic deficit in AD occurs independently of abnormalities of visuospatial function. AD Ss tended to make errors on the same items in both confrontation naming and name recognition tests, suggesting that the semantic impairment in AD involves loss of information about specific objects and their names. (30 ref).

631. Huff, F. Jacob; Collins, Chris; Corkin, Suzanne & Rosen, T. John. (1986). **Equivalent forms of the Boston Naming Test.** *Journal of Clinical & Experimental Neuropsychology,* 8(5), 556–562.
Attempted to develop a test of naming ability that is sensitive to changes in performance on repeated testing, but is unbiased by practice effects, by dividing 85 items of the Boston Naming Test (BNT) into 2 42-item forms. Both forms were given to 15 healthy adults (aged 57–84 yrs), 24 patients with a clinical diagnosis of Alzheimer's disease (aged 52–78 yrs), and 17 patients (aged 23–76 yrs) with other brain lesions. The reliability of the BNT was high, and performance on the 2 forms of the test was similar. The 2 forms of the BNT are appended. (8 ref).

632. Huff, F. Jacob & Corkin, Suzanne. (1984). **Recent advances in the neuropsychology of Alzheimer's disease.** Proceedings of the 7th Annual Meeting of the Canadian College of Neuro-Psychopharmacology: Perspectives in Canadian neuro-psychopharmacology (1984, Halifax, Canada). *Progress in Neuro-Psychopharmacology & Biological Psychiatry,* 8(4–6), 643–648.
Describes the memory, language, and visuospatial impairments that are prominent neuropsychological deficits in Alzheimer's disease (AD), noting that the neuropsychological characteristics of AD are unique and contrast with those of other brain diseases. The cholinergic hypothesis of memory dysfunction in AD—that an acetylcholine deficiency is involved—is emphasized. The neuropsychological study of patients with AD may be useful in discovering the neuronal basis of cognitive processes, in differentially diagnosing dementia, and in evaluating treatment. (33 ref).

633. Huff, F. Jacob; Mack, Lisa; Mahlmann, Jeanne & Greenberg, Sylvia. (1988). **A comparison of lexical-semantic impairments in left hemisphere stroke and Alzheimer's disease.** *Brain & Language,* 34(2), 262–278.
Compared 10 patients with aphasia due to left hemisphere stroke and 10 patients with Alzheimer's disease ([AD] aged 41–88 yrs) who were matched for severity of naming impairment on tests of lexical-semantic processing. Results suggest that lexical-semantic impairments in both groups were due to a combination of impaired access to and loss of lexical-se-

mantic information. Findings indicate that impaired access was more prominent in stroke Ss and that AD Ss suffered a greater loss of information. Results are discussed in terms of a brain model of the storage and processing of lexical-semantic information. Implications for treatment strategies are noted.

634. Hutton, J. Thomas; Nagel, J. A. & Loewenson, Ruth B. (1984). **Eye tracking dysfunction in Alzheimer-type dementia.** *Neurology,* 34(1), 99–102.
Measured performance on visual tracking tasks in 19 patients with Alzheimer-type dementia, 17 patients with pseudodementia of depression, and 17 elderly normal controls (mean ages 73, 65, and 69 yrs, respectively). Smooth-pursuit-tracking errors were identified by counting the number of catch-up saccades required to compensate for failure of the smooth-pursuit system. The group with Alzheimer-type dementia had significantly worse smooth-pursuit tracking than either pseudodementia Ss or elderly normal controls. A strong correlation (0.74) was found between severity of visual tracking abnormality and severity of dementia in Ss with Alzheimer-type dementia. (10 ref).

635. Irle, Eva; Kessler, Josef; Markowitsch, Hans J. & Hofmann, Wolfgang. (1987). **Primate learning tasks reveal strong impairments in patients with presenile or senile dementia of the Alzheimer type.** *Brain & Cognition,* 6(4), 429–449.
Tested 8 54–89 yr old Ss with the likely diagnosis of presenile or senile dementia of the Alzheimer type (SDAT) on 2 frequently used primate learning tasks: a concurrent object discrimination task and a delayed non-match-to-sample task. In addition, tests for cognitive, mnemonic, perceptual, and language functions were applied. Results suggest a severe decline of the SDAT Ss in all measures when compared with 10 control Ss matched for age, gender, and education. The 2 primate learning tasks revealed strong impairments, thus demonstrating a high sensitivity for the detection and assessment of human amnesic disorders. Implications of these findings for human neuropsychological, and especially comparative neuropsychological, research are discussed.

636. Judd, Brian W.; Meyer, John S.; Rogers, Robert L.; Gandhi, Sunil et al. (1986). **Cognitive performance correlates with cerebrovascular impairments in multi-infarct dementia.** *Journal of the American Geriatrics Society,* 34(5), 355–360.
Examined possible relationships between impairments of cognitive performance and abnormal vasomotor responsiveness in 26 patients with multi-infarct dementia (MID [mean age 67.1 yrs]), 19 with Alzheimer's dementia (AD [mean age 72.2 yrs]), and among 26 age-matched, neurologically normal, healthy volunteers. Cerebral blood flow and cognitive performance were assessed in all Ss. Significant correlations were found between cognitive capacity performance and vasomotor responsiveness in Ss with MID, but not in Ss with AD or in neurologically normal Ss. It is concluded that loss of cerebral vasomotor responsiveness among MID patients, which is a biologic marker of cerebrovascular disease, provides confirmatory evidence of the vascular etiology of MID and assists in separating MID from AD patients.

637. Kelly, Mark P.; Kaszniak, Alfred W. & Garron, David C. (1986). **Neurobehavioral impairment patterns in carotid disease and Alzheimer disease.** *International Journal of Clinical Neuropsychology,* 8(4), 163–169.
Compared 39 patients with left, right, or bilateral carotid artery disease (CAD), 17 patients with Alzheimer's disease (AD), and 17 medical-surgical controls (aged 50+ yrs) on a battery of neuropsychological tests that included the Peabody Picture Vocabulary Test (PPVT) and Wechsler Memory Scale. The groups generally showed no differences on less complex tests of language, sensory, and motor function. AD Ss were significantly more defective than all other groups on measures of attention, orientation, remote memory, recent memory,

and reasoning. In addition, all CAD groups performed significantly more poorly than controls (but better than AD Ss) on some measures of recent memory, with bilateral CAD Ss performing most poorly. CAD Ss differed from AD Ss in both pattern and the degree of cognitive impairment. (42 ref).

638. Kempler, Daniel. (1985). **Syntactic and symbolic abilities in Alzheimer's disease.** *Dissertation Abstracts International,* 45(9-A), 2859.

639. Kempler, Daniel; Curtiss, Susan & Jackson, Catherine. (1987). **Syntactic preservation in Alzheimer's disease.** *Journal of Speech & Hearing Research,* 30(3), 343–350.
Investigated the claims of the preservation of syntactic ability and the dissociation between syntactic and lexical semantic ability in 20 patients (aged 62–87 yrs) with probable Alzheimer's disease (AD). Ss' language ability was evaluated. Results show that analysis of spontaneous speech revealed a normal range and frequency of syntactic constructions but poor lexical use. A writing task showed a similar divergence. It is concluded that syntactic ability is selectively preserved in AD. Findings are consistent with a modular theory of grammar and of mental functions. It is suggested that the overlearned and automatic nature of syntactic ability may account for its resilience to cognitive dissolution and cortical degeneration.

640. Knesevich, John W.; LaBarge, Emily & Edwards, Dorothy. (1986). **Predictive value of the Boston Naming Test in mild senile dementia of the Alzheimer type.** *Psychiatry Research,* 19(2), 155–161.
Examined the prognostic implications of anomia in a group of 43 Ss with mild senile dementia of the Alzheimer type and 43 matched controls. Anomia was found to correlate with a more rapidly progressive course of illness. S's age did not account for the degree of anomia. The presence of anomia in an S with mild senile dementia of the Alzheimer type appears to indicate a more rapidly progressive course.

641. Knesevich, John W.; Martin, Ronald L.; Berg, Leonard & Danziger, Warren. (1983). **Preliminary report on affective symptoms in the early stages of senile dementia of the Alzheimer type.** *American Journal of Psychiatry,* 140(2), 233–235.
The Hamilton Rating Scale for Depression (HRSD) and the Self-Rating Depression Scale (SRDS) were administered to 30 mildly demented Ss (mean age 71.2 yrs) and to 30 nondemented controls twice at a 1-yr interval. SRDS scores of the 2 groups were not significantly different, and although demented Ss showed more depression on the HRSD than controls, the means of both groups were in the nondepressed range. The HRSD "work and activities" item accounted for some of the demented group reaching the mildly depressed range. It is suggested that depressive syndromes may be independent of and rarely associated with Alzheimer's type dementia and that any demented patient who has a depressive syndrome might therefore benefit from aggressive treatment of affective symptoms despite the fact that the usual pharmacologic agents have substantial anticholinergic activity. (10 ref).

642. Knopman, David S. & Nissen, Mary J. (1987). **Implicit learning in patients with probable Alzheimer's disease.** *Neurology,* 37(5), 784–788.
Examined whether patients with probable Alzheimer's disease (AD) were capable of implicit procedural learning. 35 52–87 yr old AD patients and 13 61–78 yr old controls were given a serial visual reaction time (RT) task with an embedded repeating sequence. The AD Ss responded more slowly than the controls, but many showed learning of the repeating sequence. The AD Ss who failed to learn the sequence were similar in age and overall severity of dementia to those who learned, but they scored lower on some tasks of nonverbal reasoning.

643. Kopelman, Michael D. (1985). **Rates of forgetting in Alzheimer-type dementia and Korsakoff's syndrome.** *Neuropsychologia,* 23(5), 623–638.
Two studies compared forgetting rates among 16 patients (aged 56–75 yrs) with Alzheimer-type dementia, 16 alcoholic Korsakoff patients (aged 38–66 yrs), and 16 normal controls (aged 38–73 yrs). After initial learning had been equated as closely as possible, Alzheimer-type Ss showed the same rate of forgetting on a picture recognition test administered at intervals over the course of a week as Korsakoff patients and controls. Results suggest that the anterograde amnesic deficit in both Alzheimer's disease and Korsakoff's syndrome is primarily an acquisition or learning deficit. The Alzheimer patients differed from both the Korsakoff patients and the healthy controls in showing diminished digit span and severely impaired performance on a test of short-term (working) memory. The variability of performance within groups on the principal tests used was also examined, and the Alzheimer results are discussed with respect to the underlying neuropathology and the implications for pharmacotherapy. (61 ref).

644. Kopelman, Michael D. (1987). **Two types of confabulation.** *Journal of Neurology, Neurosurgery & Psychiatry,* 50(11), 1482–1487.
Examined examples of confabulation in 16 Korsakoff patients, 16 Alzheimer-type dementia patients, and 17 healthy adult controls. Instances of provoked confabulation given by the Korsakoff and Alzheimer Ss in story recall were compared with those produced by the healthy Ss at a prolonged retention interval. It is argued that there may be 2 types of confabulation: spontaneous confabulation, which may result from the superimposition of frontal dysfunction on an organic amnesia; and provoked confabulation, which may reflect a normal response to a faulty memory.

645. Kopelman, Michael D. (1986). **Recall of anomalous sentences in dementia and amnesia.** *Brain & Language,* 29(1), 154–170.
16 56–74 yr old Alzheimer-type dementing patients were compared with 16 38–66 yr old amnesic (Korsakoff) patients, 16 42–74 yr old depressed patients, and 16 38–73 yr old healthy controls in the immediate recall of semantically anomalous sentences. It was found that the Alzheimer Ss were severely impaired in their recall of these sentences but that the amnesic (Korsakoff) patients were not. Alzheimer patients have a severe impairment of short-term memory, and it is argued that this deficit may make them especially dependent on the presence of semantic cues in immediate verbal recall. Thus, the removal or reversibility of these cues results in a collapse of their performance. Other research has indicated that Alzheimer patients also show impaired semantic processing, and the possible interaction of their short-term memory and semantic processing deficits is discussed. (48 ref).

646. Kopelman, Michael D. (1986). **Clinical tests of memory.** *British Journal of Psychiatry,* 148, 517–525.
Compared the performance of Alzheimer's, Korsakoff's, and depressed patients and a group of healthy controls on various clinical tests of memory. There were 16 Ss in each diagnostic group, with an age range of 38–75 yrs. The tests measured memory, orientation, paired-associate learning, digit span, and sentence recall. Wide differences were found in the discriminatory power for the different tests. The patterns of performance of the Alzheimer and Korsakoff groups differed, although this was understandable in terms of what is known about the nature of organic amnesia. Depressed patients showed relatively mild impairments, which were not correlated with the severity of their depression.

647. Koss, Elisabeth. (1986). **Olfactory dysfunction in Alzheimer's disease.** *Developmental Neuropsychology,* 2(2), 89–99.
Recent evidence suggesting involvement of the central olfactory system in Alzheimer's disease (AD) was assessed by contrasting olfactory and visual discrimination in 15 56–80 yr old probable AD Ss and 6 healthy 60–78 yr old controls. Controls performed better than AD Ss on both tasks. Mild AD Ss performed better than moderate AD Ss on visual discrimination, although the 2 groups did not differ on olfactory discrimination. Positron-emission-tomographic studies performed on 11 of the AD Ss showed no relation between olfactory performance and cerebral metabolic asymmetries, but there were relations to visual discrimination.

648. Koss, Elisabeth & Friedland, Robert P. (1987). **Neuropsychological features of early and late-onset Alzheimer's disease.** *Archives of Neurology,* 44(8), 797.
Suggests that the conclusions of C. M. Filley et al (1986), that patients with onset of Alzheimer's disease before age 65 yrs have more language impairment and that those with later onset have more visuoconstructive performance impairment, are not warranted based on their data.

649. Langhans, Joseph J. (1986). **Pantomime recognition and pantomime expression in persons with Alzheimer's disease.** *Dissertation Abstracts International,* 46(10-B), 3410–3411.

650. Largen, John W. (1981). **Memory deficit and regional cerebral blood flow in early Alzheimer's Disease.** *Dissertation Abstracts International,* 41(12-B, Pt 1), 4639.

651. Largen, John W. (1984). **Longitudinal changes in intellectual, memory, and perceptual functions in dementia of the Alzheimer's type.** *International Journal of Neuroscience,* 24(3–4), 313–314.
Investigated 2 groups of patients with dementia of the Alzheimer's type (DAT). Group 1 originally consisted of 20 Ss, 12 of whom returned the 2nd yr; 10 (mean age 65.2 yrs) of the 12 Ss completed follow-up through the 3rd yr. Group 2 consisted of 10 Ss (mean age 69.3 yrs) from an original group of 22 Ss. Results suggest that neuropsychological declines in DAT Ss may vary considerably over individuals, with some subgroups showing minimal changes in measurement periods up to 2 yrs. These data are biased in favor of minimal change due to survivor effects.

652. Larrabee, Glenn J.; Largen, John W. & Levin, Harvey S. (1985). **Sensitivity of age-decline resistant ("hold") WAIS subtests to Alzheimer's disease.** *Journal of Clinical & Experimental Neuropsychology,* 7(5), 497–504.
Evaluated the sensitivity of Wechsler Adult Intelligence Scale (WAIS) age-decline-resistant ("hold") and age-decline-sensitive ("don't hold") subtests in discriminating 25 patients (mean age 65.48 yrs) with dementia of the Alzheimer's type (DAT) from 25 normal elderly Ss (mean age 66.04 yrs) matched according to age, education, and sex. There were 13 females and 12 males in each group; both groups had an average education of 13.04 yrs. Additional test variables included the WAIS Block Design, Information, and Digit Symbol subtests and the Logical Memory and Paired Associates subtests of the Wechsler Memory Scale. Results suggest that WAIS age-decline-resistant and age-decline-sensitive subtests were both effective in discriminating the DAT from normal Ss. Global ratings of severity of dementia correlated significantly with the WAIS Information and Digit Symbol subtests, but not with memory test scores. It is concluded that the practice of estimating premorbid ability based on current "hold" test performance should be abandoned and that the utility of memory tests is greatest for an initial diagnosis of DAT, while WAIS cognitive variables may be more useful in evaluating DAT severity. (19 ref).

653. Larrabee, Glenn J.; Levin, Harvey S. & High, Walter M. (1986). **Senescent forgetfulness: A quantitative study.** *Developmental Neuropsychology,* 2(4), 373–385.

Tested 88 healthy elderly Ss (aged 60–90 yrs) on a variety of measures of cognitive function and verbal, visual, and remote memory. Data analysis by age-residualized score patterns and cluster analysis yielded Ss (10–20% of the total sample) who exhibited reduced memory efficiency with otherwise preserved cognitive abilities. However, these Ss performed at a significantly higher level than Ss with Alzheimer-type dementia. Ss with a specific decline in memory disproportionate for their age displayed features consistent with the description of benign senescent forgetfulness offered by V. A. Kral (1958; see also 1962, 1966).

654. Lauter, H. (1968). **Clinical picture and psychopathology of Alzheimer's disease.** *Psychiatria Clinica,* 1(2), 85–108.
Analyzed the case records of 203 patients wih anatomically confirmed Alzheimer's disease on symptoms and course of the disease. Despite the difficulties and inadequacies arising out of the method of the investigation, a quite uniform clinical picture emerged that could be used to discuss the relationship of the illness to Pick's disease and senile dementia. Particularly characteristic are the early appearance of mnestic disturbances and spatial disorientation as well as aphasic, apractic, and agnostic symptoms. Sometimes the cerebral atrophy cannot be demonstrated pneumoencephalographically during the early stages. EEG changes are frequent. A family history was found in 28 probands. 21 further cases who had been thoroughly investigated are discussed regarding the psychopathology of Alzheimer's disease; taking disturbances in overall spatial perception as basic, the structural links and interactions between the psychopathological symptoms are discussed.

655. Lebrun, Yvan; Devreux, Françoise & Rousseau, Jean-Jacques. (1987). **Disorders of communicative behavior in degenerative dementia.** *Folia Phoniatrica,* 39(1), 1–8.
Analyzed the verbal behavior of 4 patients (aged 62–73 yrs) with (pre-)senile dementia and moderate to severe language disorders. Two sisters diagnosed as having familial senile dementia of the Alzheimer type answered simple questions appropriately; however, some questions failed to elicit a response, and repetition of the questions resulted in inappropriate replies. They also demonstrated intelligible utterances and echolalia. The other 2 Ss did not understand any of the simple verbal instructions or questions, but the jargon they produced was often iterative with numerous repetitions of mono- and bisyllables. One S used many alliterations and assonances, whereas another had no spontaneous speech. It is concluded that a number of these features are characteristic of the verbal behavior of patients with degenerative dementia.

656. Leli, Dano A. & Scott, Linda H. (1982). **Cross-validation of two indexes of intellectual deterioration on patients with Alzheimer's disease.** *Journal of Consulting & Clinical Psychology,* 50(3), 468.
A discriminant function created from 2 indexes of intellectual deterioration was cross-validated on 17 patients with Alzheimer's disease and with nonpsychotic, nonimpaired Ss comparable in age, education, race, sex, and handedness. The Satz-Mogel short form of the WAIS was the test of intelligence. Hit rates equalled 94% for the Alzheimer's disease patients and 56% for the nonimpaired Ss. Most false-positive errors consisted of nonimpaired Ss with deterioration index ratings, indicating no deterioration being misclassified as impaired. Such errors should be minimized when the function is used with additional data sources. (2 ref).

657. Lilly, Ralph; Cummings, Jeffrey L.; Benson, D. Frank & Frankel, Michael. (1983). **The human Klüver-Bucy syndrome.** *Neurology,* 33(9), 1141–1145.
Describes 12 patients with the Klüver-Bucy syndrome (KBS) and presents case studies for 4 of these (ages 31–57 yrs). KBS occurred in head trauma, Alzheimer's disease, Pick's disease, and following herpes encephalitis. KBS was transient after head trauma but was a persistent feature of the postencephalitic syndrome. In all cases KBS was combined with aphasia, amnesia, or dementia. Human KBS resembles the monkey syndrome, but in humans there is a more elaborate complex of behavioral disturbances, including alterations in sexual behavior. The behavioral manifestations are produced by bilateral temporal lobe dysfunction. Partial expression of the syndrome may have localizing validity. (31 ref).

658. Little, A. G.; Volans, P. J.; Hemsley, D. R. & Levy, R. (1986). **The retention of new information in senile dementia.** *British Journal of Clinical Psychology,* 25(1), 71–72.
Assessed, repeatedly over 6 mo, paired-associate learning performance in 26 Ss with senile dementia of the Alzheimer type. Comparisons show that performance on changing items progressively declined, whereas performance on repeated items was maintained at initial levels. Findings indicate that these patients are able to retain some information over 1- and 2-mo intervals. (3 ref).

659. Loring, David W. & Largen, John W. (1985). **Neuropsychological patterns of presenile and senile dementia of the Alzheimer type.** *Neuropsychologia,* 23(3), 351–357.
37 patients with a presumptive diagnosis of dementia of the Alzheimer type were divided into presenile ($n = 3$ [mean age 59.5 yrs]) and senile ($n = 24$ [mean age 72.5 yrs]) groups according to the age at which they first received a clinical diagnosis. Although there were no differences in mental status, dementia rating, or chronicity of disease, multivariate analyses of Wechsler Adult Intelligence Scale (WAIS) subtests revealed the presenile Ss to be relatively impaired on Performance subtests. Univariate tests of Verbal, Performance, and Full Scale IQ were significantly lower in the presenile group. There was no group effect detected for forward digit span, adjusted for age differences based on performance of 40 age-matched controls, while the presenile group performed significantly more poorly on backward span. Significant differences were detected for an embedded figure task, as well as graphomotor speed. Data suggests that patients who develop a degenerative dementia during the presenile period are more impaired than their senile counterparts on age-adjusted measures of sustained concentration and mental tracking. (19 ref).

660. Lott, Ira T. (1982). **Down's syndrome, aging, and Alzheimer's disease: A clinical review.** *Annals of the New York Academy of Sciences,* 396, 15–27.
A literature review indicates that Down's syndrome (DS) patients aged over 35 yrs show a disproportionately high incidence of recent memory loss; short-term visual-retention deficits; aphasia-agnosia syndromes; and personality aberrations in the form of apathy, sudden personality changes, and loss of self-care skills. Age-related changes in endocrine and immunological function, other somatic indices of aging in DS, and research on chromosome 21 and aging are discussed. (105 ref).

661. MacInnes, William D. et al. (1984). **Aging, regional cerebral blood flow, and neuropsychological functioning.** Annual Meeting of American Psychological Association (1982, Washington, DC). *Journal of the American Geriatrics Society,* 32(10), 712–718.
Investigated the relationship between regional cerebral blood flow (rCBF) and performance on the Luria-Nebraska Neuropsychological Battery (LNNB) in 59 healthy and 20 Alzheimer's disease Ss, aged 56–88 yrs. Ss underwent the [133]xenon inhalation rCBF procedure described by J. S. Meyer et al (1978) and W. E. Obrist et al (1975) and were given the LNNB. Decrements in the gray-matter blood flow paralleled decrements in performance on the LNNB. Using partial correlations, a significant proportion of shared variance was observed between gray-matter blood flow and the LNNB scales. However, there was much less of a relationship between white-matter blood flow and performance on the

LNNB. Results suggest that even within a restricted-age sample, rCBF is related in a global way to neuropsychological functioning, as previously found by W. D. MacInnes et al (1983). (41 ref).

662. Mahurin, Roderick K. (1986). **Psychomotor performance in Alzheimer disease.** *Dissertation Abstracts International,* 47(3-B), 1318.

663. Mahurin, Roderick K. & Pirozzolo, Francis J. (1986). **Chronometric analysis: Clinical applications in aging and dementia.** *Developmental Neuropsychology,* 2(4), 345–362.
Reviews the use by researchers of reaction time (RT) for the evaluation of patients with Alzheimer's disease (AD) and introduces the timed card-sorting task (TCST) as a convenient measure of response time for use in the clinical setting. The clinical sensitivity of RT is discussed as well as RT in aging, patient acceptance, computer-based assessment, functional competency, longitudinal assessment, and the sensitivity of choice RT. RT performance on the TCST by 13 young controls (mean age 24.5 yrs), 12 elderly controls (mean age 65.8 yrs), and 14 AD patients (mean age 70 yrs) confirmed previously reported slowing in RT in aging and dementia. Methodological issues and hypothesized attentional mechanisms underlying RT slowing in AD are also discussed.

664. Margolis, Ronald B.; Taylor, John M. & Dunn, Edwin J. (1985). **An abbreviated Speech Sounds Perception Test with a geriatric population.** *International Journal of Clinical Neuropsychology,* 7(3), 167–169.
Examined the short form of the Speech Sounds Perception test (SSPT) of the Halstead-Reitan Neuropsychological Test Battery proposed by C. J. Golden and S. M. Anderson (1977) with groups of geriatric patients wit suspected dementia. Since even healthy elderly individuals often perform in the impaired range of the SSPT, ranges of impairment rather than the traditional impaired/unimpaired categories were used to analyze agreement between groups. 29 patients (mean age 72.1 yrs) with Alzheimer's disease, mixed dementia, and pseudodementia were randomly assigned to Group 1 and were used to establish finer ranges of classifications (mild, moderate, and severe impairment). 30 patients (mean age 71.2 yrs) with the same diagnoses as Group 1 Ss were assigned to Group 2 and were used for cross-validation of the ranges. Findings show that the number of errors on the 1st half of the SSPT were predictive of the total test score. Agreement rates for the mildly, moderately, and severely impaired ranges were 93%, 88%, and 86%, respectively, in Group 1 and 90%, 83%, and 88%, respectively, in Group 2. It is concluded that the short form of SSPT may be substituted for the original test with little loss in clinical information. (9 ref).

665. Martin, Alex. (1987). **Representation of semantic and spatial knowledge in Alzheimer's patients: Implications for models of preserved learning in amnesia.** *Journal of Clinical & Experimental Neuropsychology,* 9(2), 191–224.
Presents findings on 3 Alzheimer's disease patients (aged 50–58 yrs) with comparable levels of intellectual and memory abilities as assessed by the Wechsler Adult Intelligence Scale (WAIS). One S had a relatively circumscribed impairment of word-finding ability concurrent with intact visuospatial and constructional skill. Another S showed the opposite profile of abilities, while the 3rd S exhibited deficits in both domains. All 3 Ss were severely and globally amnesic when tested with traditional recall and recognition procedures. Corresponding profiles of preserved learning were revealed but only under conditions that limited the demands on encoding and retrieval processes. Models are offered to account for these contrasting patterns of impairment. The possibility that medial temporal structures contribute to the ability to consciously reconstruct prior experiences is discussed.

666. Martin, Alex; Brouwers, Pim; Cox, Christiane & Fedio, Paul. (1985). **On the nature of the verbal memory deficit in Alzheimer's disease.** *Brain & Language,* 25(2), 323–341.
Investigated verbal memory in 14 patients with Alzheimer's disease (AD) (aged 50–68 yrs) with previously documented deficits in word production and comprehension and in 11 normal control Ss (aged 53–71 yrs) in 2 experiments. Procedures were employed to evaluate word recall and recognition within the context of both "multistore" and "levels of processing" models of memory. In addition, memory abilities were evaluated with respect to performance on measures of verbal fluency and language comprehension. As expected, the AD Ss performed significantly worse than normal Ss on all tasks. However, in each experiment their pattern of recall across conditions was found to be qualitatively similar to that produced by normal Ss. It is argued that the memory impairment associated with AD may be largely due to an inability to encode a sufficient number of stimulus features or attributes. Furthermore, this encoding deficit includes, but is not limited to, semantic attributes. Similarities between the performance of the AD patients and reported findings with Korsakoff patients and normal Ss with "weak" memory are discussed.

667. Martin, Alex; Cox, Christiane; Brouwers, Pim & Fedio, Paul. (1985). **A note on different patterns of impaired and preserved cognitive abilities and their relation to episodic memory deficits in Alzheimer's patients.** *Brain & Language,* 26(1), 181–185.
Discusses cognitive deficits and their relation to episodic memory in patients with Alzheimer's disease (AD), noting that AD patients may present with differing patterns of cognitive impairment indicative of different regions of cortical dysfunction. These differences have implications for understanding the breakdown of specific cognitive systems and their relation to episodic and other types of memory disorders. Individual patient differences suggest that a diagnosis of AD is not sufficient justification for averaging data across patients, which may hinder neuropsychological investigation of the AD process. (11 ref).

668. Martin, Alex & Fedio, Paul. (1983). **Word production and comprehension in Alzheimer's disease: The breakdown of semantic knowledge.** *Brain & Language,* 19(1), 124–141.
Tested 14 mildly impaired patients (aged 50–68 yrs) with suspected Alzheimer's disease and 11 normal controls (aged 53–71 yrs) with tests requiring production (naming and fluency) and comprehension of single words. These included the WAIS and the Boston Naming Test. Word comprehension was assessed on a superordinate and a more specific level. The naming and fluency abilities of the Alzheimer's Ss were found to be highly correlated and impaired. Naming errors often consisted of semantic field errors that were either hierarchically or linearly related to the target name. In comparison with normals, verbal fluency was characterized by a tendency to generate proportionally more category names concurrent with reduced production of items within a category. Single-word comprehension was also impaired, except when judgments of affective meaning were required. Results suggest that Alzheimer's disease may lead to a specific disruption in semantic knowledge characterized by a difficulty in differentiating between items within the same semantic category concurrent with the relative preservation of broader categorical information. (37 ref).

669. Martin, Alex et al. (1986). **Towards a behavioral typology of Alzheimer's patients.** *Journal of Clinical & Experimental Neuropsychology,* 8(5), 594–610.
Conducted neuropsychological tests on 42 patients (aged 43–74 yrs) with Alzheimer's disease (AD) and 21 normal controls (aged 52–71 yrs). 19 of the AD Ss and 7 of the controls were also studied via positron emission tomography to obtain es-

timates of regional rates of cortical glucose metabolism. Analyses of the data indicated the presence of distinct subgroups characterized by qualitatively different profiles of cognitive impairment and corresponding patterns of cerebral hypometabolism. No subgroup differences were noted with regard to age at onset or reported duration of symptoms. Findings indicate that, in a given S, AD may initially invade a relatively circumscribed cortical region. Thus, although AD may constitute a single disease process, it does not result in a unitary neuropsychological syndrome. (65 ref).

670. Martin, E. M.; Wilson, R. S.; Penn, R. D.; Fox, J. H. et al. (1987). **Cortical biopsy results in Alzheimer's disease: Correlation with cognitive deficits.** *Neurology,* 37(7), 1201–1204.
Neuropsychologic and pathologic data are presented for a group of 11 patients (mean age 64.9 yrs) with a clinical diagnosis of probable Alzheimer's disease (AD) according to recently proposed criteria. In all cases, the diagnosis was verified by cortical biopsy. In addition, increased cortical plaque counts were associated with greater deficits in language production and comprehension and poorer performance on an index of global mental status. Results suggest that a clinical diagnosis of AD is accurate when patient selection is restricted to typical cases and that language deficits may provide a useful indicator of severity of disease in AD patients.

671. Masur, David M. (1986). **Semantic memory in normal aging and Alzheimer Type Dementia.** *Dissertation Abstracts International,* 47(3-B), 1305.

672. Masur, David M. & Fuld, Paula A. (1982). **The neuropsychological evaluation of dementia: Two case studies.** *Clinical Gerontologist,* 1(1), 23–28.
Compared behavioral and neuropsychological test findings of 2 patients (aged 57 and 73 yrs) referred for evaluation of cognitive decline and difficulty with memory. One S had a neurological diagnosis of Alzheimer's disease, and the other S was thought to have pseudodementia. The strengths and weaknesses of each are discussed in relation to those typical of many Alzheimer patients. The importance of adequate assessment of memory and learning is emphasized. (5 ref).

673. McLachlan, Donald R. et al. (1984). **Alzheimer's disease: Clinical course and cognitive disturbances.** *Acta Neurologica Scandinavica,* 69(Suppl 99), 83–89.
Describes the natural history of Alzheimer's disease (AD) and the types of psychological tests used to evaluate patients and reports on a longitudinal study of 16 outpatients (mean age at the beginning of the study 61 yrs) suspected of having AD. Cerebral functioning was assessed by repeated measures of cognitive performance (the WAIS and the Wechsler Memory Scale—Form 1), repeated administration of a signal-detection task involving a backward-masking paradigm, and repeated EEG analyses using power-spectral analysis. All evaluations were conducted over a 4–18 mo interval. Results show that cognitive function scores tended to decrease over time; increased evidence of EEG abnormalities was observed, especially in the increased variability of the resting waveforms. There was also a trend toward Ss' decreased ability to maintain performance in the signal-detection task. AD was subsequently diagnosed in 4 of the Ss. Implications for assessment and differential diagnosis are noted. (5 ref).

674. Merriam, Arnold E.; Aronson, Miriam K.; Gaston, Patricia; Wey, Su-ling et al. (1988). **The psychiatric symptoms of Alzheimer's disease.** *Journal of the American Geriatrics Society,* 36(1), 7–12.
Interviewed 175 primary family caregivers to assess the prevalence and nature of psychiatric pathology in well-diagnosed community-residing Alzheimer's disease patients. Symptoms indicative of depression were ubiquitous in the patients stud-

ied. A variety of psychotic features were also regularly reported. Implications for recognizing and treating reversible psychiatric impairment are discussed.

675. Miller, Edgar (1973). **Short- and long-term memory in patients with presenile dementia (Alzheimer's disease).** *Psychological Medicine,* 3(2), 221–224.
Examined the nature of memory disturbance in Alzheimer's disease by testing 15 presenile dementia patients and 15 nondemented controls with neurological ailments, using a simple word-list recall task. Results demonstrate that the Ss' memory disturbance was due to an impairment in short-term memory and to an additional difficulty in establishing new material in long-term storage. Results show that the 2 types of memory disorder resulting on the one hand from Alzheimer's disease and on the other from bilateral hippocampal damage are qualitatively quite different and contradict the theory that involvement of the hippocampus might explain the memory disorder of presenile dementia. Problems in obtaining a complete understanding of the nature of the amnestic phenomena in Alzheimer's disease are discussed.

676. Mitchell, David B.; Hunt, R. Reed & Schmitt, Frederick A. (1986). **The generation effect and reality monitoring: Evidence from dementia and normal aging.** *Journal of Gerontology,* 41(1), 79–84.
Investigated the role of semantic memory activation in accounting for generation effects and reality monitoring in 12 undergraduates, 12 older normal adults (mean age 65.6 yrs), and 10 patients (mean age 65.1 yrs) with dementia of the Alzheimer's type (DAT). DAT Ss were diagnosed by the Diagnostic and Statistical Manual of Mental Disorders (DSM-III) and Research Diagnostic Criteria. Older Ss were assessed on the Mini-Mental Status Exam, and all Ss completed a sentence reading and generation task, a free recall task, and a cued recall task. Both young and old normal Ss demonstrated higher recall for internally generated information than for externally presented information, whereas DAT Ss failed to demonstrate a generation effect. Similarly, reality monitoring scores (discrimination between internal and external items) were high for both age groups of normals, but near chance levels for the DAT group. Results support the hypothesis that semantic memory is an important factor in generation effects.

677. Mitsuyama, Yashio. (1985). **Delusion-hallucination, affective and personality disorders seen in the early stages of cerebrovascular dementia.** *Kyushu Neuro-psychiatry,* 31(2), 154–162.
Reports the results of clinical studies of 58 cases of cerebrovascular dementia (CD) and 43 cases of Alzheimer's disease (AD). Delusions observed in CD Ss were not pronounced and were more consistent than those of paranoid psychotics. The delusion of jealousy was more frequent in CD, and the delusion of robbery was more common in AD; these delusions usually disappeared with progressive intellectual deterioration. Affective disorder was seen more often in CD than in AD, and emotional incontinence was the most characteristic feature in CD. Findings suggest that mood change following brain infarction may not be a nonspecific psychological function but may be related to the pathophysiology of the brain. (English abstract).

678. Moberg, Paul J.; Pearlson, Godfrey D.; Speedie, Lynn J.; Lipsey, John R. et al. (1987). **Olfactory recognition: Differential impairments in early and late Huntington's and Alzheimer's diseases.** *Journal of Clinical & Experimental Neuropsychology,* 9(6), 650–664.
42 patients (mean age 72.45 yrs) with senile dementia of the Alzheimer type, 38 patients (mean age 43.73 yrs) with Huntington's disease, and 80 age-matched normal controls were administered tests of olfactory, verbal, and visual recognition after being screened for normal olfactory discrimination. Early-affected Huntington's patients with minimal chorea or cog-

nitive deficit displayed deficits in olfactory recognition despite normal verbal and visual performance, even after correction for task difficulty, suggesting involvement of olfactory brain regions early in the disease process. In the early Alzheimer's group, deficits were seen on all recognition modalities indicating more global impairment. Both overall patient groups were impaired relative to controls on all recognition tasks, with the olfactory paradigm being most affected.

679. Morris, John C.; Rubin, Eugene H.; Morris, Edward J. & Mandel, Stephen A. (1987). **Senile dementia of the Alzheimer's type: An important risk factor for serious falls.** *Journal of Gerontology*, 42(4), 412–417.
Conducted a longitudinal study of senile dementia and healthy aging, in which the occurrence of serious falls was examined in 21 male and 23 female participants (aged 64–82 yrs) with senile dementia of the Alzheimer's type (SDAT) and in 27 male and 29 female cognitively healthy elderly control participants over a 4-yr period. Falls occurred in 36% of SDAT Ss vs 11% of controls. The higher frequency of falls in demented Ss was not explained by greater neurologic deficit nor by increased drug use compared with controls. However, males with SDAT who reported falls had higher mean blood pressures and were more likely to be medicated than males with SDAT who did not fall. These differences were not observed in women. Falls in SDAT Ss were associated with an increased rate of institutionalization.

680. Morris, Robin G. (1987). **The effect of concurrent articulation on memory span in Alzheimer-type dementia.** *British Journal of Clinical Psychology*, 26(3), 233–234.
Explored the effects of concurrent articulation on memory-span performance, comparing 14 patients (mean age 77.4 yrs) with early Alzheimer-type dementia (AD) and 14 matched controls. Reduction in memory span due to concurrent articulation was the same in AD patients as controls, supporting the notion that the contribution of articulatory rehearsal to memory-span performance is undiminished in early AD.

681. Morris, Robin G. (1987). **Identity matching and oddity learning in patients with moderate to severe Alzheimer-type dementia.** *Quarterly Journal of Experimental Psychology: Comparative & Physiological Psychology*, 39(3, Sect B), 215–227.
Four patients (mean age 79.0 yrs) with moderate to severe Alzheimer-type dementia (AD) were trained to criterion on identity matching and then shifted to the same task with novel stimuli. They showed no savings in learning to match novel stimuli, whereas 4 age-matched normal controls rapidly learned the novel matching discrimination. Four other AD Ss (mean age 82.0 yrs) were initially trained on oddity, taking a similar number of trials to reach criterion as the matching group. When these Ss were subsequently shifted to the matching task with novel stimuli, they performed substantially worse than the 1st AD group. The lack of positive transfer in the shift between matching to matching suggests that the AD patients solved the identity-matching task on the basis of stimulus–response associations rather than a rule.

682. Morris, Robin G. (1986). **Short-term forgetting in senile dementia of the Alzheimer's type.** *Cognitive Neuropsychology*, 3(1), 77–97.
Explored the nature of forgetting in patients at the early stages of senile dementia of the Alzheimer's type (SDAT). Exp I tested the ability of 12 SDAT patients (mean age 77.2 yrs) to remember consonant trigrams after an interval of 0, 5, 10, or 20 sec during which they were instructed either to do nothing, articulate the word "the" repeatedly, reverse pairs of digits, or add pairs of digits together. The articulation of distractor task caused substantial forgetting with SDAT Ss in comparison with minimal forgetting in 12 healthy elderly controls. They were also clearly impaired with digit reversal and digit addition as distractor tasks, although their forgetting rates were similar to the controls. Exp II, with 9 SDAT

patients (mean age 74.1 yrs) and 9 elderly controls, showed a substantial decrement in the SDAT Ss' ability to remember consonant trigrams with both tapping and articulation as distractor tasks. Results support the hypothesis that SDAT patients have insufficient central processing resources available for maintenance rehearsal. (49 ref).

683. Morris, Robin G. (1987). **Articulatory rehearsal in Alzheimer type dementia.** *Brain & Language*, 30(2), 351–362.
Investigated the relationship between articulation rate and memory span in 21 patients with early Alzheimer type dementia ([AD] mean age 76.1 yrs), comparing their performance with that of 21 matched controls (mean age 77 yrs). Memory span was measured using auditorily and visually presented digits. AD Ss were moderately impaired in both conditions. Articulation rate was measured either by requiring Ss to read lists of random digits or repeatedly count from 1 to 10; AD Ss were slower in the counting task. Measures of memory span and articulation rate correlated significantly for the controls but not for AD Ss. Results suggest that articulatory rehearsal processes in primary memory are unimpaired at the early stages of AD.

684. Morris, Robin G. (1984). **Dementia and the functioning of the articulatory loop system.** *Cognitive Neuropsychology*, 1(2), 143–157.
Explored the functioning of the articulatory loop system in patients at the early stages of senile dementia of the Alzheimer's type. Exp I investigated the effect of phonological similarity on immediate verbal recall of letters in 17 patients (mean age 77.9 yrs) with Alzheimer's disease and 17 age-matched normal controls. Ss were presented with lists of letters drawn from 2 sets in a variety of conditions. In Exp II, in which 15 Alzheimer's patients (mean age 77.1 yrs) and 15 matched controls participated, items drawn from 2 sets of words were used, with variables of word length, mode of presentation, and articulation. Results show that, in comparison to controls, patients' memory span was clearly impaired, but the effect of phonemic confusability on immediate memory span was relatively normal and the effect of word length on span was also normal. Both effects were abolished by concurrent articulation if the stimulus material was presented visually. With auditory presentation, only the word-length effect was abolished. Results indicate that, despite overall cognitive impairment and reduced memory span, the articulatory loop system is relatively unimpaired by mild dementia. (28 ref).

685. Morris, Robin G. & Baddeley, Alan D. (1988). **Primary and working memory functioning in Alzheimer-type dementia.** *Journal of Clinical & Experimental Neuropsychology*, 10(2), 279–296.
Reviews recent neuropsychological studies of primary memory functioning in early Alzheimer-type dementia with specific reference to recent research on working memory. The deficits in primary memory follow a fairly distinct pattern with a comparatively unimpaired recency effect in free recall, a moderate impairment in memory span, and a more substantial impairment in short-term retention following distraction. The nature of these deficits is considered in relation to the working memory model of A. D. Baddeley and G. J. Hitch (1974). It is suggested that the articulatory loop system is functioning normally but that there is an impairment in the control processes of working memory.

686. Morris, Robin G. & Kopelman, Michael D. (1986). **The memory deficits in Alzheimer-type dementia: A review.** Special Issue: Human memory. *Quarterly Journal of Experimental Psychology: Human Experimental Psychology*, 38(4-A), 575–602.

Reviews and evaluates recent experimental studies of memory deficits at the early stages of Alzheimer-type dementia in relation to current theories of memory functioning in humans. While memory deficits are widespread, some aspects are more resilient to impairment. It is concluded that the deficits observed share particular features found in organic amnesia but with additional deficits that relate to impairments in other domains of functioning.

687. Moscovitch, Morris; Winocur, Gordon & McLachlan, Don. (1986). **Memory as assessed by recognition and reading time in normal and memory-impaired people with Alzheimer's disease and other neurological disorders.** *Journal of Experimental Psychology: General,* 115(4), 331–347.
Examined the dissociations in performance on 2 tests of retention—speeded reading and recognition. In Exp I, 14 undergraduates, 14 community-dwelling elderly people (CDP [mean age 68.2 yrs]), 10 institutionalized elderly people (mean age 78.6 yrs), and 8 people with memory disorders (MDP [mean age 55.3 yrs]) read sentences in normal and in geometrically transformed script at initial presentation, 1–2 hrs later, and 4–14 days later, and were required to distinguish old sentences from new ones on the latter 2 occasions. In Exp II, 12 CDP (mean age 71.4 yrs), 12 undergraduates, and 8 MDP (mean age 50.6 yrs) studied weakly-associated word pairs and sentences and were tested on recognition and speeded reading of old, new, and recombined sentences. In Exp III, 12 normal elderly people (mean age 71.4 yrs), 12 undergraduates, and 12 MDP (mean age 64.25 yrs) studied randomly-paired words and sentences. Overall results suggest that on speeded reading tests, Ss with MDs formed and retained new associations despite failing on recognition tests that required conscious recollection of a previous episode. The dissociation between these 2 ways of testing memory in normal young, elderly, and MD people is discussed in terms of a task-specific, component-process approach to memory that is contrasted with a multiple-memory-system approach. (70 ref).

688. Moss, Mark B.; Albert, Marilyn S.; Butters, Nelson & Payne, Melanie. (1986). **Differential patterns of memory loss among patients with Alzheimer's disease, Huntington's disease, and alcoholic Korsakoff's syndrome.** *Archives of Neurology,* 43(3), 239–246.
Examined the distinction between patients with Huntington's disease (HD) and Korsakoff's syndrome (KS) in recognition-memory ability. Focus was on whether these 2 patient groups can be distinguished by their performance on recognition tests using a wide range of stimuli (i.e., verbal, color, spatial, pattern, facial). 11 HD Ss (mean age 49 yrs), 10 KS Ss (mean age 58.3 yrs), 12 Ss (mean age 64.5 yrs) with Alzheimer's disease (AD), and 14 normal Ss (mean age 61.4 yrs) were compared on these tasks and also on recall of verbal stimuli at 2 delay intervals (15 sec and 2 min). Results indicate that although there was no significant difference among the 3 patient groups in their ability to recognize new spatial, color, pattern, or facial stimuli, HD Ss performed significantly better than did the other 2 groups when verbal stimuli were used. Ss with AD recalled significantly fewer words over the 15-sec delay interval than did either HD or KS Ss. Although all 3 patient groups were equally impaired relative to normal control Ss at the 15-sec delay, Ss with AD recalled significantly fewer words at the longer, as compared with the shorter, interval. Findings demonstrate that the memory impairments seen in patients with HD, KS, or AD are clearly dissociable in visual recognition and recall tasks.

689. Muramoto, Osamu. (1984). **Selective reminding in normal and demented aged people: Auditory verbal versus visual spatial task.** *Cortex,* 20(4), 461–478.
Two studies compared auditory-verbal (AV) and visual-spatial (VS) selective reminding in 60 normal 61–88 yr olds and 21 54–88 yr old inpatients and outpatients diagnosed as having either senile or presenile dementia of the Alzheimer type or multi-infarct dementia. Two selective reminding tests were devised that required Ss to process almost equal amounts of information in the AV and VS modalities. Results show that Ss' performance on VS tasks declined with age more steeply than on AV tasks. Factor analyses indicated that VS performance was factorially independent of AV performance and that VS performance accounted for most of the decline in normal Ss' performance. Demented Ss' VS performance was well correlated with the severity of dementia. A comparison between multi-infarct and Alzheimer-type Ss demonstrated that severe impairment of VS learning with relative preservation of AV learning is a distinctive pattern of Alzheimer-type dementia. Findings suggest that VS selective reminding is a useful tool in evaluating memory decline in aging and in clinically diagnosing dementia. (20 ref).

690. Murdoch, Bruce E.; Chenery, Helen J.; Wilks, Vicki & Boyle, Richard S. (1987). **Language disorders in dementia of the Alzheimer type.** *Brain & Language,* 31(1), 122–137.
The language profile of a group of 18 67–91 yr old Alzheimer (AD) patients is documented and their performance on a standard aphasia test battery compared to a group of 18 69–90 yr old institutionalized, nonneurologically impaired control Ss matched for age, sex, and educational level. AD patients scored significantly lower than controls in the areas of verbal expression, auditory comprehension, repetition, reading, and writing. Articulation abilities were the same in each group. A language deficit was evident in all AD patients. The language disorder exhibited resembled a transcortical sensory aphasia. Syntax and phonology remained relatively intact but semantic abilities were impaired. Results support the inclusion of a language deficit as a diagnostic criterion of Alzheimer's disease.

691. Naugle, Richard I. (1986). **Neuropsychological and morphological/physiological characteristics of empirically-derived dementia subgroups.** *Dissertation Abstracts International,* 47(5-B), 2177.

692. Naugle, Richard I.; Cullum, C. Munro; Bigler, Erin D. & Massman, Paul J. (1985). **Neuropsychological and computerized axial tomography volume characteristics of empirically derived dementia subgroups.** *Journal of Nervous & Mental Disease,* 173(10), 596–604.
Neuropsychological assessment data from 63 male and 75 female 39–93 yr old Alzheimer's patients were cluster analyzed to yield 5 subgroups: Cluster 1 was a low-functioning subgroup (*n* = 25) characterized by severe generalized deficits; Cluster 2 was a subgroup (*n* = 39) characterized by a higher level of visual-spatial skills relative to the other groups; Clusters 3 (*n* = 21) and 4 (*n* = 42) were virtually indistinguishable in terms of verbal ability and memory but differed with regard to visual-spatial skills; and Cluster 5 was a subgroup (*n* = 11) that presented with relatively better preserved verbal abilities. Despite their different neuropsychological profiles, the subgroups did not differ significantly with regard to those complaints that were noted early in the course of the disease process. However, they differed significantly in terms of Ss' educational backgrounds, the distribution of males and females, and the age of the Ss at the onset of the disease. Analysis of the degree and lateralization of cortical atrophy using volumetric techniques suggested little relationship with neuropsychological examination results. Ventricular volume differences among the 5 subgroups were not significant after the effect of age had been partialled out. Results are discussed in relation to the multiple factors relating to brain structure and cognition in Alzheimer's disease. (42 ref).

693. Neary, D.; Snowden, J. S.; Bowen, D. M.; Sims, N. R. et al (1986). **Neuropsychological syndromes in presenile dementia due to cerebral atrophy.** *Journal of Neurology, Neurosurgery & Psychiatry,* 49(2), 163–174.

In a prospective study of 24 patients (aged 43–69 yrs) with presenile dementia associated with cerebral atrophy, clinical and psychological characteristics of Ss' disorder were examined in relation to pathological and chemical findings obtained from tissue analysis following cerebral biopsy. The histological features of Alzheimer's disease (AD) were found in 75% of cases. Distinctive patterns of neuropsychological breakdown allowed clinical grouping of patients (e.g., AD or non-AD), but there was no absolute concordance between clinical and patho-chemical groupings. (37 ref).

694. Nebes, Robert D. & Boller, François. (1987). **The use of language structure by demented patients in a visual search task.** *Cortex,* 23(1), 87–98.
Investigated whether knowledge of the sequential letter dependencies present in spelling remains intact in demented patients, using 20 patients (mean age 67.2 yrs) with mild to moderate Alzheimer's disease (AD), 20 normal controls (mean age 23.6 yrs), and 20 normal controls (mean age 67.2 yrs). Each patient was matched with a young control in sex and education and with an older control in sex, education, and age. Speed searching an array of letters for a target was measured. Results show that despite differing in overall speed of response, Ss were affected equally by the approximation to English of the stimuli (i.e., both normal and demented Ss searched words faster than low-order approximations). It is concluded that knowledge of the probability patterns of spelling remained intact and accessible in the semantic memory of the demented patients studied.

695. Nebes, Robert D.; Boller, François & Holland, Audrey. (1986). **Use of semantic context by patients with Alzheimer's disease.** *Psychology & Aging,* 1(3), 261–269.
Used semantic-priming procedures to examine limitations in the use of semantic context by 18 patients (mean age 68.9 yrs) with Alzheimer's disease (AD) and to determine whether any such contextual effects were mediated solely through automatic processes or whether attentional processes were also involved. Three tasks were applied to examine the effect of semantic context on the performance of 18 normal elderly Ss (mean age 67.2 yrs), 18 normal young Ss (mean age 24.1 yrs), and the AD Ss. When normal and AD Ss were asked to decide whether a given item was a member of a certain category, their response times were equally affected by the item's dominance in the category. The time that AD Ss took to recognize a word was actually affected more by the semantic context provided by a priming sentence than was that of normal Ss. When asked to generate the final word of an incomplete sentence, AD Ss performed very poorly unless potential responses were highly constrained by sentence context. (31 ref).

696. Nebes, Robert D. & Madden, David J. (1988). **Different patterns of cognitive slowing produced by Alzheimer's disease and normal aging.** *Psychology & Aging,* 3(1), 102–104.
Aging has previously been shown to produce a generalized proportional slowing of all cognitive operations. In contrast, the present results suggest that Alzheimer's disease produces a disproportionate reduction in the speed with which patients carry out one or more mental operations. The tasks that demented patients found particularly difficult involved either a self-directed search of their lexicon or the use of familiarity information.

697. Nebes, Robert D.; Martin, David C. & Horn, Lisa C. (1984). **Sparing of semantic memory in Alzheimer's disease.** *Journal of Abnormal Psychology,* 93(3), 321–330.
A number of investigators have suggested that unlike the normal elderly population, patients with Alzheimer's disease have a severe semantic-memory deficit. However, the semantic-memory tasks used in previous studies have been confounded by the heavy demands they placed on effortful processing. In the present study, 20 demented (mean age 71 yrs)

and 20 normal (mean age 69.8 yrs) elderly Ss were given a battery of episodic-memory tasks and 3 tasks that examined how intact and accessible their semantic memory was under conditions that did not require effortful processing. Although the demented Ss were greatly inferior to the normal Ss on the episodic-memory tests, they performed equally well on the semantic-memory test: The naming latency of both groups was equally facilitated by a semantic prime; the recall accuracy of both normal and demented Ss for a string of letters was similarly affected by the degree to which the string approximated English orthography; and recall accuracy for a string of words was affected equally in the 2 groups by the degree to which the word string obeyed syntactic and semantic rules. (42 ref).

698. Nestor, Paul G. (1987). **The attentional cost of preserved mental operations in normal aging and in early Alzheimer's disease.** *Dissertation Abstracts International,* 47(12-B, Pt 1), 5074–5075.

699. Nicholas, Marjorie; Obler, Loraine K.; Albert, Martin L. & Helm-Estabrooks, Nancy. (1985). **Empty speech in Alzheimer's disease and fluent aphasia.** *Journal of Speech & Hearing Research,* 28(3), 405–410.
Examined 14 measures of empty speech during a picture description task in 19 48–80 yr olds with Alzheimer's dementia (ADM), 16 48–82 yr olds with Wernicke's aphasia (WA), 8 46–65 yr olds with anomic aphasia (AAP), and 30 37–79 yr old normal controls to determine whether these groups could be distinguished on the basis of their discourse. Results show that ADM Ss were distinguished from WA Ss by their production of more empty phrases and conjunctions, whereas WA Ss produced more neologisms and more verbal and literal paraphasias. ADM Ss shared many empty speech characteristics with AAP Ss. Naming deficits, as measured by confrontation naming tasks, did not correlate with empty discourse production. (19 ref).

700. Nissen, Mary J. et al. (1985). **Spatial vision in Alzheimer's disease: General findings and a case report.** Meeting of the Association for Research in Vision and Ophthalmology (1983, Sarasota, Florida). *Archives of Neurology,* 42(7), 667–671.
Investigated whether 15 patients (aged 53–76 yrs) with Alzheimer's disease who presented with symptoms that are typical of the disease (amnesia, aphasia, and apraxia) would also show defects in visual sensitivity. Contrast sensitivity to 5 spatial frequencies was measured in Ss and in 8 normal control Ss (aged 55–75 yrs). Results indicate that Alzheimer's disease was associated with reduced sensitivity to spatial contrast, even in Ss whose primary symptoms did not involve vision. It appears that Alzheimer's disease produces a loss in sensitivity that affects thresholds for detecting coarse and fine patterns alike. A dramatic low frequency loss in an S with a severe disorder of object and face recognition confirms the importance attributed to low spatial frequency information for object and face recognition. (18 ref).

701. Norberg, Astrid; Melin, Else & Asplund, Kenneth. (1986). **Reactions to music, touch and object presentation in the final stage of dementia: An exploratory study.** *International Journal of Nursing Studies,* 23(4), 315–323.
Studied 2 Ss in the final stage of dementia of the Alzheimer type to assess the effects of music, touch, and object presentation as means of stimulation. Each S experienced 16 sessions over 12 consecutive days. Reactions of Ss were recorded via direct observations, analyses of videotape recordings, and measurement of pulse and rate of respiration. Study results indicate that the Ss had different behavioral repertoires and that they both reacted differently to music than to touch and object presentation. Future studies should investigate means of interpreting reactions of Alzheimer patients.

702. Ober, Beth A. et al. (1986). **Retrieval from semantic memory in Alzheimer-type dementia.** *Journal of Clinical & Experimental Neuropsychology,* 8(1), 75–92.
Investigated retrieval from semantic memory (measured by tasks requiring Ss to name items from a given category) in 10 mild Alzheimer-type dementia (Mild-ATD) Ss (mean age 62.3 yrs), 9 moderate-to-severe Alzheimer-type dementia (MS-ATD) Ss (mean age 64.7 yrs), and 11 normal controls (mean age 64.27 yrs). Semantic retrieval performance was shown to be highly sensitive to both the presence and the severity of ATD. Retrieval from both semantic categories and letter categories showed differences in the rate of production of correct responses between groups. These rate differences were not due to differences in accessibility of low-dominance semantic category members or low-frequency letter category members. An increase in errors and decrease in correct responses contributed to the deficits of the ATD Ss. The pattern of errors changed from Mild- to MS-ATD. Qualitative and quantitative differences were also observed in the performance of Mild- vs MS-ATD groups on a 3rd type of semantic retrieval task—the supermarket task. As performance of the ATD Ss declined on these tasks, so did their performance on other tasks assessing attention, language, and memory. Findings are discussed in terms of the progressive breakdown in both attentional and semantic memory functions that are associated with ATD. (37 ref).

703. Ober, Beth A.; Koss, Elisabeth; Friedland, Robert P. & Delis, Dean C. (1985). **Processes of verbal memory failure in Alzheimer-type dementia.** *Brain & Cognition,* 4(1), 90–103.
Compared multiple aspects of verbal learning and memory performance in 12 Ss (mean age 63.8 yrs) with mild Alzheimer-type dementia (ATD), 5 Ss (mean age 63.3 yrs) with moderate ATD, and 10 healthy Ss (mean age 63.8 yrs). H. Buschke's (1973) selective-reminding paradigm was used. Results show the following: (1) Both groups of ATD Ss depended less on long-term memory (LTM) and more on short-term memory relative to control Ss. (2) Mild-ATD Ss showed less LTM encoding than moderate-ATD Ss. (3) Moderate-ATD Ss retrieved a smaller portion of the items presumed to be encoded into LTM than did mild-ATD Ss. (4) High-imagery words increased LTM encoding and retrieval as compared to low-imagery words for moderate-ATD Ss only. Findings are explained by the inability of ATD Ss to attend to more than 1 component of the list-learning task, in conjunction with differences in the deployment of attention between mild- and moderate-ATD Ss. (44 ref).

704. O'Carroll, Ronan E. & Gilleard, C. J. (1986). **Estimation of premorbid intelligence in dementia.** *British Journal of Clinical Psychology,* 25(2), 157–158.
Administered a neuropsychological test battery to 30 Ss (aged 65–86 yrs) with dementia. 18 Ss had Alzheimer's disease, 9 Ss had multi-infarct dementia, and 3 Ss had dementia of mixed etiology. Four cognitive and behavioral measures of severity of dementia revealed no significant relationships between National Adult Reading Test or Mill Hill Vocabulary Scale—Synonym section scores and measures of severity. No differences were observed on any of the measures when Ss with Alzheimer's disease were compared with those adjudged to have multi-infarct dementia. (14 ref).

705. Østergaard, Peter K. (1985). **Capgras syndrome in senile dementia of the Alzheimer type.** *Journal of the American Geriatrics Society,* 33(11), 811.
Presents the cases of 2 women (aged 72 and 81 yrs) with senile dementia of the Alzheimer type who developed Capgras syndrome. One of the Ss believed her husband to be an imposter, while the other believed that her own body had been replaced. Pharmacological treatment (dosulepin [dothiepin HCl; 25 mg] and clomipramine and haloperidol [30 and 1 mg/day, respectively]) reduced both the syndrome and concomitant depressive symptoms. (5 ref).

706. Oyebode, J. R.; Barker, W. A.; Blessed, G.; Dick, D. J. et al. (1986). **Cognitive functioning in Parkinson's disease: In relation to prevalence of dementia and psychiatric diagnosis.** *British Journal of Psychiatry,* 149, 720–725.
43 patients (aged 53–77 yrs) with idiopathic Parkinson's disease (PD) underwent detailed cognitive assessment. Cognitive deficits typical of senile dementia of Alzheimer's type (SDAT) were found in 7% of the Ss, but most showed definite impairments not typical of SDAT. Cognitive impairment was significantly more likely in Ss with more severe PD symptoms. There was substantial agreement between the psychiatric diagnosis and the psychological picture of SDAT, and some links were found between other diagnostic categories and nature of cognitive functioning. Cognitive deficits were also found in two-thirds of the Ss with no psychiatric diagnosis.

707. Perez, F. I. et al. (1975). **Analysis of intellectual and cognitive performance in patients with multi-infarct dementia, vertebrobasilar insufficiency with dementia, and Alzheimer's disease.** *Journal of Neurology, Neurosurgery & Psychiatry,* 38(6), 533–540.
Used the WAIS to investigate the performance of a total of 42 patients, 45–85 yrs old, with multi-infarct dementia (MID), dementia due to Alzheimer's disease (AD), and vertebrobasilar insufficiency (VCI) with dementia. Significant differences in cognitive and intellectual performance were found between patients with dementia due to VBI and MID vs neuronal atrophy of the AD type. The group with AD performed significantly and consistently lower on all measures. There were no significant differences between the 2 cerebrovascular disease groups, even though the MID group performed consistently more poorly than the VBI. A discriminant function analysis classified 74% of the patients correctly based on the individual WAIS scores. The diagnosis was more easily made when tasks measuring visual motor coordination and abstract reasoning were included in the analysis. (15 ref).

708. Perez, Francisco I.; Gay, Joe R. & Taylor, Ronald L. (1975). **WAIS performance of neurologically impaired aged.** *Psychological Reports,* 37(3, Pt 2), 1043–1047.
Investigated the WAIS performance of 42 45–85 yr old inpatients with multi-infarct dementia, dementia due to Alzheimer's disease, or vertebrobasilar insufficiency with dementia. Significant differences were found between patients with vertebrobasilar insufficiency and multiple infarctions vs neuronal atrophy of the Alzheimer type. The group with Alzheimer's disease performed significantly lower on all subtests. There were no significant differences between the 2 cerebrovascular disease groups. A discriminant function analysis classified 74% of the patients correctly based on the individual WAIS scores. A step-wise regression analysis ranked Block Design and Similarities as the best discriminators.

709. Pillon, Bernard; Dubois, Bruno; Lhermitte, François & Agid, Yves. (1986). **Heterogeneity of cognitive impairment in progressive supranuclear palsy, Parkinson's disease, and Alzheimer's disease.** *Neurology,* 36(9), 1179–1185.
Analyzed patterns of cognitive and behavioral impairment in 8 patients (mean age 63.7 yrs) with progressive supranuclear palsy (PSP), Parkinson's disease (PD), and senile dementia of the Alzheimer's type (SDAT) and in controls matched for age, sex, manual laterality, educational level, and degree of intellectual deterioration. The scores of the patients were significantly lower than those of controls and were comparable on tests of verbal and visuospatial functions as well as global memory. SDAT Ss could be distinguished by the severity of verbal memory disorders, patients with PSP, and to a lesser degree those with PD, by impaired performances on tests sensitive to frontal lobe dysfunction.

710. Reisberg, Barry. (1985). **Alzheimer's disease update.** *Psychiatric Annals,* 15(5), 319–322.
Reviews the results of cross-sectional and longitudinal observations of the nature of normal aging and Alzheimer's disease (AD). Findings indicate 5 distinct phases of AD: forgetfulness, early confusion, late confusion, early dementia, and middle dementia. A global deterioration scale (GDS) for age-associated cognitive decline and AD is presented, and functional assessment staging of AD is discussed. The functional assessment stages are divided into 7 major concordant stages with the GDS as well as into further subdivisions. It is contended that the recognition of these phases represents a considerable advance in the understanding of AD since the stages enable clinicians and scientists to accurately quantify the precise magnitude of impairment in AD more readily. They also represent an advance in enabling clinicians to differentially diagnose AD. In vivo concomitants of normal aging and AD are discussed. Previous research indicates that a variety of pathological changes that occur in the normal aged brain occur to a greater extent in the brains of people with AD; these include senile plaques, neurofibrillary tangles, granulovacuolar degeneration, and cortical atrophy. (16 ref).

711. Reisberg, Barry et al. (1984). **Functional staging of dementia of the Alzheimer type.** New York Academy of Sciences: First colloquium in biological sciences (1983, New York, New York). *Annals of the New York Academy of Sciences,* 435, 481–483.
Presents data indicating 7 distinct global clinical stages of progressive cognitive decrement in normal aging and dementia of the Alzheimer's type (DAT) and 7 corresponding functional assessment (FA) stages. Two investigations, using samples of 50 and 40 outpatients (mean ages 71.2 and 70.7 yrs), correlated FA stages with Ss' performance on psychometric test measures and scores on a mental-status test. Results indicate that FA stages may assist in the rapid, accurate clinical staging of DAT. (6 ref).

712. Reisberg, Barry; Borenstein, Jeffrey; Franssen, Emile; Shulman, Emma et al. (1986). **Remediable behavioral symptomatology in Alzheimer's disease.** *Hospital & Community Psychiatry,* 37(12), 1199–1201.
The behavioral symptoms of Alzheimer's disease stem from neurochemical changes and from the psychological impact of the cognitive losses. They include paranoid and delusional ideation, hallucinations, activity disturbances (e.g., wandering, purposeless activity), aggressivity, diurnal rhythm disturbance, affective disturbance (e.g., tearfulness), and anxieties and phobias. Low-dosage neuroleptic treatment may aid in symptom relief and postpone the need to institutionalize the patient.

713. Reisberg, Barry; Ferris, Steven H.; Shulman, Emma; Steinberg, Gertrude et al. (1986). **Longitudinal course of normal aging and progressive dementia of the Alzheimer's type: A prospective study of 106 subjects over a 3.6 year mean interval.** *Progress in Neuro-Psychopharmacology & Biological Psychiatry,* 10(3–5), 571–578.
Community-residing Ss (aged 60–83 yrs) with normal aging or dementia of the Alzheimer's type (DAT) were assessed on a global deterioration scale (GDS) reflecting the continuum of cognitive dysfunction from normal aging to severe DAT. At 3½-yr follow-up, Ss were reassessed with respect to mortality, institutionalization, and clinical change (defined as at least a 2-point change on the 7-point GDS). Results suggest that patients at deterioration levels GDS greater than or equal to 4 were more likely to show negative outcomes, specifically, institutionalization, death, or clinical deterioration, than Ss from less impaired S groups. 76% of Ss at deterioration levels 4 or greater had negative outcomes at follow-up, whereas 90% of Ss with deterioration levels less than 4 did not.

714. Reisberg, Barry; Ferris, Steven H.; Franssen, Emile; Kluger, Alan et al. (1986). **Age-associated memory impairment: The clinical syndrome.** *Developmental Neuropsychology,* 2(4), 401–412.
Demonstrated mental status boundaries between age-associated memory impairment (AAMI) and progressive dementia, particularly Alzheimer's disease (AD), as suggested by M. F. Folstein et al (1975). Clinically distinguishable stages of progressive cognitive impairment in AAMI and in AD were delineated by the present 1st author and colleagues (1982). Longitudinal investigations of 106 AAMI or AD Ss (aged 60–83 yrs) by the present 1st author and colleagues (1986) suggest clinical and mental status boundaries between these conditions.

715. Rezek, Donald L. (1987). **Olfactory deficits as a neurologic sign in dementia of the Alzheimer type.** *Archives of Neurology,* 44(10), 1030–1032.
Evaluated the sense of smell of 18 patients (mean age 70 yrs) with mild dementia of the Alzheimer type (DAT), 6 "questionably" demented Ss (mean age 71.4 yrs), and 28 controls (mean age 70.4 yrs). Patients' threshold estimates for identifying 5 fragrances were higher than that of controls. When given a multiple-choice list of the test fragrances and 5 other odors, identification of odors improved in both demented and normal Ss. It is concluded that olfactory deficits are a sensitive, although nonspecific, indicator of mild DAT. Practical and diagnostic implications of testing smell in the elderly are noted.

716. Ripich, Danielle N. & Terrell, Brenda Y. (1988). **Patterns of discourse cohesion and coherence in Alzheimer's disease.** *Journal of Speech & Hearing Disorders,* 53(1), 8–15.
Compared patterns of discourse (use of propositions, cohesion devices, and judgments of coherence) in the speech of 6 well elderly and 6 patients with senile dementia of the Alzheimer type (SDAT) during topic-centered interviews. SDAT Ss used significantly more words and conversational turns. Although significant differences in propositional form and cohesion devices were not found, a pattern of cohesion disruptions in SDAT Ss was identified that is consistent with previously noted patterns of language dissolution. Coherence judgments by 4 listeners showed significant differences between the 2 groups. Breakdowns in coherence were related to 1 subtype of cohesion disruption, missing element. It is argued that SDAT results not only in the impairment of linguistic abilities but also in the impairment of discourse abilities.

717. Rosen, Wilma G.; Mohs, Richard C. & Davis, Kenneth L. (1984). **A new rating scale for Alzheimer's disease.** *American Journal of Psychiatry,* 14(11), 1356–1364.
Proposes a new rating instrument, the Alzheimer's Disease Assessment Scale, designed to evaluate the severity of cognitive and noncognitive behavioral dysfunctions characteristic of persons with Alzheimer's disease. Item descriptions, administration procedures, and scoring are outlined. 27 Ss with Alzheimer's disease (aged 54–80 yrs) and 28 normal Ss (aged 55–73 yrs) were administered the scale. Findings indicate that 21 items, 60% of which consisted of cognitive items and memory tasks, achieved significant interrater reliability and test–retest reliability and thus constituted the final scale. Scale items are appended. (32 ref).

718. Rosswurm, Mary H. (1986). **Perceptual processing deficits and short-term memory in persons with Alzheimer's disease.** *Dissertation Abstracts International,* 47(4-A), 1257.

719. Rubin, Eugene H.; Morris, John C. & Berg, Leonard. (1987). **The progression of personality changes in senile dementia of the Alzheimer's type.** *Journal of the American Geriatrics Society,* 35(8), 721–725.
Evaluated 44 patients (aged 64–81 yrs) with mild senile dementia of the Alzheimer's type (SDAT) over a 50-mo period.

Passive, agitated, and self-centered behavioral changes were noted on initial evaluation in two-thirds, one-third, and one-third, respectively, of Ss. Over the follow-up period, the percentage of Ss who exhibited agitated and self-centered behaviors doubled. The percentage of Ss who demonstrated all 3 behavioral changes increased from 11% at entry to the study (mild SDAT) to over 50% when the dementia had reached a severe stage. The presence of personality changes at a mild stage of dementia did not predispose Ss to more rapid progression to a more advanced stage of illness.

720. Rubin, Eugene H.; Morris, John C.; Storandt, Martha & Berg, Leonard. (1987). **Behavioral changes in patients with mild senile dementia of the Alzheimer's type.** *Psychiatry Research,* 21(1), 55–62.
Behavioral changes in 44 Ss with well-characterized mild senile dementia of the Alzheimer's type (SDAT) and 16 Ss with only questionable SDAT were compared with those in a control group of 58 Ss. Answers to open-ended questions and personality items from a dementia scale indicated 4 clinically useful groups: passive, agitated, self-centered, and suspicious. 75% of Ss with mild SDAT had behavioral changes compared with 10% of controls. Passive symptoms were the most common, occurring in two-thirds of mild SDAT Ss. Agitated and self-centered symptoms were common, occurring half as frequently as passive symptoms. Passive symptoms occurred alone in 25% of those with mild SDAT, whereas passive symptoms, together with agitated and/or self-centered symptoms, were present in 11–16% of Ss with mild SDAT. Agitated or self-centered symptoms rarely occurred alone.

721. Sagar, H. J.; Cohen, N. J.; Corkin, Suzanne & Growdon, J. H. (1985). **Dissociations among processes in remote memory.** *Annals of the New York Academy of Sciences,* 444, 533–535.
Examined selectivity of deficit in remote memory processes in patients with Alzheimer's disease (AD), Parkinson's disease (PD), and long-standing focal brain trauma, and in healthy controls and a patient with bilateral medial temporal-lobe resection. Remote memory for personal events and for famous public events over a 50-yr period was assessed. Results show dissociations between remote memory processes for content and temporal context in PD Ss and for encoding, storage, or retrieval of memories from different time periods in AD Ss and the resection patient; there was no dissociation between memory functions for personal and public events or between recall and recognition deficits.

722. Salmon, David P.; Shimamura, Arthur P.; Butters, Nelson & Smith, Stan. (1988). **Lexical and semantic priming deficits in patients with Alzheimer's disease.** *Journal of Clinical & Experimental Neuropsychology,* 10(4), 477–494.
In Exp I, lexical priming was assessed in 28 patients with dementia of the Alzheimer type (DAT), Huntington's disease (HD), or alcoholic Korsakoff's syndrome (KS) and in 27 intact controls. Although all 3 patient groups were impaired on tests of recall and recognition, only the DAT Ss exhibited a priming deficit on a stem-completion task. In Exp II, 38 DAT, HD, and control Ss were administered a semantic priming test. Results for this association task showed that DAT Ss were significantly less likely to produce the 2nd word of a semantically related pair than were the other S groups. It is suggested that the memory capacities of DAT patients are characterized by a breakdown in the structure of semantic memory.

723. Sano, Mary. (1987). **Attentional processes in aging and Alzheimer's disease.** *Dissertation Abstracts International,* 47(12-B, Pt 1), 5077.

724. Satz, Paul; Van Gorp, Wilfred G.; Soper, Henry V. & Mitrushina, Maura. (1987). **WAIS—R marker for dementia of the Alzheimer type? An empirical and statistical induction test.** *Journal of Clinical & Experimental Neuropsychology,* 9(6), 767–774.
Wechsler Adult Intelligence Scale—Revised (WAIS—R) scores (age-corrected) were analyzed on 149 healthy volunteers (aged 60–94 yrs) who were part of an ongoing aging study. Because only 12% of the sample revealed a specific WAIS—R subtest pattern that has been shown to occur more frequently in dementia of the Alzheimer's type (DAT) than in cases of multi-infarct dementia, the pattern's utility as a conditional marker of DAT in 3 different hypothetical clinical base rate settings was evaluated. Results provide some support for the application of this marker in certain clinical settings.

725. Schlotterer, George R. (1979). **Changes in visual information processing with normal aging and progressive dementia of the Alzheimer type.** *Dissertation Abstracts International,* 39(7-B), 3564.

726. Schultz, Kathryn A.; Schmitt, Frederick A.; Logue, Patrick E. & Rubin, David C. (1986). **Unit analysis of prose memory in clinical and elderly populations.** *Developmental Neuropsychology,* 2(2), 77–87.
Analyzed the Logical Memory subtest of the Russell revision of the Wechsler Memory Scale in older adult groups. Patients' neuropsychological test data were reviewed, and the paragraphs from the Logical Memory subtest were analyzed using unit analysis. Ss were 69 clinically diagnosed Alzheimer's patients, 13 multi-infarct dementia (MID) patients, 15 metabolic-disorder patients, 14 head-injury cases, 14 affective disorder patients, and 37 healthy adults (mean ages 62.81, 58.77, 51.43, 40.29, 50.29, and 66.51 yrs respectively). Quantitative analyses of recall revealed group differences, with normal and affective disorder patients having the best recall scores and MID and Alzheimer patients the poorest. Qualitative analysis of which memory units were recalled, however, showed similarities in memory processing among the groups.

727. Sciara, Anthony D. (1986). **Hospital-based neuropsychological services.** *Psychiatric Hospital,* 17(3), 140–142.
Contends that hospital-based neuropsychological testing services may offer the opportunity of evaluating patients with brain damage and concomitant emotional problems, those with Alzheimer's disease, and those with substance abuse induced deficits. In addition, services may be marketed to attorneys, neurologists, and neurosurgeons.

728. Serby, Michael. (1986). **Olfaction and Alzheimer's disease.** *Progress in Neuro-Psychopharmacology & Biological Psychiatry,* 10(3–5), 579–586.
Suggests that disturbances in the sense of smell may be important both clinically and theoretically in Alzheimer's disease. The neuroanatomical and neurochemical bases for this disturbance are discussed. It is concluded that the effect of aging per se on olfactory performance cannot be assessed without rigorous control for cognitive dysfunction in sampled populations.

729. Shekim, Lana O. (1985). **Production of discourse in individuals with Alzheimer's disease.** *Dissertation Abstracts International,* 45(7-B), 2127.

730. Shimamura, Arthur P.; Salmon, David P.; Squire, Larry R. & Butters, Nelson. (1987). **Memory dysfunction and word priming in dementia and amnesia.** *Behavioral Neuroscience,* 101(3), 347–351.
Memory performance of patients with the clinical diagnosis of Alzheimer's disease was compared with performance of patients with alcoholic Korsakoff's syndrome and patients with Huntington's disease. Although all patient groups exhibited impairment on tests of verbal memory, only patients

with Alzheimer's disease exhibited priming. Priming is an unconscious expression of recently encountered material, and it is intact even in severely amnesic patients. Because mildly demented patients with Alzheimer's disease exhibited impaired priming, damage to brain structures in addition to those damaged in the amnesic syndrome must occur at a relatively early stage of the disease process.

731. Shindler, Andrea G.; Caplan, Louis R. & Hier, Daniel B. (1984). **Intrusions and perseverations.** *Brain & Language,* 23(1), 148–158.
22 Ss with presumed senile dementia of the Alzheimer's type (SDAT), 22 with dementia other than SDAT, 20 with aphasia, and 17 healthy controls over 50 yrs of age were examined for intrusions and perseverations. Perseverations were defined as the immediate inappropriate repetition of a prior response, whereas intrusions were defined as the inappropriate repetition of prior responses after intervening stimuli. Results indicate that intrusions and perseverations occurred in demented and aphasic Ss, but were rare in controls. Intrusions occurred most often in Ss with SDAT or Wernicke aphasia, but also in Ss with dementia other than SDAT. Intrusions were not correlated with dementia severity. It is asserted that intrusions cannot be considered pathognomonic of SDAT: They occurred when Ss were unable to access correct responses from long-term memory and instead substituted erroneous responses selected from short-term memory. Perseverations were most common in the Wernicke aphasics and Ss with dementia due to communicating hydrocephalus. Although frontal lobe dysfunction is prominent in communicating hydrocephalus, it was absent in cases of Wernicke aphasia. Findings confirm prior suggestions that perseveration can occur in the absence of frontal lobe injury. Low correlations were found between intrusions and perseverations, suggesting that these seemingly similar behaviors are distinct and are probably produced by separate neuropsychological mechanisms. (27 ref).

732. Shomaker, Dianna. (1987). **Problematic behavior and the Alzheimer patient: Retrospection as a method of understanding and counseling.** *Gerontologist,* 27(3), 370–375.
Examined continuity of behaviors across a lifespan in 9 patients (aged 60–90 yrs) with Alzheimer's disease. Interviews with family members of the patients revealed, not as expected by the families, continuity of behavior patterns from before until after onset of dementia. Frequency and intensity of some past behaviors apparently increased, and their expression became inappropriate. It is suggested that an understanding of the relationship between behavior before the onset of disease and afterwards is helpful in counseling patients' families.

733. Shore, David; Overman, Carol A. & Wyatt, Richard J. (1983). **Improving accuracy in the diagnosis of Alzheimer's disease.** *Journal of Clinical Psychiatry,* 44(6), 207–212.
Describes the cases of 3 patients (aged 48–64 yrs) incorrectly diagnosed as having Alzheimer's disease. Certain objective tests of dementia (the Extended Scale for Dementia, Mini-Mental Status) and language functions (the Porch Index of Communicative Ability), as well as the London Psychogeriatric Rating Scale (completed by a family member), have been found useful and are described briefly. The importance of reevaluating demented patients to document the course of their illness is emphasized to improve the accuracy of diagnosis in suspected cases of Alzheimer's disease. (34 ref).

734. Shuttleworth, Edwin C. & Huber, Steven J. (1988). **The naming disorder of dementia of Alzheimer type.** *Brain & Language,* 34(2), 222–234.
Investigated the characteristics of the naming disorder (anomia) of dementia of the Alzheimer type (DAT) in 20 patients (mean age 66.8 yrs) divided into a mild and a moderate-severe group. Ss' difficulties in naming real objects and object drawings were examined. Results indicate the presence of a progressive anomia that was sensitive both to word frequency and to image quality. Although the proportion of perceptual-recognition and aphasic errors in the DAT Ss was similar to that in 25 age- and education-matched normal controls, evidence suggests that variations in the character of the anomia existed among individual DAT Ss.

735. Skelton-Robinson, M. & Jones, S. (1984). **Nominal dysphasia and the severity of senile dementia.** *British Journal of Psychiatry,* 145, 168–171.
Investigated the relationship between the degree of senile dementia and the severity of naming difficulties in order to determine whether naming problems are caused principally by agnosia. 20 Ss, aged 69–88 yrs, who had been diagnosed as suffering from dementia participated. Two were males, and 18 were females. The Ss were assessed using the Behavior Rating scale of the Clifton Assessment Procedures for the Elderly, an information/memory/concentration test, and a confrontation-naming test. Results indicate that the degree of nominal dysphasia shown by a patient may be a reliable index of the severity of dementia, as measured by both behavioral and cognitive rating scales. The confrontation-naming test approach to the assessment and severity of senile dementia (Alzheimer's type) may avoid 2 confounding factors (premorbid intellectual ability and cooperation of the S at interview) that influence the results of current psychological tests of dementia. (17 ref).

736. Skurla, Ellen; Rogers, Joan C. & Sunderland, Trey. (1988). **Direct assessment of activities of daily living in Alzheimer's disease: A controlled study.** *Journal of the American Geriatrics Society,* 36(2), 97–103.
Studied the relationship between severity of dementia and performance in 4 experimental tasks in 9 patients (aged 45–73 yrs) with Alzheimer's disease (AD) and 9 age-, gender-, and education-matched controls. The experimental tasks were developed in order to establish a direct measure of functional performance in common activities of daily living. In the AD Ss, significant but moderate positive associations were found between a clinical dementia rating scale (CDR), a comprehensive rating tool designed specifically for AD, and performance on the experimental tasks. A significant correlation was also found between the results of the Short Portable Mental Status Questionnaire (SPMSQ), a less specific dementia assessment instrument, and the CDR but not between the SPMSQ and the performance measure. When compared to normal Ss, the cognitively impaired Ss required more assistance and time in completing the tasks. The findings support the conclusion that severity of dementia and performance on activities of daily living tasks are related but distinct concepts and should be measured separately.

737. Smith, Wanda L. (1986). **An examination of reinforcer identification and stimulus discrimination in elderly individuals with Alzheimer's disease.** *Dissertation Abstracts International,* 47(4-B), 1764.

738. Snodgrass, Joan G. & Corwin, June. (1988). **Pragmatics of measuring recognition memory: Applications to dementia and amnesia.** *Journal of Experimental Psychology: General,* 117(1), 34–50.
This article has 2 purposes: The first is to describe 4 theoretical models of yes–no recognition memory and present their associated measures of discrimination and response bias. These models are then applied to a set of data from normal Ss to determine which pairs of discrimination and bias indices show independence between discrimination and bias. The 2nd purpose is to use the indices from the acceptable models to characterize recognition memory deficits in dementia and amnesia. Young normal Ss, Alzheimer's disease patients, and parkinsonian dementia patients were tested with

80

picture recognition tasks with repeated study–test trials. Huntington's disease patients, mixed etiology amnesics, and age-matched normals were tested by Butters, Wolfe, Martone, Granholm, and Cermak (1985) using the same paradigm with word stimuli. Three major points are emphasized: First, any index of recognition memory performance assumes an underlying model. Second, even acceptable models can lead to different conclusions about patterns of learning and forgetting. Third, efforts to characterize and ameliorate abnormal memory should address both discrimination and bias deficits.

739. Sokolchik, E. I. (1986). **Affective disturbances in Alzheimer's disease.** *Zhurnal Nevropatologii i Psikhiatrii,* 86(9), 1376–1380.
Studied the course and clinical picture of depressive and other affective disorders in 21 54–75 yr olds with Alzheimer's disease and in 11 67–83 yr olds with senile dementia. The age at disease onset, circumstances surrounding the appearance of depressive symptoms, and the rate of development and severity of affective disorders were studied in the 2 groups. (English abstract).

740. Spear, Susan E. (1985). **Breakdown of the use of names in Alzheimer's Disease: An information-processing approach.** *Dissertation Abstracts International,* 45(7-B), 2344.

741. Sreenivasan, Shoba. (1987). **A longitudinal examination of electrophysiological and neuropsychological variables as predictors of decline in Senile Dementia Alzheimer's type.** *Dissertation Abstracts International,* 48(3-B), 891.

742. Steffes, Robert & Thralow, Joan. (1987). **Visual field limitation in the patient with dementia of the Alzheimer's type.** *Journal of the American Geriatrics Society,* 35(3), 198–204.
Investigated the existence of a visual field limitation and its effect on the patient with advanced Alzheimer's disease (AD), using 12 AD patients and 12 control patients demented from causes secondary to reasons other than AD. Ss were aged 37–86 yrs. Results indicate that Ss demented due to AD had visual field losses significantly greater than other demented Ss. It is suggested that the significant visual loss is of importance in assisting in differential diagnosis, performing patient care, and planning patient environments.

743. Storandt, Martha et al. (1984). **Psychometric differentiation of mild senile dementia of the Alzheimer type.** *Archives of Neurology,* 41(5), 497–499.
Describes the development of a battery of 4 psychological tests that can be administered in 10 min and that was developed to successfully classify 98% of patients with mild dementia of the Alzheimer's type and healthy older persons matched for age, sex, and social position. Only 2 of 84 persons (ages 63–84 yrs) were misclassified. The 4 tests are the Logical Memory and Mental Control subtests of the Wechsler Memory Scale, the Trailmaking Test—Form A, and word fluency for the letters *S* and *P*. (17 ref).

744. Storrie, Michael C. & Doerr, Hans O. (1980). **Characterization of Alzheimer Type Dementia utilizing an abbreviated Halstead-Reitan battery.** *Clinical Neuropsychology,* 2(2), 78–82.
An abbreviated version of the Halstead-Reitan Neuropsychological Test Battery can be administered successfully to patients with an Alzheimer-type dementia (ATD). The battery provides quantitative documentation of neuropsychological impairment manifested clinically by these individuals. While WAIS subscores were not particularly helpful in the characterization of ATD relative to other types of diffuse brain damage, ATD patients exhibited particular difficulty with the Category Test but showed well-preserved finger-tapping ability. (10 ref).

745. Strauss, Milton E.; Weingartner, Herbert & Thompson, Karen. (1985). **Remembering words and how often they occurred in memory-impaired patients.** *Memory & Cognition,* 13(6), 507–510.
Examined memory in 7 Korsakoff's (KD), 13 Huntington's (HD), and 9 Alzheimer's (SDAT) patients (aged 31–69 yrs) and 17 50–67 yr old normal controls, using measures that permit the separate examination of aspects of cognitive operations that are effort-demanding and those that appear to occur more automatically in learning and memory operations. All 3 of the clinical groups demonstrated dysfunctions in memory-learning processes that normally can be accomplished automatically. The effort-demanding memory performance of KD and HD Ss, but not of SDAT Ss, reflected how often an event occurred in a manner similar to that of normal age-matched controls. Data indicate that SDAT Ss were unable to monitor event frequency and unable to make use of repetition as aid in encoding. Data also indicate that each of the patient groups demonstrated obvious and profound disturbance in memory under attention-effort demanding conditions. (15 ref).

746. Sulkava, Raimo & Amberla, Kaarina. (1982). **Alzheimer's disease and senile dementia of Alzheimer type: A neuropsychological study.** *Acta Neurologica Scandinavica,* 65(6), 651–660.
Investigated neuropsychological performance in 36 presenile patients with Alzheimer's disease and 35 patients with senile dementia of Alzheimer type by using the Finnish version of the Luria Neuropsychological Test Battery. The most deteriorated performances in both groups were in memory, intellectual functions, higher visual and motor functions, and orientation. The neuropsychological functions deteriorated gradually in the course of the disease process so that the shape of the performance profile was preserved. The progression of the disease seemed to be more rapid in senile patients; but neuropsychologically, there were no significant differences between Alzheimer's disease and senile dementia of Alzheimer type. They seemed to form a continuum of one disease. In early stages, the disease is characterized by lowered activity, disorientation, and paranoia. Apraxic, agnosic, and aphasic disorders appear next. In the advanced stages, only some basic automatic functions are preserved. (20 ref).

747. Sullivan, Edith V.; Corkin, Suzanne & Growdon, John H. (1986). **Verbal and nonverbal short-term memory in patients with Alzheimer's disease and in healthy elderly subjects.** *Developmental Neuropsychology,* 2(4), 387–400.
Examined the component processes of deteriorating short-term memory in patients with Alzheimer's disease (AD). 14 AD Ss (aged 57–76 yrs), whose dementia ranged from mild to severe, and 10 healthy Ss (aged 52–76 yrs) received a distractor task used by J. Brown (1958) and L. R. Peterson and M. J. Peterson (1959), in which class of material, number of memoranda, and agent of forgetting were manipulated. AD Ss showed significant forgetting with shorter intervals and smaller memory loads than healthy Ss when distraction was present; without distraction, AD Ss' recall of nonverbal material was impaired, which may be attributable to greater task difficulty and to a diminished rehearsal capacity. Data from individual Ss suggest that verbal and nonverbal systems can deteriorate independently.

748. Swindell, Carol S. (1986). **Expressive language disturbance in probable Alzheimer's disease.** *Dissertation Abstracts International,* 47(6-B), 2400–2401.

749. Tamminga, C. A.; Foster, N. L.; Fedio, P.; Bird, E. D. et al. (1987). **Alzheimer's disease: Low cerebral somatostatin levels correlate with impaired cognitive function and cortical metabolism.** *Neurology,* 37(1), 161–165.
Somatostatinlike immunoreactivity in the cerebrospinal fluid (CSF) from 24 Alzheimer patients (mean age 60 yrs) was

significantly lower than in that from 24 controls (mean age 59 yrs). The degree of reduction correlated with indices of intellectual impairment and decline in cortical glucose utilization as determined by positron emission tomography. There was a close association between reduction in CSF somatostatin and glucose hypometabolism in the parietal lobe. In postmortem cortical tissue from 8 Alzheimer Ss somatostatin levels were lower in posterior parietal but not in anterior frontal cortex, suggesting that loss of somatostatin-containing neurons, especially in the parietal association cortex, may be a critical determinant for Alzheimer dementia.

750. Tariot, Pierre et al. (1985). **How memory fails: A theoretical model.** Special Issue: Alzheimer's disease. *Geriatric Nursing,* 6(3), 144–147.
Discusses memory impairment and relates it to the broad definition of dementia. There are numerous theories about how memory fails—the approach of the present article is to identify systems that may be distinct physiologically, biologically, and theoretically. The breakdown is necessarily schematic, emphasizing distinctions for clarity while recognizing that these symptoms presumably overlap. A theoretical outline (model) of some component processes that affect memory functions (episodic and semantic memory, failures of episodic memory, and effortful and automatic processes) is applied to show how memory fails in different ways in illnesses (Alzheimer's disease, Korsakoff's disease, and depression) in which superficially similar kinds of memory failure can occur. Conclusions regarding these diseases and memory function are presented, and therapeutic and rehabilitative implications of this model are discussed. (3 ref).

751. Teng, Evelyn L.; Chui, Helena C.; Schneider, Lon S. & Metzger, Laura E. (1987). **Alzheimer's dementia: Performance on the Mini-Mental State Examination.** *Journal of Consulting & Clinical Psychology,* 55(1), 96–100.
The performance of 141 Alzheimer's patients on the Mini-Mental State Examination was analyzed. Performance on all items showed significant negative correlation with the duration of illness. The most difficult item was "recall," and little improvement in recall was obtained with cuing. The second-most-difficult item was "copy a design." Only 3% of the patients passed both items. The early-onset group (age < 65 yrs) performed more poorly than the late-onset group (aged ≥ 65 yrs) on items that tested for language and visuoconstructive abilities, but scores for both groups showed comparable rates of decline with the duration of illness. (16 ref).

752. Teri, Linda. (1986). **Severe cognitive impairments in older adults.** *Behavior Therapist,* 9(3), 51–54.
Discusses (1) general information regarding severe cognitive impairment in older adults, (2) assessment of cognition in senile dementia of the Alzheimer's type (SDAT), and (3) behavioral assessment of SDAT. Recent research findings are also discussed with regard to the presence of behavioral disturbance in SDAT and the relationship of such disturbance to disease characteristics. Behavioral problems affected a significant portion of patients and seemed related to severity of cognitive impairment rather than to other disease or patient characteristics.

753. Teri, Linda; Larson, Eric B. & Reifler, Burton V. (1988). **Behavioral disturbance in dementia of the Alzheimer's type.** *Journal of the American Geriatrics Society,* 36(1), 1–6.
Investigated the relationship between level of cognitive impairment and nature of behavioral disturbance in 127 60–94 yr old patients with dementia of the Alzheimer's type. A standardized dementia rating scale and a checklist of behavioral problems were employed. Results indicate that (a) problems significantly increased with increased cognitive impairment; (b) problems reported varied with cognitive severity; and (c) behavioral problems were not significantly associated

with age, gender, duration, or age at onset of dementia. It is suggested that problems associated with impairment (such as wandering, agitation, and incontinence) are characteristic of the disease and should be incorporated into education and intervention programs; problems not associated with impairment (such as hallucinations and irrational suspicions) should be addressed on an individual basis.

754. Thal, Leon J.; Grundman, Michael & Golden, Robert. (1986). **Alzheimer's disease: A correlational analysis of the Blessed Information-Memory-Concentration Test and the Mini-Mental State Exam.** *Neurology,* 36(2), 262–264.
Conducted a correlational analysis of the scores on G. Blessed and colleagues' (1968) Information-Memory-Concentration Test and the Mini-Mental State Exam in 40 patients (aged 50–90 yrs) with Alzheimer's disease. The average product moment correlation coefficient between the 2 tests on repeated administration over 6 wks ranged from –0.73 to –0.83. Both tests demonstrated test–retest reliability coefficients of 0.75 and above. A formula was developed to convert one test score to the other. (8 ref).

755. Tierney, Mary C.; Snow, William G.; Reid, David W.; Zorzitto, Maria L. et al. (1987). **Psychometric differentiation of dementia: Replication and extension of the findings of Storandt and coworkers.** *Archives of Neurology,* 44(7), 720–722.
Analyzes data derived from a 2-yr, prospective study using measures similar to those of M. Storandt et al (1984) to test 72 patients (mean age 74.4 yrs) with senile dementia of the Alzheimer type (SDAT), 52 patients (mean age 73.6 yrs) with other dementias, and 42 normal controls (mean age 69.9 yrs). Ss were administered 4 neuropsychological tests (2 subtests of the Wechsler Memory Scale and measures of trailmaking and word fluency). Results replicate the findings of Storandt and colleagues in that the 4 tests distinguished Ss with SDAT from normal controls. To a lesser extent, the tests also accurately distinguished between the controls and Ss with other dementias.

756. Tsushima, William T. & Pang, Dawn B. (1987). **Neuropsychological test performance in Alzheimer's disease: An 11-year case study.** *International Journal of Clinical Neuropsychology,* 9(3), 120–124.
Presents an 11-yr case study of a woman who initially reported memory difficulties at age 66 yrs and who was finally diagnosed as having Alzheimer's disease at age 77 yrs. The S submitted to annual medical examinations and 4 neuropsychological examinations, as well as other neurodiagnostic procedures. Neuropsychological tests were found to be more sensitive to changes in her condition than other neurodiagnostic techniques. It is suggested that a comprehensive examination, test–retest data, and behavioral observation are needed in the early evaluation of Alzheimer's disease.

757. Tuokko, H. & Crockett, D. (1987). **Central cholinergic deficiency WAIS profiles in a nondemented aged sample.** *Journal of Clinical & Experimental Neuropsychology,* 9(2), 225–227.
P. A. Fuld (1984) described a Wechsler Adult Intelligence Scale (WAIS) profile associated with drug-induced cholinergic deficiency in young adults and dementia of the Alzheimer's type. The frequency of occurrence of this profile was examined in 74 healthy elderly persons (aged 50–90 yrs) who were administered the WAIS. Results suggest that the profile rarely occurs in independently functioning elderly persons, thus lending support to Fuld's findings that the profile may be relatively specific to dementia of the Alzheimer's type. Hypotheses as to the significance of this index of pathology are discussed.

758. Uhlmann, Richard F.; Larson, Eric B. & Koepsell, Thomas D. (1986). **Hearing impairment and cognitive decline in senile dementia of the Alzheimer's type.** *Journal of the American Geriatrics Society,* 34(3), 207–210.
Tested the hypothesis that auditory status is a predictor of cognitive functional decline in senile dementia of the Alzheimer's type (SDA) in 156 SDA patients, aged 60+ yrs, who received a comprehensive medical evaluation including baseline screening for hearing impairment with the finger friction test and serial assessment of cognitive function with the Mini-Mental State Examination. Age and cognitive function at entry to the study were greater among 36 Ss with impaired hearing than among 120 normal Ss. The demographic profiles of the impaired and normal hearing groups were otherwise similar, as was the prevalence of depression. Intervening mortality rates were nearly identical. Decline in cognitive function 1 yr later was nearly twice as great in the impaired hearing group, even when controlled for age and initial cognitive function. Results suggest that hearing impairment may be a prognostic indicator for subsequent cognitive dysfunction in SDA and are consistent with the hypothesized relationship between hearing impairment and dementia in SDA. (22 ref).

759. Van der Loos, Judy I. (1987). **The structure of spontaneous language production in Alzheimer's, Huntington's and Parkinson's Disease.** *Dissertation Abstracts International,* 47(12-B, Pt 1), 4783.

760. Vitaliano, Peter P. et al. (1984). **Memory, attention, and functional status in community-residing Alzheimer type dementia patients and optimally healthy aged individuals.** *Journal of Gerontology,* 39(1), 58–64.
Two investigations examined patterns of cognitive performance in 23 healthy elderly controls, 18 mildly impaired patients with senile dementia of the Alzheimer type (SDAT), and 16 moderately impaired SDAT patients. All Ss were aged 53–88 yrs. The degree to which cognitive test scores could predict functional performance was also examined. The Mini-Mental State Examination and the Dementia Rating Scale were used to assess attention, calculation, recognition memory, recall, and orientation. Functional competence measures included maintenance, communication, and recreational abilities. Exp I showed that the attention and memory factors that best distinguished controls from mildly impaired Ss (recall and orientation) differed from those that best distinguished mildly from moderately impaired Ss (recognition and attention). Exp II indicated that it was possible to predict behavioral competence in Ss with dementia from knowledge of their attentional and memory deficits. (24 ref).

761. Vitaliano, Peter P. et al. (1986). **Functional decline in the early stages of Alzheimer's disease.** *Psychology & Aging,* 1(1), 41–46.
Reports a 2-yr follow-up of 15 Alzheimer's disease (AD) patients (mean age 67.8 yrs) characterized by mild functional impairment and 22 age-, sex-, and education-matched controls. In a previous cross-sectional study by P. Prinz et al (1982) of these 37 Ss and 16 AD patients (mean age 70.2 yrs) with moderate functional impairment, measures of memory and attention deficits accounted for much of the impairment observed in functional competence. The current longitudinal study found that these same initial assessments could be used to predict functional decline in the 15 mildly impaired Ss, who were observed to decline to levels similar to those of the 16 moderate patients. In contrast, the controls exhibited little decline during the same period. Results affirm that it is possible to diagnose AD in its mild form and demonstrate the validity of the initial diagnosis. (21 ref).

762. Volicer, Ladislav; Seltzer, Benjamin; Rheaume, Yvette; Fabiszewski, Kathy et al. (1987). **Progression of Alzheimer-type dementia in institutionalized patients: A cross-sectional study.** *Journal of Applied Gerontology,* 6(1), 83–94.
Evaluated 88 institutionalized patients (aged 57–87 yrs) with dementia of the Alzheimer type (DAT). Ratings of speech, cooperation, social contact, and communication were in the very low range in Ss with DAT duration of 3 yrs or longer, while the rating of mood was similar regardless of DAT duration. Half of the Ss were unable to dress themselves 5 yrs after onset of symptoms and unable to sleep regularly 6 yrs after onset. By 7 yrs, 50% had developed rigidity on passive movement, and by 8 yrs half were unable to feed themselves and walk without assistance. By 9 to 10 yrs, 50% had developed contractures of the limbs and were mute.

763. Warner, M. Dhyanne; Peabody, Cecilia A.; Flattery, Jennifer J. & Tinklenberg, Jared R. (1986). **Olfactory deficits and Alzheimer's disease.** *Biological Psychiatry,* 21(1), 116–118.
17 Ss (aged 55–82 yrs) with primary degenerative dementia (Alzheimer's disease) at an early stage and 17 normal controls were administered a scratch-and-sniff test of olfactory function. Results suggest that an olfactory deficit may be one of the earlier symptoms of Alzheimer's disease. Problems that can be caused by an olfactory deficit are discussed. (11 ref).

764. Weiner, Mark J.; Hallett, Mark & Funkenstein, H. Harris. (1983). **Adaptation to lateral displacement of vision in patients with lesions of the central nervous system.** *Neurology,* 33(6), 766–772.
Studied the visual-motor adaptation to lateral displacement of vision by prism glasses in 25 normal individuals and 52 patients with cerebellar dysfunction, Parkinson's disease, right or left cerebral hemisphere lesions, Alzheimer's disease, or Korsakoff's syndrome. Adaptation was analyzed in 2 phases: the return to normal pointing with prism glasses in place (the "error reduction portion") and the mispointing in the opposite direction after the glasses were removed (the "negative aftereffect portion"). Negative aftereffect, which seems to be the best measure of true adaptation, was significantly reduced only for the Ss with cerebellar dysfunction. This poor performance supports the involvement of the cerebellum in motor learning. (23 ref).

765. Weingartner, Herbert et al. (1983). **Forms of memory failure.** *Science,* 221(4608), 380–382.
Contrasted aspects of episodic and semantic memory by comparing the determinants of 8 patients (mean age 57 yrs) with Korsakoff's disease (KD) with 8 patients (mean age 58 yrs) with progressive degenerative dementia (PD), probably of an Alzheimer's type. Ss and 8 controls (mean age 61 yrs) completed the Wechsler Memory Scale and experimental measures of episodic memory. Ss with KD demonstrated global memory deficits similar to those seen in PD Ss. KD Ss could recall rules and principles for organizing information and gain access to their previously acquired knowledge (semantic memory), whereas recent memory was grossly impaired. In contrast, PD Ss had little access to previously acquired knowledge and therefore great difficulty in organizing and encoding ongoing events. Implications for the development of therapeutic strategies for cognitive impairments are discussed. (34 ref).

766. Weingartner, Herbert. (1986). **The roots of failure.** *Psychology Today,* 20(1), 6–7.
Discusses the present authors' studies of people with a variety of different forms of memory impairment that have been conducted in the hope of discovering some of the relationships between changes in brain function and the specific ways memory can fail. These studies include comparing people with Alzheimer's, Huntington's, and Korsakoff's diseases; ex-

amining how drugs that disrupt specific brain systems change cognitive processes; and investigating how drugs might be useful in reversing the types of memory failure associated with various diseases.

767. Weinstein, Barbara E. & Amsel, Lynn. (1987). **Hearing impairment and cognitive function in Alzheimer's disease.** *Journal of the American Geriatrics Society,* 35(3), 274–275.
Comments on R. Uhlmann and colleagues' (1986) article on hearing impairment and cognitive decline in senile dementia of the Alzheimer's type, by arguing that due to the study's methodological limitations, the relationship between hearing impairment and cognitive function in Alzheimer's disease remains open to question.

768. Welden, S. & Hall, D. (1986). **Dementia differentiation: AD & SDAT.** *Clinical Gerontologist,* 4(3), 66–69.
Describes a test of linguistic behaviors for distinguishing what is claimed to be an overdiagnosed group of patients with Alzheimer's disease (AD) or senile dementia of the Alzheimer type (SDAT). It is argued that approximately 67% of presently diagnosed Alzheimer patients are actually members of a 2nd group whose prognosis is much more benign and who appear amenable to psychotherapeutic or pharmacological intervention.

769. Wilson, Robert S. et al. (1982). **Facial recognition memory in dementia.** *Cortex,* 18(3), 329–336.
Previous investigations of memory in senile dementia of the Alzheimer's type (SDAT) have focused on verbal learning and memory. The aim of the present study was to determine whether the amnesia of SDAT is limited to verbal material. 29 patients with SDAT (mean age 69.3 yrs) and 41 healthy normal controls (mean age 69.3 yrs) were given a test of facial perception and 2 recognition memory tasks, one for words and the other for faces. Results indicate that dementia Ss showed a deficit in the retention of facial information. This deficit could not be attributed to faulty initial perception or to a response bias. The verbal and facial memory deficits in SDAT differed: Performance on tests of verbal and facial memory was relatively independent, and substantial encoding and linguistic defects contributed to only the verbal memory disorder resulting in more severe impairment on verbal memory tests. Implications for research on the neuropharmacology and pathophysiology of SDAT are discussed. (20 ref).

770. Wilson, Robert S. et al. (1983). **Word frequency effect and recognition memory in dementia of the Alzheimer type.** *Journal of Clinical Neuropsychology,* 5(2), 97–104.
Normal persons show better recognition memory for rare than for common words. Exp I examined this word frequency effect in 17 patients (mean age 69.9 yrs) with dementia of the Alzheimer type (DAT) and 20 normal controls (mean age 68 yrs). DAT Ss showed a normal tendency to false alarm to common words but failed to show the normal rare-word advantage in their hit rate. In Exp II, memory was studied in 19 normal Ss, aged 20–60 yrs, immediately following list presentation and after a delay of 1 wk, when it was approximately equivalent to that of DAT Ss. There was no attenuation of the usual rare-word advantage. Findings suggest that DAT Ss fail to encode the featural and intrastructural elements of to-be-remembered verbal information and that this processing deficit may contribute to their impaired recognition memory performance. (24 ref).

771. Wilson, Robert S.; Bacon, Lynd D.; Fox, Jacob H. & Kaszniak, Alfred W. (1983). **Primary memory and secondary memory in dementia of the Alzheimer type.** *Journal of Clinical Neuropsychology,* 5(4), 337–344.
Investigated free recall of word lists in 47 patients (mean age 68.2 yrs) with dementia of the Alzheimer type (DAT) and 31 normal controls of equivalent age and education. Recall was divided into primary memory (PM) and secondary memory

(SM) components based on the number of items intervening between presentation and recall. Patients showed a greater deficit on the SM than on the PM measure, and there was little evidence of proactive interference in the patient group. The PM and SM measures were independent in the controls but not in the patient group, and the size of patients' PM deficit increased linearly with greater numbers of items between presentation and attempted recall. Findings suggest that the memory disorder of DAT is partially the result of defective PM, which also places limits on the input available for SM processing. (29 ref).

772. Winogrond, Iris R. & Fisk, Albert A. (1983). **Alzheimer's disease: Assessment of functional status.** *Journal of the American Geriatrics Society,* 31(12), 780–785.
Assessed the cognitive, psychologic, and behavioral functioning of 17 adults with Alzheimer's disease who were enrolled in a daycare program for Alzheimer's patients. Measures included assessments of Ss' orientation, attention and concentration, global cognitive and language functions, global cognitive function and psychomotor speed, abstract thinking, judgment and information, and overall cognitive functioning. It is noted that such data are useful in determining realistic expectations of patient function by family and staff. Results show that testing established a statistically significant association between cognitive and behavioral functions, and between morale and behavioral function; however, only modest correlations between cognitive and psychologic functions emerged. (38 ref).

773. Zigman, Warren B.; Schupf, Nicole; Lubin, Robert A. & Silverman, Wayne P. (1987). **Premature regression of adults with Down syndrome.** *American Journal of Mental Deficiency,* 92(2), 161–168.
Compared the adaptive skills of 2,144 Ss (aged 20–69 yrs) with Down's syndrome (DS) with those of 4,172 age-matched, developmentally disabled Ss without DS. Activities of daily living and cognitive skills were examined across etiology, age group, and level of mental retardation. Results show that for DS Ss at all levels of retardation, adaptive competence declined with increasing age to a greater extent than for controls. Clear age-related deficits associated with DS were observed only in Ss aged 50+ yrs. Findings support previous evidence of an increased risk for the clinical signs of Alzheimer's disease among people with DS; however, signs of dementia appeared later in life than would be predicted from available neuropathological data.

Physiological Aspects

774. Abalan, François; Barberger-Gateau, Pascale; Maciet, Gérard & Dartigues, Jean-François. (1987). **Plasma volume in senile and presenile Alzheimer's disease.** *Biological Psychiatry,* 22(1), 114–115.
Among 30 72–95 yr old patients with senile dementia of the Alzheimer type (SDAT), hematocrit, hemoglobin, and plasma protein levels differed between the 1st and 3rd week of hospitalization. The possible role of dehydration or malnutrition as a cause or consequence of SDAT is discussed.

775. Adem, Abdu; Nordberg, Agneta; Bucht, Gösta & Winblad, Bengt. (1986). **Extraneural cholinergic markers in Alzheimer's and Parkinson's disease.** *Progress in Neuro-Psychopharmacology & Biological Psychiatry,* 10(3–5), 247–257.
Analyzed muscarinic and nicotinic binding sites in lymphocytes from 30 patients with Alzheimer's disease, multi-infarct dementia, and Parkinson's disease and from 13 age-matched controls. A significant decrease in the number of both muscarinic and nicotinic binding sites was obtained in lymphocytes from Alzheimer Ss, while in Parkinson Ss a

significant decrease was found only in the nicotinic binding sites. No change was observed in cholinesterase activity in plasma from Alzheimer Ss, whereas a significant decrease in plasma cholinesterase activity was found in Parkinson Ss.

776. Bajalan, A. A.; Wright, C. E. & Van der Vliet, V. J. (1986). **Changes in the human visual evoked potential caused by the anticholinergic agent hyoscine hydrobromide: Comparison with results in Alzheimer's disease.** *Journal of Neurology, Neurosurgery & Psychiatry,* 49(2), 175–182.
Investigated the effect of the anticholinergic drug of hyoscine hydrobromide (HHB) on the visual evoked potential (VEP) of 10 normal Ss (aged 21–37 yrs). The flash and pattern reversal VEP was compared before injecting Ss with HHB (0.6 mg, subcutaneously), during the period of maximum effect and 24 hrs after injection. HHB produced a slowing of P2 and N3 components of the flash VEP in Ss but did not affect the pattern reversal VEP. Results, which are similar to those found in Alzheimer's disease, may be explained by an underlying defect of the cholinergic system. (32 ref).

777. Balldin, Jan et al. (1983). **Dexamethasone suppression test and serum prolactin in dementia disorders.** *British Journal of Psychiatry,* 143, 277–281.
Performed the dexamethasone suppression test (DST) on 21 patients with dementia of the Alzheimer type (DAT), 11 patients with multi-infarct dementia (MI), and 14 healthy controls. 12 of the DAT Ss and 8 MI Ss showed abnormal lack of suppression, compared with just 1 member of the control group. Abnormal DST was related to dementia as such and not to age or depression or to levels of CSF monoamine metabolites. (18 ref).

778. Berg, Leonard. (1985). **Does Alzheimer's disease represent an exaggeration of normal aging?** *Archives of Neurology,* 42(8), 737–739.
Presents evidence in gross anatomy, histology, chemistry, physiology, clinical assessment, psychometrics, and epidemiology in order to compare younger and older Alzheimer's disease (AD) Ss. The lack of increased amount of lipofuscin in the brain, the loss of dendritic arborization, and the suggested qualitative difference in AD suggest that it does not represent an exaggeration of normal aging. (11 ref).

779. Bertholf, Roger L. (1986). **Aluminum binding to plasma proteins: A study of the speciation of aluminum in the sera of healthy, uremic, and Alzheimer's diseased individuals.** *Dissertation Abstracts International,* 46(10-B), 3423.

780. Blackwood, D. H.; St. Clair, D. M.; Blackburn, I. M. & Tyrer, G. M. (1987). **Cognitive brain potentials and psychological deficits in Alzheimer's dementia and Korsakoff's amnesic syndrome.** *Psychological Medicine,* 17(2), 349–358.
Analyzed auditory event-related potentials, including the P300 response, in 20 patients with Alzheimer-type dementia ([ATD] aged 54–67 yrs), 17 patients with Korsakoff's syndrome ([KS] aged 49–75 yrs), and 23 controls (aged 51–78 yrs), using a version of A. R. Luria's (1966) neuropsychological investigation. Prolonged P300 latency and reduced P300 amplitude, which are features of normal aging, and ATD correlated significantly with impaired language ability in ATD patients and controls. There was a significant negative correlation between P300 latency and visual memory in ATD and a significant positive correlation in KS. Findings indicate that P300 changes associated with ATD and aging are not related to visual or verbal memory loss.

781. Blass, John P. et al. (1985). **Red blood cell abnormalities in Alzheimer disease.** *Journal of the American Geriatrics Society,* 33(6), 401–405.
Conducted a prospective, double-blind study of 84 unselected persons in a dementia clinic. Red blood cell/plasma choline ratios were found to be significantly higher in 47 Ss (mean age 72 yrs) with clinically defined Alzheimer's disease (DAT)

than in 37 non-DAT, nondepressed Ss (mean age 73 yrs) The latter group included intellectually intact Ss and Ss with other dementias who were comparable to the Ss with DAT age, sex, and degree of cognitive impairment. The elevated mean ratio reflected the greater proportion of DAT Ss with high red blood cell plasma choline ratios. These elevated ratios appeared to be related to both increases in red cell content and decreases in plasma choline. Results confirm and extend those previously reported in several, but not all series, examining Ss with DAT and agree with other evidence that DAT has systemic manifestations in nonneural cells that may be useful in further investigations of the disease's cellular pathophysiology. (53 ref).

782. Borda, Robert P. (1985). **The 40/sec middle-latency auditory response in Alzheimer's disease, Parkinson's disease, and age-matched normals.** *Dissertation Abstracts International,* 45(9-B), 3062.

783. Branconnier, Roland J.; Dessain, Eric C.; McNiff, Maureen E. & Cole, Jonathan O. (1986). **Blood ammonia and Alzheimer's disease.** *American Journal of Psychiatry,* 143(10), 1313.
Elaborates on findings presented by M. Fisman et al (1985) that demonstrate a significantly higher postprandial blood concentrations of ammonia in Alzheimer's disease patients than in hospitalized and normal control Ss by presenting the present authors' findings from a pilot study of 12 primary degenerative dementia patients (mean age 67.4 yrs) that corroborate the findings of Fisman et al, suggesting that hyperammonemia may occur frequently in patients with Alzheimer's disease. (4 ref).

784. Brenner, Richard P.; Ulrich, Richard F.; Spiker, Duane G.; Sclabassi, Robert J. et al. (1986). **Computerized EEG spectral analysis in elderly normal, demented and depressed subjects.** *Electroencephalography & Clinical Neurophysiology,* 64(6), 483–492.
Studied the EEG in 35 patients with Alzheimer's disease (AD), 23 with major depression, and 61 healthy controls (ages 51–89, 55–87, and 51–82 yrs, respectively). Compared to other groups, AD patients had a significant increase in the theta and alpha$_1$ bandwidths as well as an increased theta-beta difference. The parasagittal mean frequency, beta$_1$, and beta$_2$ activity were significantly decreased. In AD patients, there was a high correlation between spectral parameters (parasagittal mean frequency, delta and theta activity, and the theta–beta difference) and the Folstein score. EEG measures were more accurate in identifying AD patients who had lower Folstein scores.

785. Charles, G.; Mirel, J. & Lefevre, A. (1986). **Suppression du cortisol après dexaméthasone chez des patients déments. / Dexamethasone suppression in dementia.** *Encéphale,* 12(3), 105–110.
Studied the validity of the dexamethasone suppression test (DST) in 64 male and female Belgian adults (aged 69–92 yrs) with Alzheimer's disease or vascular dementias without depression. Ss underwent 2 1-mg overnight DSTs separated by 7 days. The Sandoz Clinical Assessment Geriatric Scale by R. D. Venn (1983), modified Ischemic Score, and International Classification of Diseases-IX criteria for Alzheimer's disease were used to separate the Ss into Alzheimer's and multi-infarct types of dementia. (English abstract).

786. Charles, Gerard A.; Lefevre, Andre; Mirel, Jean & Rush, A. John. (1986). **Suppression of cortisol following dexamethasone in demented patients.** *Psychiatry Research,* 17(3), 173–182.
Evaluated the behavior of the dexamethasone suppression test (DST) in 64 nondepressed dementia patients, aged 69–92 yrs, who had been in a clinically stable and drug-free state for at least 6 mo. Ss underwent 2 1-mg overnight DSTs separated

by 7 days. An ischemic score and the International Classification of Diseases—Ninth Revision criteria for Alzheimer's disease were used to dichotomize Ss into Alzheimer's and multi-infarct types of dementia. Ss with vascular dementias were significantly more likely to evidence DST nonsuppression, and DSTs in this group were less reproducible from week to week than DSTs in Alzheimer's patients. Results suggest that a positive DST in drug-free, stable, mildly demented cases with a few depressive symptoms justifies an empirical trial of antidepressant medication.

787. Christie, J. E.; Whalley, Lawrence J.; Bennie, J.; Dick, H. et al. (1987). **Characteristic plasma hormone changes in Alzheimer's disease.** *British Journal of Psychiatry,* 150, 674–681.
A systematic endocrine investigation in 9 dementia, 16 depression, and 37 control Ss showed that plasma growth hormone (GH) was higher in the morning and plasma thyroid stimulating hormone (TSH) concentrations were higher throughout the day in 18 patients with Alzheimer-type dementia (ATD) than in 7 age-matched depressed patients (MDD), and plasma TSH concentrations were also higher throughout the day in female ATD compared with age-matched female controls. Plasma concentrations of estrogen-stimulated neurophysin (ESN) were lower throughout the day in ATD compared with MDD and controls and lower in the morning compared with other dementias. It is suggested that the high plasma GH and TSH concentrations in ATD may reflect the reduced hypothalamic content of somatostatin ATD, and the reduced concentrations of ESN may reflect reduced cholinergic activity in ATD brain. The authors conclude that these selective hormonal changes provide a useful diagnostic test for Alzheimer's disease.

788. Coben, Lawrence A.; Danziger, Warren & Storandt, Martha. (1985). **A longitudinal EEG study of mild senile dementia of Alzheimer type: Changes at 1 year and at 2.5 years.** *Electroencephalography & Clinical Neurophysiology,* 61(2), 101–112.
Compared resting EEGs in 40 Ss (aged 64.2–81.5 yrs) with senile dementia of Alzheimer type (SDAT) and 41 healthy controls (aged 64.6–82.8 yrs) at 3 times of testing over a 2.5 yr period. Measures included mean EEG frequency and percentage of power in alpha, beta, theta, and delta frequency bands. Occipital to vertex derivation values were averaged for left and right hemispheres. In controls, delta increased, and beta and mean frequency decreased over the study period with no significant change in theta or alpha. In the SDAT group, all 5 EEG measures changed significantly. Theta distinguished between all 4 stages of dementia. In the mild stage of SDAT, theta, beta, and mean frequency were already different from control values. In the moderate stage, these differences persisted, and alpha became different. Delta was the last to change. It is suggested that EEG changes may be related to rate as well as to stage of deterioration, raising concerns about the psychometric and global rating scales used to measure clinical degree of dementia. (French abstract) (38 ref).

789. Coben, Lawrence A.; Danziger, Warren L. & Hughes, Charles P. (1983). **Visual evoked potentials in mild senile dementia of Alzheimer type.** *Electroencephalography & Clinical Neurophysiology,* 55(2), 121–130.
Recorded visual EPs (VEPs) to chessboard shift and to flash stimulation from 40 Ss (aged 64.2–82.5 yrs) with mild senile dementia of Alzheimer type and 40 matched controls. Demented Ss had longer latency of Peaks P3 and N3 and larger amplitude of segment N2–P3. These 3 are the earliest reported changes in the VEP in Alzheimer disease. Implications for the study of cortical EPs and intracortical loss of inhibitory potentials are discussed. (French abstract) (37 ref).

790. Coben, Lawrence A.; Danziger, Warren L. & Berg, Leonard. (1983). **Frequency analysis of the resting awake EEG in mild senile dementia of Alzheimer type.** *Electroencephalography & Clinical Neurophysiology,* 55(4), 372–380.
Recorded spontaneous resting EEGs in 40 Ss (aged 64.2–82.5 yrs) with senile dementia of Alzheimer type (SDAT) and 40 individually matched controls without SDAT. All of the demented Ss had only a mild degree of dementia, and all were still living in the community. Several measures of EEG activity were calculated, based on the power spectra of the EEG samples from left and right occipital-to-vertex derivations. Paired *t* tests showed significant differences between demented and control group means for measures of theta and beta activity, but not for measures of alpha and delta activity. The earliest changes in the resting EEG in SDAT were increased theta and decreased beta power. These changes are different from those reported in normal aging, in which a decrease in alpha activity accompanies the changes in theta and beta. The absence of increased delta and the presence of decreased beta in demented Ss are consistent with the early stages of SDAT in which the disease is largely confined to the gray matter of the cerebral cortex. (French abstract) (30 ref).

791. Cohen, Bruce M.; Zubenko, George S. & Babb, Suzann M. (1987). **Abnormal platelet membrane composition in Alzheimer's-type dementia.** *Life Sciences,* 40(25), 2445–2451.
Studied platelet membrane composition in Ss with Alzheimer-type dementia and in neurologically healthy volunteers. Findings suggest that there is no general abnormality of membrane lipids in Ss suffering from Alzheimer-type dementia. In fact, it appears that such patients have an increase in internal membranes.

792. Davis, Kenneth L. et al. (1986). **Cortisol and Alzheimer's disease: I. Basal studies.** *American Journal of Psychiatry,* 143(3), 300–305.
16 patients with Alzheimer's disease (mean age 64.1 yrs) and 19 nondemented controls (mean age 65.6 yrs) participated in studies of cortisol secretion during sleep and at 9 AM and were given dexamethasone suppression tests (DSTs) and lumbar punctures. Nocturnal and 9 AM cortisol concentrations were significantly higher in the demented Ss. Cerebrospinal fluid (CSF) 3-methoxy-4-hydroxyphenylglycol negatively correlated with mean nocturnal cortisol. The most severely demented Ss had the highest 9 AM and mean nocturnal cortisol concentrations. DST results did not distinguish samples with substantially different nocturnal cortisol concentrations. Findings suggest that measurements of basal plasma cortisol concentrations and dexamethasone suppression provide different information but support the notion of somewhat higher than normal cortisol concentrations in Alzheimer's disease patients. (36 ref).

793. Davous, Patrick. (1987). **Cortisol and Alzheimer's disease.** *American Journal of Psychiatry,* 144(4), 533–534.
Compares results of the present author's research with the dexamethasone suppression test (DST) in 27 nondepressed patients (aged 71–95 yrs) affected by senile dementia of the Alzheimer type with findings by K. L. Davis et al (see PA, Vol 73:17577) and B. S. Greenwald et al (see PA, Vol 73: 22266). Contrary to those studies, the present author found a relation between nonsuppression and dementia severity but no age difference between suppressors and nonsuppressors or association between depression and dementia.

794. de Ajuriaguerra, J. et al. (1976). **Alimentary behavior in degenerative or mixed dementias, with a predominance of the degenerative processes of old age.** *Annales Médico-Psychologiques,* 2(2), 213–241.
The integration of the complex function of alimentation, which is genetic and instinctual at its base (but also incorporates learned and social components) is detailed to provide

information through a systematic study of its dissolution in the presence of CNS deterioration. 19 patients 61–96 yrs old (mean age 82) with simple senile dementias and 15 with Alzheimer's disease (almost all females) were studied by 3 methods: questionnaire, observation of basic eating behaviors, and observation of eating-related behaviors (e.g., use of utensils, sequencing of food consumed, and reactions to skipped meals). The most characteristic symptomatic behaviors were modification of eating behaviors linked to changes in biological rhythms, lack of competence in the skills required for eating, and the intrusion of disturbances that interfered with alimentary acts. The chronology of disintegration reflected, at first, considerable individual differences in alimentary capacities, followed by greater similarity as deterioration increased. A hypothesis regarding the mechanism of these changes is offered.

795. Deary, Ian J.; Hendrickson, Alan E. & Burns, Alistair. (1987). **Serum calcium levels in Alzheimer's disease: A finding and an aetiological hypothesis.** *Personality & Individual Differences,* 8(1), 75–80.
Tested the hypothesis that individual differences in calcium levels in patients suffering from senile dementia of the Alzheimer type (SDAT) would correlate with individual differences in cognitive test scores, using 10 SDAT inpatients (with a mean Mini-Mental State score of 1.1) and 10 SDAT outpatients (with a mean Mini-Mental State score of 20.8). Results show lower serum Ca^{2+} levels in severely demented patients when compared with mildly affected individuals. Findings are discussed in relation to the theory of the biological basis of psychometric intelligence developed by A. E. Hendrickson (1982).

796. de Leon, Mony J.; la Regina, Mary E.; Ferris, Steven H.; Gentes, Cynthia I. et al. (1986). **Reduced incidence of left-handedness in clinically diagnosed dementia of the Alzheimer type.** *Neurobiology of Aging,* 7(3), 161–164.
Used the Edinburgh Handedness Inventory to study handedness patterns in 3 elderly (aged 60–80 yrs) groups: 217 normal Ss, 73 depressed, and 73 with Alzheimer's disease (AD). The Global Deterioration Scale was used to assess dementia. Results indicate a reduced frequency of left handedness in AD (2.6%) relative to control (11.1%) and depression (13.7%) groups. Within the limited age range studied, no relationships were found between age and handedness preference either within or across the groups. For the AD group there was no relationship between severity of global impairment and strength of handedness. Results suggest that compared to right handers, left handers are less vulnerable to the cognitive changes associated with AD. Nevertheless, it is also possible that left handers are overrepresented among early onset dementia patients and die before entering the pool of senile dementia patients.

797. Ebstein, Richard P.; Oppenheim, Gerald; Ebstein, Bonnie S.; Amiri, Zamir et al. (1986). **The cyclic AMP second messenger system in man: The effects of heredity, hormones, drugs, aluminum, age and disease on signal amplification.** *Progress in Neuro-Psychopharmacology & Biological Psychiatry,* 10(3–5), 323–353.
Reviews the literature concerning the effect of various vectors (e.g., heredity, endogenous catecholamines, steroid hormones, drugs) on adenylate cyclase activity in humans. It is asserted that the intracellular effects of a number of hormonal signals are mediated by the cyclic adenosine 3,5-monophosphate (AMP) 2nd-messenger system, and the ubiquitous distribution of hormone-stimulated adenylate cyclase suggests the importance of this enzyme complex in normal aging and pathophysiological states (e.g., Alzheimer's disease).

798. Ebstein, Richard P.; Oppenheim, Gerald; Zlotogorski, Zoli; Van Dijk, Yehuda et al. (1986). **Age related decline in aluminum-activated human platelet adenylate cyclase: Post-receptor changes in cyclic AMP second messenger signal amplification in normal aging and dementia of the Alzheimer type.** *Life Sciences,* 39(13), 1167–1175.
Studied the effect of normal aging and disease state on 2nd messenger activity in 17 healthy human Ss (aged 17–87 yrs) and 8 Ss with Alzheimer's disease (AD). A significant decline in aluminum-stimulated platelet adenylate cyclase (AC) activity in older, healthy Ss was observed. An age-associated decline in NaF-stimulated cyclic adenosine monophosphate (AMP) synthesis was also demonstrated for normal, nondemented Ss. Findings suggest an age-associated lesion at the level of the guanine nucleotide regulatory protein/catalytic subunit of the AC complex. For AD Ss, no such decline in platelet AC activity was detected, and increased sensitivity to aluminum and NaF was demonstrated.

799. Ebstein, Richard P.; Oppenheim, Gerald & Stessman, Jochanan. (1984). **Alzheimer's disease: Isoproterenol and prostaglandin E_1-stimulated cyclic AMP accumulation in lymphocytes.** *Life Sciences,* 34(23), 2239–2243.
Compared the isoproterenol and prostaglandin E_1 $(PGE)_1$-stimulated cyclic adenosine monophosphate (AMP) accumulation in lymphocytes obtained from 10 patients (aged 74–87 yrs) with senile dementia of the Alzheimer type (SDAT), 10 elderly Ss (aged 73–85 yrs) with no significant cognitive decline, and 10 young Ss (aged 21–36 yrs). Data indicate reduced lymphocyte beta-adrenergic receptor activity in SDATs and in aged controls; a parallel decline in lymphocytic prostaglandin E_1 receptor activity was seen in the aged controls. In SDATs, however, such lymphocytic prostaglandin E_1 receptor activity was significantly raised and correlated with a rating scale for severity of dementia. Results lend support to the concept that involvement of the immunological systems may be important in the pathogenesis of Alzheimer's disease. (27 ref).

800. Eikelenboom, Piet; Vink-Starreveld, M. L.; Jansen, W. & Pronk, J. C. (1984). **C_3 and haptoglobin polymorphism in dementia of the Alzheimer type.** *Acta Psychiatrica Scandinavica,* 69(2), 140–142.
Investigated the C_3 and haptoglobin phenotype distribution in 60 patients (mean age 73.5 yrs) with dementia of the Alzheimer type. In contrast with previous research, results indicate no significant association between dementia of the Alzheimer type and certain C_3 or haptoglobin phenotypes. In addition, there was no indication of an excess of haptoglobin type 1-1 or C_3 type FF in Ss with early onset of dementia. (14 ref).

801. Elovaara, I.; Maury, C. P. & Palo, J. (1986). **Serum amyloid A protein, albumin and prealbumin in Alzheimer's disease and in demented patients with Down's syndrome.** *Acta Neurologica Scandinavica,* 74(3), 245–250.
Measured the concentrations of serum amyloid A (SAA) protein, albumin, and prealbumin in 22 patients (aged 61–95 yrs) with Alzheimer's disease (AD), 21 demented patients (aged 35–54 yrs) with Down's syndrome, and 16 age-matched controls with other neurological diseases. Both patient groups evidenced an increase in the SAA level and a decrease in albumin and prealbumin. Results suggest an association between increased SAA levels and the pathogenesis of AD.

802. El Sobky, A.; El-Shazly, M.; Darwish, A. K.; Davies, T. et al. (1986). **Anterior pituitary response to thyrotropin releasing hormone in senile dementia (Alzheimer type) and elderly normals.** *Acta Psychiatrica Scandinavica,* 74(1), 13–17.
Compared 16 patients (aged over 65 yrs) with senile dementia of the Alzheimer type (SDAT) with 11 age-matched normal Ss with respect to their responses of thyrotropin (TSH) and prolactin (PRL) to thyrotropin-releasing hormone challenge.

Both groups showed a continuing rise in TSH response at 60 min, and no difference was found between the groups. A significantly exaggerated PRL response at 20 min was found in the SDAT group. There was no difference between sexes with respect to either the TSH or PRL response.

803. Endo, Hidetoshi; Yamamoto, Takayuki & Kuzuya, Fumio. (1986). **HLA system in senile dementia of Alzheimer type and multi-infarct dementia in Japan.** *Archives of Gerontology & Geriatrics,* 5(1), 51–56.
Studied the human lymphocyte antigens (HLAs) of 122 patients (aged 41–96 yrs) with senile dementia of the Alzheimer type (SDAT) and 92 patients (aged 58–93 yrs) with multi-infarct dementia. Measurements were also taken for 66 age-matched normal controls (aged 54–100) and 31 younger normal controls (aged 22–58 yrs). Data show a significant association between HLA B16 and SDAT. A significant difference was observed in the occurrence of HLA Cw 3 between SDAT Ss and controls. It is noted that in the general population, the frequency of B16 is higher in Europe and the US than in Japan. It is suggested that the difference in the prevalence of SDAT between Japan and other countries is caused by genetic factors. (15 ref).

804. Erkinjuntti, T.; Partinen, Markku; Sulkava, R. & Salmi, T. (1985). **Sleep related respiratory disturbances in dementia: SCSB-recording as a new method to analyse nocturnal respiration of demented patients.** World Psychiatric Association Symposium: Psychopathology of dream and sleeping (1983, Helsinki, Finland). *Psychiatria Fennica,* Suppl, 106–110.
Investigated the occurrence of sleep-related respiratory disturbances in 13 patients with vascular dementia (mean age 66 yrs) and in 11 patients with Alzheimer's disease (mean age 68 yrs), using the static charge sensitive bed method. The method enables continuous monitoring of respiratory movements, the ballistocardiogram, and body movements. Analysis showed a correlation between age and total sleeping time, severity of dementia, and restlessness of sleep; a pattern indicating sleep apnea syndrome was found more often in Ss with vascular dementia. (12 ref).

805. Essa, Mohsain; Gibbs, Helen & Chojnacki, Michael. (1984). **Zinc and copper in dementia.** Special Issue: Dementia assessment. *Clinical Gerontologist,* 3(2), 43–45.
Reports on a study of zinc and copper levels in 15 Alzheimer's patients. Findings suggest that zinc and copper are not affected by and are not factors in dementia. (8 ref).

806. Fisman, Michael et al. (1985). **Hyperammonemia in Alzheimer's disease.** *American Journal of Psychiatry,* 142(1), 71–73.
Measured fasting and 3-hr postprandial blood ammonia levels in 22 61–87 yr old hospitalized Alzheimer patients, 13 64–77 yr old hospitalized patients with schizophrenia or Korsakoff's psychosis, and 24 53–88 yr old normal adults. Results show that the blood ammonia levels were significantly higher in the Alzheimer Ss than in the 2 control groups. In Alzheimer Ss, fasting blood ammonia levels were significantly higher in those whose EEGs showed triphasic waves than in Ss without this change. Alzheimer and control Ss also differed in the direction of change from fasting to postprandial blood ammonia levels. (8 ref).

807. Fisman, Michael et al. (1986). **"Blood ammonia and Alzheimer's disease": Dr. Fisman and associates reply.** *American Journal of Psychiatry,* 143(10), 1313–1314.
Responds to the report by R. J. Branconnier et al (1986) of findings that parallel the present authors' (1985) findings of hyperammonemia in Alzheimer's disease patients by agreeing with Branconnier et al that it is unlikely that a high ammonia level causes Alzheimer's disease and by proposing altered hepatic metabolism secondary to hypothalamic involvement in Alzheimer's disease as an alternative explanation along with other potential explanations. (5 ref).

808. Fowler, Clare J. & Harrison, M. J. (1986). **EEG changes in subcortical dementia: A study of 22 patients with Steele-Richardson-Olszewski (SRO) syndrome.** *Electroencephalography & Clinical Neurophysiology,* 64(4), 301–303.
Compared the EEGs of 22 SRO patients (20 of whom had mild-to-severe subcortical dementia) with those of 22 patients who had a comparable degree of dementia due to cortical atrophy due to Alzheimer's disease. Results show that SRO Ss with dementia did not have characteristic EEG changes, and EEGs were generally within normal limits or only mildly abnormal. It is concluded that it may not be possible in a case of mild-to-moderate dementia to distinguish between a subcortical or cortical pathogenesis from the EEG. (French abstract).

809. Fu, Tsu-ker; Matsuyama, Steven S.; Kessler, John O. & Jarvik, Lissy F. (1986). **Philothermal response: Microtubules and dementia.** *Neurobiology of Aging,* 7(1), 41–43.
Examined the role of microtubules in the philothermal response of polymorphonuclear leukocytes (PMNs) using colchicine in 12 21–74 yr olds. Findings indicate that colchicine inhibited PMN migration in a dose dependent fashion. Spatial distribution analysis of the responding cell population revealed a preferential inhibition of distal cell migration, a pattern similar to that found for PMNs obtained from patients with dementia of the Alzheimer type (DAT). The result is consistent with the known role of microtubules in directed cell migration and the hypothesized microtubular defect in DAT. It is suggested that further investigations of microtubules may provide insight into the etiology and pathogenesis of DAT. (17 ref).

810. Giannelli, A. et al. (1985). **Oligoelementi nella demenza senile tipo Alzheimer—Prospettive eziopatogenetiche, possibilità diagnostiche e terapeutiche. / On oligoelements in Alzheimer's disease: Etiopathogenetic perspectives and possibilities at the diagnostic-therapeutic level.** *Rivista Sperimentale di Freniatria e Medicina Legale delle Alienazioni Mentali,* 109(2), 376–389.
Measured the serum concentrations of copper and zinc and the plasma concentrations of aluminum in a group of 29 patients (aged 52–87 yrs), 18 with Alzheimer's type senile dementia (ATSD) and 11 with multi-infarct disease (MID) and other psychiatric pathologies such as depression and paranoid syndrome. Results show that there was no significant difference in serum copper concentration between the 2 groups and that in the ATSD group, serum zinc concentration was diminished and plasma aluminum concentration was increased as compared with the MID group. These data are in accord with previous studies of samples of central nervous system (CNS) tissue (biopsy or autopsy). It is suggested that the measurement of blood concentrations of zinc and aluminum could be a simple, complementary method for the diagnosis of ATSD. The therapeutic possibilities of zinc and chelation of aluminum in the treatment of ATSD are suggested. (24 ref).

811. Giaquinto, S. & Nolfe, G. (1986). **The EEG in the normal elderly: A contribution to the interpretation of aging and dementia.** *Electroencephalography & Clinical Neurophysiology,* 63(6), 540–546.
Studied 47 normal elderly (aged 60–80 yrs), 16 normal Ss (aged 40–60 yrs), and 14 patients (mean age 67 yrs) affected by primary dementia using EEG recordings from different brain areas. Results show that there was persistence of the regional distribution of the alpha frequency that was higher in

occipital than in frontal leads in the normal elderly and that spectral composition in the same group kept its typical profile with age. Alpha-dominant tracings formed 68%. (French abstract).

812. Gibson, Gary E.; Nielsen, Pamela E.; Sherman, Kathleen A. & Blass, John P. (1987). **Diminished mitogen-induced calcium uptake by lymphocytes from Alzheimer patients.** *Biological Psychiatry,* 22(9), 1079–1086.
Assessed calcium homeostasis in mitogen-stimulated lymphocytes in 9 patients with Alzheimer's disease (AD). Calcium uptake by lymphocytes was 10–15% lower than that of lymphocytes from age-matched controls. However, neither superficially bound nor total calcium was altered by AD. It is suggested that the small differences in uptake may reflect larger differences in cytosolic calcium, in later calcium-mediated events, or in the response of particular subsets of lymphocytes.

813. Grady, Cheryl L.; Haxby, James V.; Schlageter, N. L.; Berg, G. et al. (1986). **Stability of metabolic and neuropsychological asymmetries in dementia of the Alzheimer type.** *Neurology,* 36(10), 1390–1392.
Examined right/left asymmetries in cerebral glucose utilization and neuropsychological performance in 16 right-handed patients (aged 45–77 yrs) with dementia of the Alzheimer type (DAT) twice over a mean interval of 15 mo. Neuropsychological asymmetry was expressed as the difference between performances on visuoconstructive and language tasks. Test/retest comparisons showed significant declines on the neuropsychological measures but no significant changes in the neuropsychological and metabolic asymmetry indices. Significant correlations were found between neuropsychological and metabolic asymmetry in frontal and parietal cortex. Individual patterns of asymmetry in these DAT patients appear stable over time.

814. Greenwald, Blaine S. et al. (1985). **Red blood cell choline: I. Choline in Alzheimer's disease.** *Biological Psychiatry,* 20(4), 367–374.
Studied red blood cell (RBC) and plasma choline values in 17 48–77 yr old drug-free patients with Alzheimer's disease (AD) and in 15 47–76 yr old normal elderly controls in an investigation that included 13 age- and sex-matched pairs. Results from RBC and plasma analyses indicate that mean values for RBC choline, plasma choline, and the ratio of RBC/plasma choline did not differ between the AD and control groups. Degree of dementia did not correlate with any blood choline measure. A correlation was found between age and RBC choline and the RBC/plasma choline ratio in normals, but not in AD Ss. RBC choline correlated with plasma choline in AD Ss only. Results do not support the use of RBC and plasma choline concentrations as either a diagnostic tool to identify AD patients or an antemortem index of the cholinergic deficit in brains of patients with Alzheimer's disease. (28 ref).

815. Greenwald, Blaine S. et al. (1986). **Cortisol and Alzheimer's disease: II. Dexamethasone suppression, dementia severity, and affective symptoms.** *American Journal of Psychiatry,* 143(4), 442–446.
Conducted dexamethasone suppression tests (DSTs) with 22 nondepressed Alzheimer's disease patients (aged 53–80 yrs) to determine whether the DST can help distinguish patients with coexisting dementia and depression from those with dementia alone. Dexamethasone (1 mg) was administered orally, and postdexamethasone cortisol levels were obtained the next day 9, 17, and 24 hrs following the initial dexamethasone administration. Results indicate that 11 Ss were nonsuppressors. Nonsuppressors tended to be older than suppressors but did not differ in depression or dementia scores on a memory and information test and a dementia rating scale. Postdexamethasone cortisol levels measured 9 hrs following the administration of dexamethasone correlated with depressive

symptoms. A relationship was also demonstrated between the severity of dementia and depressive symptoms. Findings indicate that symptoms of depression can be found in patients with Alzheimer's disease who do not meet the criteria for major depressive episode, suggesting that depressive symptoms are an intrinsic part of the Alzheimer's disease syndrome. (34 ref).

816. Greenwald, Blaine S.; Mohs, Richard C. & Davis, Kenneth L. (1987). **"Cortisol and Alzheimer's disease": Dr. Greenwald and associates reply.** *American Journal of Psychiatry,* 144(4), 534–535.
Comments on P. Davous's (1987) report on the dexamethasone suppression test (DST) in dementia patients and the apparently disparate findings with regard to the relation between DST results and dementia. It is suggested that the discrepancies may be due to inconsistent methodological variables across studies, including differences in homogeneity of clinical samples and diagnostic criteria, rating scales and raters, and dose of dexamethasone.

817. Hanin, Israel et al. (1984). **Elevated red blood cell/ plasma choline ratio in dementia of the Alzheimer type: Clinical and polysomnographic correlates.** *Psychiatry Research,* 13(2), 167–173.
In a prospective study, a shift was observed in distribution of red blood cell (RBC)/plasma choline ratios among 22 55–81 yr old patients with probable dementia of the Alzheimer type (DAT), compared with 26 58–82 yr old healthy controls and 20 55–81 yr old depressed patients. 15 DAT patients showed RBC/plasma choline ratios greater than 1.9, in contrast to 9 controls and 7 depressives. The subgroup of DAT Ss with elevated RBC/plasma choline ratios was older and more cognitively impaired, showed later onset of dementia, and had less REM sleep than the DAT subgroup with normal RBC/ plasma choline ratios. Within the entire group of DAT Ss, the RBC/plasma choline ratio showed a significant inverse correlation with REM sleep latency. Findings are discussed in relation to abnormalities in other nonneural Alzheimer tissues and within the context of cholinergic involvement in both DAT and the timing of REM sleep. (27 ref).

818. Hendrie, High C.; Wellman, Henry N.; Hall, Kathleen S.; Farlow, Martin R. et al. (1987). **Single photon emission tomographic brain images in dementia of the Alzheimer type.** *American Journal of Psychiatry,* 144(3), 387–388.
Single photon emission tomographic brain images in 12 patients (mean age 63.3 yrs) with dementia of the Alzheimer type and in 5 normal Ss (mean age 69.4 yrs) revealed regional deficits in the patients' cerebral blood flow that were not revealed by magnetic resonance imaging and computerized axial tomography scans done in the neurological evaluation phase of the study.

819. Hirsch, Betsy A. (1983). **A cytogenetic investigation of DNA repair mechanisms in Alzheimer disease.** *Dissertation Abstracts International,* 43(11-B), 3769.

820. Hoch, Carolyn C.; Reynolds, Charles F.; Kupfer, David J.; Houck, Patricia R. et al. (1986). **Sleep-disordered breathing in normal and pathologic aging.** *Journal of Clinical Psychiatry,* 47(10), 499–503.
In a study of sleep-disordered breathing among 139 49–85 yr olds, sleep apnea occurred in 10 of 34 Alzheimer's Ss compared with 3 of 56 healthy controls, 5 of 35 depressive Ss, and 4 of 24 Ss with mixed symptoms of both cognitive impairment and depression. Alzheimer's Ss had a significantly higher proportion of nonrapid eye movement (NREM)-related than REM-related apnea. Moreover, a significant positive correlation between the apnea index and severity of dementia was found in apnea-positive Alzheimer's Ss, as well as in the entire sample of Alzheimer's Ss. Clinical and neuropathologic implications are discussed.

821. Hutton, John T. (1981). **Smooth pursuit and saccadic eye movements in dementia.** *Dissertation Abstracts International,* 41(7-B), 2555–2556.

822. Jagust, William J.; Friedland, Robert P. & Budinger, Thomas F. (1985). **Positron emission tomography with [^{18}F]Fluorodeoxyglucose differentiates normal pressure hydrocephalus from Alzheimer-type dementia.** *Journal of Neurology, Neurosurgery & Psychiatry,* 48(11), 1091–1096.
Studied 3 patients (55–62 yrs old) with normal pressure hydrocephalus, 17 patients (55–75 yrs old) with Alzheimer-type dementia, and 7 healthy elderly controls (59–68 yrs old), using positron emission tomography and [^{18}F]Fluorodeoxyglucose (FDG). Both Alzheimer-type dementia and normal pressure hydrocephalus groups showed lower cortical rates of FDG utilization than controls. However, the patterns of metabolic abnormality were distinctly different in the 2 dementia groups, with Alzheimer-type dementia Ss demonstrating bilateral temporoparietal hypometabolism, while normal pressure hydrocephalus Ss showed globally diminished glucose use. (34 ref).

823. Jenike, Michael A. (1984). **The dexamethasone suppression test in geriatric patients: Jenike responds.** Special Issue: Dementia assessment. *Clinical Gerontologist,* 3(2), 36.
Responds to comments made by M. Carnes and N. H. Kalin (1984) concerning the author's (1983) report on the use of the dexamethasone suppression test to diagnose depression in elderly patients. Additional data on the use of the test with Alzheimer's patients are noted. (1 ref).

824. Jolkkonen, Jukka; Soininen, Hilkka; Halonen, Toivo; Ylinen, Aarne et al. (1986). **Somatostatin-like immunoreactivity in the cerebrospinal fluid of patients with Parkinson's disease and its relation to dementia.** *Journal of Neurology, Neurosurgery & Psychiatry,* 49(12), 1374–1377.
Measured acetylcholinesterase, somatostatinlike immunoreactivity, and homovanillic acid levels in the cerebrospinal fluid (CSF) of 36 patients (aged 44–81 yrs) with early stages of Parkinson's disease and in 19 control patients (aged 38–78 yrs) undergoing lumbar puncture for other conditions. In patients with Parkinson's disease the levels of somatostatin-like immunoreactivity were lower than in the controls; these values were lowest in demented Parkinsonian patients. Concentrations of homovanillic acid were also significantly lower in Parkinsonian patients. The reduced somatostatinlike immunoreactivity in the CSF agrees with previous postmortem studies and indicates that Parkinson's disease and Alzheimer's disease may have some neurochemical features in common.

825. Jonker, C.; Eikelenboom, P. & Tavenier, P. (1982). **Immunological indices in the cerebrospinal fluid of patients with presenile dementia of the Alzheimer type.** *British Journal of Psychiatry,* 140, 44–49.
In 10 patients (53–68 yrs old) with presenile dementia of the Alzheimer type and in 10 controls (20–66 yrs old), the levels of different immunoglobulins were determined in both serum and cerebrospinal fluid (CSF). Gel electrophoretic techniques were used to determine possible oligoclonal bands in the gamma-globulin region. There was no indication that Ss with Alzheimer disease produced globulins within the CNS. (17 ref).

826. Kanof, Philip D.; Greenwald, Blaine S.; Mohs, Richard C. & Davis, Kenneth L. (1985). **Red blood cell choline: II. Kinetics in Alzheimer's disease.** *Biological Psychiatry,* 20(4), 375–383.
Compared the kinetic parameters of choline uptake into red blood cells from 15 Alzheimer's disease (AD) patients (aged 48–77 yrs) and 13 normal controls (aged 47–74 yrs). The K_d and V_{max} values for choline uptake into red cells were determined based on a kinetic analysis of choline uptake at 6 concentrations of labeled extracellular choline. The theoretical choline uptake, representing the initial rate of choline influx into choline-depleted red cells given the plasma choline concentration and the kinetic parameters of choline uptake, was also calculated. Results reveal that AD Ss and controls did not differ in any kinetic parameter of choline uptake. K_d and V_{max} values for red cell choline uptake were strongly correlated among normal controls, but not among AD Ss. The theoretical choline uptake was strongly correlated with the severity of dementia in AD Ss. Findings support the hypothesis that the enhanced vulnerability of cholinergic neurons in AD may be due to altered choline metabolism. Findings are discussed in relation to altered choline metabolism in Alzheimer's disease. (28 ref).

827. Katz, Paul R. & Chutkow, Jerry G. (1986). **Dementia, myoclonus, and EEG findings typical of Jakob-Creutzfeldt disease in a patient with Alzheimer's disease.** *New York State Journal of Medicine,* 86(3), 157–158.
Presents the case of a 62-yr-old man who 11 yrs prior to death manifested dementia, myoclonus, and periodic EEG complexes, which resulted in a diagnosis of Jakob-Creutzfeldt disease (JCD). S was subsequently diagnosed with Alzheimer's disease (AD), based on a computed tomographic scan. It is suggested that differentiation between AD and JCD may be difficult at times. (14 ref).

828. Keller, William J. (1986). **Forty hertz EEG activity in the elderly: Dementia, depression, and normal aging.** *Dissertation Abstracts International,* 46(7-B), 2492–2493.

829. Krankenhagen, B. & Kohler, G. K. (1973). **Alzheimer's disease.** *Fortschritte de Neurologie, Psychiatrie und ihrer Grenzgebiete,* 41(3), 141–165.
Studied the course of Alzheimer's disease in 16 female and 5 male 46–65 yr old patients wih anamneses of 4–120 mo duration prior to admission at a clinic. Ss also were examined in order to investigate the connections between pneumoencephalographic, EEG, and brain-electric-psychopathological correlations. Ss underwent neurological and psychopathological examinations and cerebrospinal fluid tests. Results are presented in several graphs and tables and discussed in detail. (English summary).

830. Lawlor, Brian A.; Sunderland, Trey; Mellow, Alan M. & Murphy, Dennis L. (1988). **Thyroid disease and dementia of the Alzheimer type.** *American Journal of Psychiatry,* 145(4), 533–534.
Medical records of 50 patients with primary degenerative dementia and 25 age-matched controls revealed no significant differences between the 2 groups in terms of thyrotropin-stimulating hormone level or history of prior thyroid disease, questioning the hypothesis that abnormal thyroid function is a risk factor in dementia.

831. Leppler, John G. (1981). **The P_3 potential and its clinical usefulness in the objective classification of dementia.** *Dissertation Abstracts International,* 41(7-B), 2548–2549.

832. Leuchter, Andrew F.; Spar, James E.; Walter, Donald O. & Weiner, Herbert. (1987). **Electroencephalographic spectra and coherence in the diagnosis of Alzheimer's-type and multi-infarct dementia: A pilot study.** *Archives of General Psychiatry,* 44(11), 993–998.
Investigated EEG differences in 12 patients with dementia of the Alzheimer's type (DAT [mean age 75 yrs]), 6 patients with multi-infarct dementia (MID [mean age 75 yrs]), and 6 healthy controls (mean age 73 yrs), using computer-based topographic analysis. Demented Ss were distinguished from controls by a diminished ratio of high- to low-frequency electrical activity in the left temporal region. Using this variable, all controls and 15 demented Ss were correctly classified. The 3 misclassified Ss were among the least impaired DAT patients. Examination of coherence distinguished between DAT and MID Ss. Discriminant analysis of EEG fre-

quency and coherence resulted in accurate classification of 22 Ss.

833. Loring, David W. (1983). **Forty Hz EEG in Alzheimer's disease, multi-infarct dementia, and normal aging.** *Dissertation Abstracts International,* 43(12-B), 4153.

834. Loring, David W.; Sheer, Daniel E. & Largen, John W. (1985). **Forty hertz EEG activity in dementia of the Alzheimer type and multi-infarct dementia.** *Psychophysiology,* 22(1), 116–121.
Examined high frequency EEG activity within the 40-Hz band at rest and during 2 problem-solving tasks in 12 patients (mean age 69.1 yrs) with presumptive diagnoses of dementia of the Alzheimer type (DAT) in 12 patients (mean age 69.7 yrs) with multi-infarct dementia (MID), and in 12 normal SS (mean age 67.9 yrs). The DAT Ss differed significantly from normal Ss and MID Ss, exhibiting both decreased rates of 40-Hz EEG activity and no task-appropriate pattern of cerebral lateralization. There was significantly less 40-Hz activity present in MID Ss during performance of a sentence repetition task than in controls. Results suggest that patterns of 40-Hz EEG activity may be of utility in the early diagnosis of DAT and that the 40-Hz rhythm appears able to discriminate between patient populations that present with similar patterns of dementia. (26 ref).

835. Markand, Omkar N. (1986). **Electroencephalogram in dementia.** *American Journal of EEG Technology,* 26(1), 3–17.
Suggests that EEG changes in elderly Ss suspected to have dementia are different from those in normally aging Ss and that EEG is helpful in separating organic dementia from pseudodementia. In the early stages of dementia due to degenerative disorders of the central nervous system (CNS) (e.g., Alzheimer's disease), the EEG is either normal or shows scattered theta-delta activities and decreasing frequency of the alpha rhythm; as the disease progresses the EEG is almost always abnormal. In toxic-metabolic causes of intellectual impairment the EEG abnormalities are more pronounced. Different forms of abnormal EEG may be observed in patients with dementia due to focal CNS injury, Jakob-Creutzfeldt disease, and Huntington's disease.

836. Martin, Peter R. et al. (1986). **Sleep EEG in Korsakoff's psychosis and Alzheimer's disease.** *Neurology,* 36(3), 411–414.
Compared all-night sleep EEGs in 7 patients (aged 53–66 yrs) with Korsakoff's psychosis (KP), 8 patients (mean age at onset 60.9 yrs) with presumptive Alzheimer's disease (AD), and 9 healthy controls (aged 52–69 yrs). After 1 night of adaptation, Ss were studied 2–8 nights with polygraphic recording of EEG, electrooculogram (EOG), and electromyogram (EMG). KP Ss had significantly increased intermittent time awake compared to both controls and AD Ss and shorter REM latency minus time awake compared to controls. AD Ss had significantly reduced delta sleep compared to controls. It is suggested that differences in the pattern of sleep EEG abnormalities may be due to different pathogenic mechanisms but that their utility in differential diagnosis requires further study. (25 ref).

837. Mayeux, R.; Stern, Y.; Sano, M.; Cote, L. et al. (1987). **Clinical and biochemical correlates of bradyphrenia in Parkinson's disease.** *Neurology,* 37(7), 1130–1134.
Compared the performance of 3 groups consisting of 15 patients with Parkinson's disease (PD), 12 age-matched controls, and 21 mildly impaired patients (mean age range 59.3–68.1 yrs) with probable Alzheimer's disease (AD) on tests of general intellect, memory, and reaction time (RT) and on a continuous performance task (CPT) measuring attention and vigilance. The PD Ss formed 2 distinct groups: One group had significantly more omission errors and fewer correct responses on the CPT than did controls or AD Ss. This group

was considered to have bradyphrenia. Their performance on measures of general intellectual and memory function was similar to that of the AD Ss. Cerebrospinal fluid (CSF) 3-methoxy-4-hydroxyphenylglycol (MHPG) correlated with the CPT and RT in all PD Ss; those with bradyphrenia had the highest CSF-MHPG levels.

838. Miller, Bruce L.; Jenden, Donald J.; Cummings, Jeffrey L.; Read, Stephen et al. (1986). **Abnormal erythrocyte choline and influx in Alzheimer's disease.** *Life Sciences,* 38(6), 485–490.
When choline transport and levels were studied in erythrocytes from 13 patients (mean age 71.5 yrs) with Alzheimer's disease (DAT) and 11 age-matched controls (mean age 66.6 yrs), mean levels were significantly higher in the DAT group. Findings suggest that erythrocyte choline is elevated in a subset of patients with DAT and that the low affinity transport system is also abnormal in these patients.

839. Newhouse, Paul A.; Sunderland, Trey; Tariot, Pierre N.; Mueller, Edward A. et al. (1986). **Prolactin response to TRH in Alzheimer's disease and elderly controls.** *Biological Psychiatry,* 21(10), 963–967.
Found a blunted prolactin response to thyrotropin-releasing hormone (TRH) in 11 43–71 yr old patients with dementia of the Alzheimer type compared to that in 11 age- and sex-matched normal controls. Data suggest a disturbed endocrine regulation in Alzheimer's disease that appears to be related directly to the underlying brain disorder and not to measured depressive symptoms, age, or weight.

840. Partanen, Juhani V.; Soininen, H. & Riekkinen, P. J. (1986). **Does an ACTH derivative (Org 2766) prevent deterioration of EEG in Alzheimer's disease?** *Electroencephalography & Clinical Neurophysiology,* 63(6), 547–551.
44 patients (mean age range 69–76 yrs) with Alzheimer's disease served as Ss in a double-blind, no crossover study of the effect of a synthetic adrenocorticotropic hormone (ACTH) analog (Org 2766) on the EEG. Results of quantitative EEG power spectrum analysis show no improvement that could be related to Org 2766, either by comparing the successive EEG sessions or by comparing the drug-treated group with the placebo-treated group. (French abstract).

841. Patterson, Julie V. (1985). **Auditory evoked potentials in dementia.** *Dissertation Abstracts International,* 45(8-B), 2713.

842. Peabody, Cecilia A.; Minkoff, Jerome R.; Davies, Helen D.; Winograd, Carol H. et al. (1986). **Thyrotropin-releasing hormone stimulation test and Alzheimer's disease.** *Biological Psychiatry,* 21(5–6), 553–556.
Measured levels of thyrotropin-stimulating hormone (TSH), prolactin (PRL), growth hormone (GH), and cortisol before and after injection with thyrotropin-releasing hormone (TRH) in 9 men (55–74 yrs old) with Alzheimer-type dementia and 9 age-matched controls. The Alzheimer group had a lower PRL baseline and a greater PRL response to TRH, a finding inconsistent with other studies. GH and TSH responses to TRH did not differ between groups.

843. Penttilä, M.; Partanen, Juhani V.; Soininen, H. & Riekkinen, P. J. (1985). **Quantitative analysis of occipital EEG in different stages of Alzheimer's disease.** *Electroencephalography & Clinical Neurophysiology,* 60(1), 1–6.
Studied EEG frequency analysis in 42 patients (mean age 73 yrs) in different stages of Alzheimer's disease (AD), 11 same-age healthy controls, and 11 young healthy controls (mean age 33 yrs). Selected findings show that the percentage power of the alpha band, the occipital peak frequency, and the ratio of powers in the alpha and delta bands decreased linearly in different stages of AD. The generally accepted EEG criteria

for AD, including slowing of the dominant occipital rhythm and accentuation of the diffuse irregular slow waves, were found to describe advanced, not mild, disease. (French abstract) (13 ref).

844. Philpot, M. et al. (1985). **Prolactin cell autoantibodies and Alzheimer's disease.** *Journal of Neurology, Neurosurgery & Psychiatry,* 48(3), 287–288.
Sera were collected from 20 63–95 yr old Alzheimer patients with clinically diagnosed Alzheimer's type senile dementia and 3 patients (mean age 61 yrs) with Down's syndrome who had had intellectual deterioration. None of the sera from either group contained autoantibodies to prolactin cells, although 6 had gastric parietal cell, 5 had thyroglobulin autoantibodies, and 5 were positive for thyroid microsomal autoantibody. Findings are discussed in terms of the study by A. Pouplard et al (1983) showing sera positive for prolactin cell autoantibodies in similar Ss. (9 ref).

845. Prinz, Patricia N. et al. (1982). **Sleep, EEG and mental function changes in senile dementia of the Alzheimer's type.** *Neurobiology of Aging,* 3(4), 361–370.
Studied sleep, EEG, and mental function variables in 44 Ss diagnosed as having probable senile dementia of the Alzheimer's type (SDAT) and 22 controls matched for age and minimal depression. Results indicate that sleep, EEG, and mental function variables all undergo significant change even in the early, mild stage of SDAT, with further change in the moderate and severe stages of dementia. Mental function variables also underwent significant decline across levels of dementia. Sleep and mental function variables had strong power in correctly classifying Ss into control vs mild dementia groups (90 and 100%, respectively). Dominant occipital rhythm frequency, a clinical EEG measure, also discriminated as well (75%). Results indicate that sleep and EEG variables discriminate well for early, mild SDAT in minimally depressed aged individuals. (60 ref).

846. Rae-Grant, Alex; Blume, Warren; Lau, Catherine; Hachinski, Vladimir C. et al. (1987). **The electroencephalogram in Alzheimer-type dementia: A sequential study correlating the electroencephalogram with psychometric and quantitative pathologic data.** *Archives of Neurology,* 44(1), 50–54.
Assessed sequential EEGs in 139 50–90 yr old patients with dementia of the Alzheimer's type (DAT) and 148 47–90 yr old controls, enabling documentation of sequential and specific EEG parameters in the population and correlation with psychometric and morphometric data. It was found that a large proportion of the DAT Ss showed a tendency to remain stable in their EEG patterns, and even in some cases to improve over 2–3 yrs. Correlations were found between EEG grade and psychometric scores, and morphometric neuron loss and EEG severity, which suggest that EEG findings can indicate whether DAT is more or less likely when clinical evaluation leaves doubt.

847. Renvoize, E. B. (1984). **An HLA and family study of Alzheimer's disease.** *Psychological Medicine,* 14(3), 515–520.
Examined histocompatibility antigens in 37 45–64 yr old White patients with a clinical diagnosis of presenile dementia of the Alzheimer's type and 87 65–89 yr old White patients with senile dementia of the Alzheimer's type. All Ss were typed for 20 of the main human lymphocyte antigen (HLA)-A and -B group antigens. The next of kin of 10 HLA-B15 positive and 10 HLA-B15 negative Alzheimer's disease (AD) Ss matched for sex and age at onset of AD and 14 other unmatched AD patients were interviewed. Cases of AD occurring among 1st-degree relatives were then identified. A diagnosis of AD was made in relatives if a history of progressive dementia in the absence of strokes or other significant disease was found. Relatives affected with AD were traced and HLA-typed. The HLA-A and -B antigen frequencies in the Ss were compared with frequencies found in 458 unrelated blood donors and healthy hospital staff drawn from similar ethnic and geographical backgrounds. Results suggest that AD is not strongly associated with any particular HLA antigen, although there may be a weak association with HLA-A2, B15, and Cw3. (30 ref).

848. Reynolds, Charles F. et al. (1985). **Sleep apnea in Alzheimer's dementia: Correlation with mental deterioration.** *Journal of Clinical Psychiatry,* 46(7), 257–261.
In a prospective study of sleep-disordered breathing among 23 58–82 yr old healthy controls, 17 55–81 yr old major depressives, and 21 49–85 yr old nondepressed demented patients with probable Alzheimer's disease, sleep apnea (defined as an apnea index of 5 or more) was found in 42.9% of demented patients, 17.6% of depressives, and 4.3% of controls. A significant association between sleep apnea and dementia of the Alzheimer type was found in women but not in men. Moreover, severity of dementia was significantly correlated with apnea index. Neuropathologic and clinical implications are discussed. (12 ref).

849. Reynolds, Charles F.; Kupfer, David J.; Hoch, Carolyn C.; Houck, Patricia R. et al. (1987). **Sleep deprivation as a probe in the elderly.** *Archives of General Psychiatry,* 44(11), 982–990.
Examined recovery from sleep deprivation (SD) in 15 Alzheimer's dementia (AD) patients (mean age 73.3 yrs), 15 depressed patients (mean age 72 yrs), and 15 healthy controls (mean age 72.6 yrs). Results indicate that depression or AD compromised the augmentation of sleep continuity and slow wave sleep seen in healthy elderly following SD. REM latency decreased during recovery sleep (RS) in controls but increased in the patients. Compared with AD patients, depressed patients had more sleep continuity disturbance before and after SD, a more protracted course of RS, and increased slow-wave density in the 2nd non-REM sleep period during recovery.

850. Reynolds, Charles F.; Kupfer, David J.; Houck, Patricia R.; Hoch, Carolyn C. et al. (1988). **Reliable discrimination of elderly depressed and demented patients by electroencephalographic sleep data.** *Archives of General Psychiatry,* 45(3), 258–264.
67 nondemented depressed patients, 49 patients with probable Alzheimer-type dementia, 42 patients with depression and dementia, and 77 healthy controls (aged 49–89 yrs) were kept psychotropic drug free for 14 days before EEG sleep study protocols were obtained. Analyses of sleep alterations in depression and dementia were performed. Four measures contributed to the discrimination of depressed and demented Ss: REM sleep percent (higher in depressives), NREM sleep percent (higher in demented Ss), REM sleep latency (lower in depressives), and sleep maintenance or early morning awakening. 80% and 81% of the diagnostically pure patients were correctly identified by backward and general stepwise discriminant function analysis, respectively.

851. Robbins, Jay H. et al. (1985). **Parkinson's disease and Alzheimer's disease: Hypersensitivity to X rays in cultured cell lines.** *Journal of Neurology, Neurosurgery & Psychiatry,* 48(9), 916–923.
Lymphoblastoid lines were irradiated from 24 patients (31–72 yrs old) with sporadic Parkinson's disease (PD), Alzheimer's disease (AD), amyotrophic lateral sclerosis (ALS), and multiple sclerosis. The mean survival values of the 8 PD and of the 6 AD lines, but not of the 5 ALS lines, were less than that of the lines from 28 normal controls (12–71 yrs old). Results can be explained by a genetic defect arising as a somatic mutation during embryogenesis causing defective repair of the X-ray type of DNA damage. Such a DNA repair defect could cause an abnormal accumulation of spontaneously occurring DNA damage in PD and AD neurons in vivo, resulting in their premature death. (43 ref).

852. Rogers, Robert L. et al. (1986). **Decreased cerebral blood flow precedes multi-infarct dementia, but follows senile dementia of Alzheimer type.** *Neurology,* 36(1), 1–6.
Conducted a 7-yr prospective study, using annual checkups, neurologic examinations, and questionnaires, of 181 neurologically normal elderly volunteers (aged 50–99 yrs) to examine the onset of senile dementia. Results show that 6 Ss developed senile dementia of the Alzheimer type (SDAT) in 7 yrs, a rate of 0.47% new cases each year, and that 10 Ss had multi-infarct dementia (MID), a rate of 0.78% new cases each year. The high incidence of MID was thought to reflect preselection of Ss (48.6%) with risk factors for, but without symptoms of, atherothrombotic stroke. Of 88 Ss at risk of stroke, 11.4% developed MID. In MID Ss, cerebral blood flow (CBF) values began to decline approximately 2 yrs before onset symptoms, while in SDAT patients, CBF levels remained normal until symptoms of dementia appeared. (44 ref).

853. Rosan, Robert C. (1987). **Physical complications of Alzheimer's disease.** Special Issue: The physician's guide to counseling the elderly. *Medical Aspects of Human Sexuality,* 21(3), 77–88.
Reviews the common physical complications of Alzheimer's disease (AD) by presenting 4 cases and describing the measures used in treatment and prevention. Complications illustrated include altered sleeping habits and sundowning syndrome, thyroid dysfunction, unsuspected urinary tract infection, and progressive septicemia. The patient's history, laboratory findings, and the differentiation of AD from concomitant illness are discussed. It is suggested that early detection and prompt, effective management can prevent family crises and improve the quality of the AD patient's life.

854. Sanders, David J. (1987). **Event-related potentials and cognition in Alzheimer's disease.** *Dissertation Abstracts International,* 48(2-B), 593.

855. Scileppi, Kenneth P.; Blass, John P. & Baker, Herman G. (1984). **Circulating vitamins in Alzheimer's dementia as compared with other dementias.** *Journal of the American Geriatrics Society,* 32(10), 709–711.
Compared blood levels of 12 vitamins in 55 patients with Alzheimer's disease (AD) and 58 control Ss (10 intellectually alert, 12 depressed, 28 with multi-infarct dementias, and 8 with other specific dementias). No significant differences in vitamin blood levels were found between the AD group and the control groups, either individually or collectively. Conventional parenteral vitamin treatment of 7 Ss with vitamin deficits did not benefit their cognitive states. It is concluded that conventional vitamin malnutrition did not contribute to the disability in these Ss. (8 ref).

856. Scott, Linda H. (1982). **Regional cerebral blood flow and verbal and nonverbal memory in Alzheimer's disease and normal aging.** *Dissertation Abstracts International,* 43(4-B), 1268.

857. Seltzer, Benjamin; Burres, J. K. & Sherwin, Ira. (1984). **Left-handedness in early and late onset dementia.** *Neurology,* 34(3), 367–368.
In 65 males with the diagnosis of dementia of the Alzheimer type, left-handedness was significantly more frequent among Ss with an age at onset (AAO) of 47–64 yrs than among Ss with an AAO of 65–90 yrs. It is suggested that some factor present in early-AAO dementia might lead to both exaggerated left hemisphere vulnerability and reduced life span, while the absence of this factor would lead to a population that is long-lived and has a low prevalence of both language disturbance and left-handedness, as observed in late-AAO Ss. (14 ref).

858. Sherman, Kathleen A.; Gibson, Gary E. & Blass, John P. (1986). **Human red blood cell choline uptake with age and Alzheimer's disease.** *Neurobiology of Aging,* 7(3), 205–209.
Temperature-dependent choline uptake at low and high choline concentrations increased in red blood cells (RBCs) from 11 elderly controls (mean age 71.6 yrs) and 11 Alzheimer's patients (mean age 77.3 yrs) compared to 9 young controls (mean age 31.8 yrs). These changes in transport were not directly related to altered RBC choline content. However, plasma choline content was significantly elevated in elderly controls and Alzheimer's Ss compared to young control values. The RBC to plasma ratio of choline was reduced in elderly compared to young controls, whereas the ratio in Alzheimer's Ss was between the 2 other groups.

859. Shore, David & Wyatt, Richard J. (1983). **Aluminum and Alzheimer's disease.** *Journal of Nervous & Mental Disease,* 171(9), 553–558.
Measured Al concentrations in the nuclei of paired-helical filaments in the brains of 10 patients (mean age 63.6 yrs) with Alzheimer's disease and 10 controls (mean age 62.2 yrs). No differences were found. However, controls only were found to have elevations of Al concentrations in the serum, CSF, and hair. Findings suggest that Al alone is not a cause of Alzheimer's disease. (48 ref).

860. Shore, David et al. (1984). **Hair and serum copper, zinc, calcium, and magnesium concentrations in Alzheimer-type dementia.** *Journal of the American Geriatrics Society,* 32(12), 892–895.
Analyzed serum and hair concentrations of copper, zinc, magnesium, and calcium; serum concentrations of albumin; and hair concentrations of manganese in 10 55–79 yr old outpatients in the early-to-middle stages of Alzheimer's disease (AD) and their 10 55–72 yr old healthy spouses. No differences in serum or hair concentrations were found. Thus, determinations of these hair and serum mineral concentrations do not appear to be of use in the diagnosis of AD. (18 ref).

861. Sims, N. R.; Finegan, J. M. & Blass, J. P. (1985). **Altered glucose metabolism in fibroblasts from patients with Alzheimer's disease.** *New England Journal of Medicine,* 313(10), 638–639.
Fibroblasts from 6 Ss (mean age 62 yrs) with Alzheimer's disease and from 7 matched controls (mean age 63 yrs) were grown in minimal essential medium. Observations of the results suggest that (1) the major difference in $^{14}CO_2$ production occurred during a period of rapid metabolism within the 1st 190 min, whereas the difference in lactate production occurred after this initial period; and (2) alterations in glucose metabolism may be expressed in other tissues. Findings also suggest pathophysiologically plausible mechanisms for selective neuronal cell death. (12 ref).

862. Singh, Vijendra K. & Fudenberg, H. Hugh. (1986). **Can blood immunocytes be used to study neuropsychiatric disorders?** *Journal of Clinical Psychiatry,* 47(12), 592–595.
Discusses evidence that demonstrates a structural and functional interrelationship between the immune system and central nervous system (CNS). Based on analogies between these 2 systems, the proposal is made that at least some neuropsychiatric diseases can be evaluated by functional studies of peripheral blood immunocytes. This hypothesis is supported by the results of immunologic function studies of various subpopulations of immunocytes obtained from patients with Alzheimer's disease and retinitis pigmentosa.

863. Skias, Demetrios et al. (1985). **Senile dementia of Alzheimer's type (SDAT): Reduced T8⁺-cell-mediated suppressor activity.** *Neurology,* 35(11), 1635–1638.

Compared 16 patients (aged 60–85 yrs) with SDAT and 14 controls (aged 57–84 yrs) with respect to T8⁺-cell-mediated suppressor function using a pokeweed mitogen-induced immunoglobulin secretion assay. Suppressor function was lower in both SDAT and elderly controls than in 5 young adults (aged 20–40 yrs). In SDAT Ss, there seemed to be an exaggeration of the age-related decline in suppressor-cell function. Whether such changes reflect accelerated changes of intrinsic lymphocyte properties or aberrant neural influences on lymphocytes remains to be resolved. (21 ref).

864. Small, Gary W. et al. (1985). **Thyroid disease in patients with dementia of the Alzheimer type.** *Journal of the American Geriatrics Society,* 33(8), 538–539.
Compared the frequencies of prior thyroid disease, thyroid medication use, and abnormal serum thyroxine levels in 61 patients (average age 71.7 yrs) with dementia of the Alzheimer type (DAT) with those of 38 controls (average age 73.6 yrs). It was found that the 33 women with DAT had a 24.2% frequency of prior thyroid disease, comparable with that found in a previous epidemiologic study by H. Heyman et al (1984). The 19 female controls, however, had a similar frequency, failing to support Heyman and colleagues' finding of an association between DAT and thyroid disease. (9 ref).

865. Smallwood, Robert G.; Vitiello, Michael V.; Giblin, Elizabeth C. & Prinz, Patricia N. (1983). **Sleep apnea: Relationship to age, sex, and Alzheimer's dementia.** *Sleep,* 6(1), 16–22.
Examined the relationship of sleep apnea to age, sex, and Alzheimer's dementia in 10 young male controls (aged 23–38 yrs), 24 elderly male controls (aged 50–80 yrs), 6 elderly female controls (aged 58–75 yrs), 11 elderly males (aged 56–81 yrs) with Alzheimer's disease, and 4 elderly females (aged 61–82 yrs) with Alzheimer's disease. Ss were monitored during their regular bedtime hours for breathing patterns and nondominant limb movement and using an EEG, EMG, EOG, and EKG. Mean apnea/hypopnea index [(AH)I] was significantly greater in elderly males than in young males or elderly females. Mean (AH)I and percentage of Ss with an (AH)I > 5 in the Alzheimer groups were not significantly different from age and sex-matched controls. Results were similar when the apnea index was substituted for (AH)I. The data from this preliminary study indicate that healthy, elderly males with no sleep complaints and elderly males with Alzheimer's disease experience a significant, subclinical ventilatory impairment during sleep. Data from the 10 elderly females and 10 young males indicated no such impairment. The physiological significance of this degree of sleep apnea in otherwise healthy elderly males is unclear at present. (French abstract) (25 ref).

866. Soininen, H.; Partanen, V. J.; Helkala, Eeva-Liisa & Riekkinen, Paavo J. (1982). **EEG findings in senile dementia and normal aging.** *Acta Neurologica Scandinavica,* 65(1), 59–70.
Compared EEGs of 62 patients (mean age 78.1 yrs) with senile dementia of the Alzheimer type (SDA), 22 patients (mean age 76.6 yrs) with multi-infarct dementia (MID), and 90 age- and sex-matched normal controls. SDA Ss differed significantly from controls in EEG normality, overall disturbance, dominant occipital rhythm, accentuation of theta and delta, fluctuations in alertness, paroxysmal activity, and H-reaction. With increasing intellectual impairment in the SDA group, the dominant occipital rhythm became slower. The MID group differed from controls in all EEG parameters and from SDA Ss only in asymmetric findings, which were more common in MID Ss. 29% of the controls had mild EEG alterations. Asymmetric findings, mainly theta activity in left temporal region, were common. H-reaction was well preserved. It is concluded that the EEG is valuable in differentiating dementia patients from normal elderly people, but it is not reliable by itself in the differentiation between MID and SDA. (22 ref).

867. Spydell, John D. (1982). **Forty hertz EEG activity in normal elderly and in elderly with dementia of the Alzheimer's type.** *Dissertation Abstracts International,* 42(8-B), 3483.

868. Spydell, John D. & Sheer, Daniel E. (1983). **Forty Hertz EEG activity in Alzheimer's type dementia.** *Psychophysiology,* 20(3), 313–319.
EEG activity within the 40-Hz band was monitored during several tasks and during a nontask condition. 12 right-handed 46–77 yr old Ss diagnosed as having Alzheimer's type dementia were compared to 12 51–77 yr old neurologically normal Ss of comparable IQ; WAIS scores ranged from 94 to 120. While the normal group exhibited appropriate increases in 40-Hz activity during problem solving, the Alzheimer's type dementia group did not. The task appropriate lateralization of 40-Hz activity seen in the normal group was absent in the Alzheimer's group. (23 ref).

869. St. Clair, D. & Whalley, L. J. (1983). **Hypertension, multi-infarct dementia and Alzheimer's disease.** *British Journal of Psychiatry,* 143, 274–276.
Conducted a retrospective review and postmortem examination of the cases of 89 patients with presenile dementia. Results indicate significant differences between subtypes of dementia. The 27 Ss with multi-infarct dementia more often had cardiovascular abnormalities than the 46 Ss with Alzheimer's disease. 23 Alzheimer Ss and 3 of 16 Ss with mixed features had a systolic pressure below 140 mm Hg. (10 ref).

870. St. Clair, David M.; Blackwood, Douglas H. & Christie, Janice E. (1985). **P3 and other long latency auditory evoked potentials in presenile dementia Alzheimer type and alcoholic Korsakoff syndrome.** *British Journal of Psychiatry,* 147, 702–706.
Measured the P300 (P3) and other long latency auditory evoked potentials in 15 patients (aged 54–67 yrs) with presenile dementia Alzheimer type (ATD), 16 patients (aged 49–72 yrs) with alcoholic Korsakoff syndrome (KS), and 23 control Ss (aged 51–72 yrs) drug free for at least 4 wks before testing. Results indicate that the latency of the P3 was significantly longer and the amplitude significantly smaller in the ATD group than in both the KS and control groups. The KS group did not differ significantly from the control group in either latency or amplitude of P3, but both the KS and ATD groups had reduced N1 and P2 compared to controls. Using a combination of P3 latency and amplitude, 70% of the ATD Ss could be separated from the other groups with no false positives. Findings suggest that evoked potential recording may be of value in the diagnosis of early ATD. (17 ref).

871. Sulkava, Raimo; Nordberg, U.-R.; Erkinjuntti, Timo & Westermarck, T. (1986). **Erythrocyte glutathione peroxidase and superoxide dismutase in Alzheimer's disease and other dementias.** *Acta Neurologica Scandinavica,* 73(5), 487–489.
Activities of 2 enzymes (erythrocyte glutathione peroxidase and superoxide dismutase) were measured in 4 patients (aged 58–74 yrs) with Alzheimer's disease (AD), 4 Ss (aged 57–83 yrs) with multi-infarct dementia, a 33-yr-old with Huntington's disease, and a 44-yr-old with Hakola-Nasu disease. No significant differences were found between the Ss with AD and controls.

872. Sunderland, Trey et al. (1986). **Thyrotropin-releasing hormone and dementia.** *American Journal of Psychiatry,* 143(10), 1318.
Comments on a report by C. A. Peabody et al (1986) regarding their pilot experience administering thyrotropin-releasing hormone (TRH) to 4 Alzheimer's disease patients by noting that a much higher dose of the peptide or a TRH-drug combination is required to achieve substantial brain levels. The present authors present their own findings with Alz-

heimer's disease patients, which suggest an abnormality in the pituitary response to TRH similar to that found in some other neuropsychiatric conditions (including depression). (5 ref).

873. Sunderland, Trey; Tariot, Pierre N.; Cohen, R. M.; Newhouse, P. A. et al. (1987). **Dose-dependent effects of deprenyl on CSF monoamine metabolites in patients with Alzheimer's disease.** *Psychopharmacology,* 91(3), 293–296.
Administered deprenyl, a monoamine oxidase (MAO) inhibitor to 13 patients (mean age 57.1 yrs) with dementia of the Alzheimer type (DAT). Three monoamine metabolites, homovanillic acid (HVA), 5-hydroxyindoleacetic acid (5-HIAA), and 3-methoxy-4-hydroxyphenylglycol (MHPG) were measured. Deprenyl treatment (10 mg/day) for 3–4 wks was associated with reductions in HVA and 5-HIAA and deprenyl (40 mg/day) for 3–4 more wks led to greater reductions in HVA and MHPG than 5-HIAA. Results are consistent with in vitro biochemical and anatomical data from primate brain suggesting that at low doses of deprenyl, MAO-B inhibition might be expected to selectively affect dopamine and serotonin-containing neurons, while at higher doses noradrenergic neurons may become relatively more affected by the drug.

874. Suranyi-Cadotte, B. E. et al. (1985). **Platelet ³H-imipramine binding distinguishes depression from Alzheimer dementia.** *Life Sciences,* 37(24), 2305–2311.
Investigated the usefulness of [³H]-imipramine binding and serotonin uptake in diagnosing depression in the elderly. Ss were 10 patients (mean age 63 yrs) with idiopathic Parkinson's disease, 9 patients (mean age 69 yrs) with primary degenerative dementia of the Alzheimer type, and 17 patients (mean age 65 yrs) with major depressive disorder. Two control groups consisted of 11 younger (mean age 34 yrs) and 11 elderly (mean age 66 yrs) healthy Ss. Whereas the maximum rate of platelet serotonin uptake was significantly reduced in all patient groups compared to age matched normal Ss, the density of [³H]-imipramine binding was reduced in depressed patients only. The lower maximum binding values in depressed patients was independent of patient age. These data suggest that platelet [³H]-imipramine binding may be a useful laboratory index that discriminates depression from dementia in the elderly. (48 ref).

875. Tavy, D. L.; Van Woerkom, T. C.; Morré, H. H. & Slaets, J. P. (1986). **Alteration of the visual blink reflex in patients with dementia.** *Journal of Neurology, Neurosurgery & Psychiatry,* 49(6), 718.
Demonstrated that the latency of the visual blink reflex (VBI) of 12 patients (mean age 77.2 yrs) with senile dementia (Alzheimer type dementia or multi-infarct dementia) was significantly increased compared to 12 controls (mean age 70.5 yrs). It is suggested that the alteration of the VBI in senile dementia is due to lesions or functional disturbances at the level of the brain stem.

876. Taylor, G. R. et al. (1984). **Herpes simplex virus and Alzheimer's disease: A search for virus DNA by spot hybridisation.** *Journal of Neurology, Neurosurgery & Psychiatry,* 47(10), 1061–1065.
Used a sensitive hybridization screening technique (spot hybridization) to search postmortem brain DNA extracts for herpes simplex I-virus (HSV) sequences in 9 human non-neurological controls (mean age 75 yrs at death), 8 human Alzheimer's disease cases (mean age 71 yrs at death), and HSV-infected mice. A reconstruction experiment showed that .1 herpes genome equivalents/cell could be detected in 100 μg tissue extracts. Although herpes sequences were readily detected in infected mice, none of the human brains contained such sequences. Results do not support the findings of N. W. Fraser et al (1981) that HSV DNA is commonly found in the human CNS. (20 ref).

877. Thal, Leon J. (1985). **Changes in cerebrospinal fluid associated with dementia.** *Annals of the New York Academy of Sciences,* 444, 235–241.
Discusses changes in cerebrospinal fluid (CSF) as a biological marker of Alzheimer's disease (AD) and other dementias. Routine analysis of CSF glucose, protein, and cell count does not distinguish AD patients from age-matched controls, although some investigators have reported a decrease in total protein. More recently, several reports of abnormal proteins in the CSF of dementia patients have appeared. Of all the neurotransmitter changes in AD, the decrease in presynaptic cholinergic markers is the most profound. A large number of neuropeptides have been measured in brain tissue from AD patients, including somatostatin, cholecystokinin, vasoactive intestinal peptide, enkephalin, thyrotropin-releasing hormone, neurotensin, vasopressin, oxytocin, and substance P. A number of other peptides have also been examined in the CSF of AD patients. (43 ref).

878. Thienhaus, Ole J.; Cliffe, Charles; Zemlan, Frank P. & Bosmann, H. Bruce. (1986). **Superoxide dismutase, chromosome 21, and Alzheimer's disease.** *Biological Psychiatry,* 21(11), 1106–1107.
Compared the superoxide dismutase (SOD-1) activity in skin fibroblasts from a 53-yr-old man with familial Alzheimer's disease and in those from a 14-yr-old girl with Down's syndrome and a healthy 55-yr-old man. Fibroblasts from the Alzheimer's and the Down's Ss revealed significantly greater SOD-1 activity than those of the normal control.

879. Thienhaus, Ole J.; Hartford, James T.; Skelly, Michael F. & Bosmann, H. Bruce. (1985). **Biologic markers in Alzheimer's disease.** *Journal of the American Geriatrics Society,* 33(10), 715–726.
Discusses efforts to find a biologic marker of Alzheimer's disease that is more accessible than the brain, such as a constituent of circulating blood, cerebrospinal fluid (CSF), or urine. It is suggested that if marker assays were quantifiable, prognostic predictions might become possible, permitting monitoring of the course of disease and providing an important diagnostic complement to psychometric assessment methods. A brief overview of diagnostic approaches to dementing illness, including etiological, pathogenesis, cerebral change, and clinical syndrome levels of intervention, is presented. Efforts to obtain a biologic marker in the cholinergic system, somatostatin levels, biogenic amines, and metabolic and endocrine parameters of Alzheimer's patients are described along with the potential use of immunologic factors, genetic markers, and computed axial tomography scans and evoked potentials to identify Alzheimer's disease patients. It is suggested that, while studies that have attempted to identify a peripheral correlate to the central transmitter pathology are characterized by inconsistency, several promising areas of research are currently being investigated. (108 ref).

880. Thienhaus, Ole J.; Zemlan, Frank P.; Bienenfeld, David; Hartford, James T. et al. (1987). **Growth hormone response to edrophonium in Alzheimer's disease.** *American Journal of Psychiatry,* 144(8), 1049–1052.
Studied the suggestion that neuropathologic data from patients with Alzheimer's disease indicate the presence of neurofibrillary tangles in hypothalamic regions associated with regulation of pituitary hormone release. Explored was the hypothesis that cholinergic projections to hypothalamic nuclei controlling pituitary growth hormone (GH) release degenerate in Alzheimer's disease. Integrity of cholinergic regulation was tested by assaying the GH response to a presynaptic cholinergic challenge. After administration of the choline esterase inhibitor edrophonium, the peak GH response was 14 ng/ml in 8 healthy elderly control Ss (mean age 63 yrs) and only 2 ng/ml in 14 Alzheimer's patients (mean age 71 yrs). The magnitude of GH blunting was correlated with cognitive and functional deficits. Possible implications of

these data for enhanced accuracy in the diagnosis of dementia are discussed.

881. Thomas, D. R.; Hailwood, R.; Harris, B.; Williams, P. A. et al. (1987). **Thyroid status in senile dementia of the Alzheimer type (SDAT).** *Acta Psychiatrica Scandinavica,* 76(2), 158–163.
Investigated thyroid function in 21 patients (mean age 76.4 yrs) with severe senile dementia of the Alzheimer type (SDAT) and in 17 age- and sex-matched normal controls. Free thyroid hormone levels of triiodothyronine (T_3) and thyroxine (T_4) were measured, as were the thyrotrophin (TSH), prolactin (PRL), and growth hormone (GH) responses to thyrotrophin releasing hormone (TRH). When compared to controls, Ss demonstrated a significantly lower free T_3 value (but not free T_4), a blunted TSH response to TRH, slightly elevated basal PRL and GH values, and a small GH response to TRH. Results show the relative normality of neuroendocrine function, particularly thyroid status, in SDAT.

882. Thomas, D. R.; Jones, E.; Warner, N.; Harris, B. et al. (1988). **Peripheral serotoninergic receptor sensitivity in senile dementia of the Alzheimer type.** *Biological Psychiatry,* 23(2), 136–140.
Platelet aggregation induced by 5-hydroxytryptamine (5-HT) was used as a measure of the functional responsiveness of peripheral 5-HT receptors in 18 drug-free patients (mean age 77.06 yrs) suffering from senile dementia of the Alzheimer type (SDAT) and 18 age- and sex-matched controls. No significantly different aggregatory response was noted between the 2 groups. The response mediated by platelet release products did not appear to be abnormal in Ss with SDAT.

883. Trappler, B.; Viswanathan, R. & Sher, J. (1986). **Alzheimer's disease in a patient on long-term hemodialysis: A case report.** *General Hospital Psychiatry,* 8(1), 57–60.
Describes a progressive dementia in a 49-yr-old Black male on long-term hemodialysis, in which the initial presentation simulated depression. Typical features of dialysis dementia were lacking. Autopsy revealed a ruptured cerebral aneurysm, polycystic kidneys, moderately severe atherosclerosis, military tuberculosis, and neurofibrillary degeneration of the hippocampus. The significance of a possible relationship between end-stage renal disease hemodialysis and Alzheimer's disease in this case is discussed. (22 ref).

884. Tresch, Donald D.; Folstein, Marshal F.; Rabins, Peter V. & Hazzard, William R. (1985). **Prevalence and significance of cardiovascular disease and hypertension in elderly patients with dementia and depression.** *Journal of the American Geriatrics Society,* 33(8), 530–537.
Compared the prevalence and significance of clinical heart disease and hypertension in 3 groups of elderly patients (94 Alzheimer's dementia [AD] Ss [aged 60–91 yrs], 37 multi-infarct dementia [MID] Ss [aged 60–89 yrs], and 52 Ss [aged 60–91 yrs] with major depression). Results support previous studies that have shown a low prevalence of cardiac disease and hypertension in AD Ss. In comparison, cardiac disease and hypertension were quite common in MID Ss and Ss with major depression. (50 ref).

885. Van Dorp, T. A. et al. (1985). **Prolactin cell autoantibodies and Alzheimer's disease.** *Journal of Neurology, Neurosurgery & Psychiatry,* 48(12), 1308–1309.
Attempted to replicate a study by A. Pouplard et al (1983) that suggested evidence of autoimmune dysfunction in Alzheimer's disease. The postmortem blood sera from 15 Alzheimer's patients and 29 psychiatric controls (schizophrenics, cyclic psychotics, and depressives [aged 65+ yrs]) were analyzed for prolactin cell autoantibodies. The high frequency of antibodies reacting to prolactin cells reported by Pouplard et al was not confirmed. (4 ref).

886. Van Tiggelen, Cees J. (1984). **Alzheimers disease/alcohol dementia: Association with zinc deficiency and cerebral vitamin B12 deficiency.** *Journal of Orthomolecular Psychiatry,* 13(2), 97–104.
Elderly patients (mean age 74 yrs) with senile dementia of the Alzheimer's type (SDAT [$n = 24$]), alcohol-related brain damage and alcohol dementia (AD [$n = 9$]), and multi-infarct dementia (MID [$n = 10$]) were compared to 28 normal age-matched controls to examine the connection between zinc deficiency and copper toxicity, as measured by the ratio of serum copper (se-Cu) to serum zinc (se-Zn), and a discrepancy between normal serum B12 and low CSF B12 in the dementia Ss. It was found that the SDAT and AD Ss showed a significant increase in the se-Cu/se-Zn ratio compared to the MID Ss and the controls, indicating the presence of zinc deficiency and relative copper toxicity in SDAT and AD, but not in MID. A high incidence of pathologically low CSF B12 levels was found in the SDAT and AD Ss despite normal serum B12 levels. Normal levels of CSF B12 and serum B12 were found in the MID Ss. Results indicate abnormal function of the choroid plexus and possibly of the blood–brain barrier in SDAT and AD Ss but not in MID Ss. It is suggested that the combination of zinc deficiency and copper toxicity causes limbic disinhibition and defective central noradrenergic neurotransmission. The neuroendocrine effects of the limbic disinhibition and the impaired regulation of cerebral microcirculation by a defective noradrenergic system is exacerbated by depression. Such a syndrome is disguised as dementia because of the reduced plasticity of the aging brain. (66 ref).

887. Visser, S. L. et al. (1985). **Visual evoked potentials (VEPs) in senile dementia (Alzheimer type) and in non-organic behavioural disorders in the elderly: Comparison with EEG parameters.** *Electroencephalography & Clinical Neurophysiology,* 60(2), 115–121.
42 patients (mean age 76 yrs) with senile dementia of the Alzheimer type were compared with 51 normal Ss (mean age 73.3 yrs) and with 40 elderly patients (mean age 73.7 yrs) with nonorganic psychiatric disorders. All Ss were examined by EEG (routine visual inspection and power spectrum density analysis) and VEP (pattern reversal) testing. In dementia the late components (N130, P165, and N220) of the VEP were delayed, but the EEG was abnormal more often than was the VEP. It is concluded that the EEG (visual inspection and power spectrum density analysis) detects abnormalities in dementia more than does the VEP, so VEPs cannot replace the EEG in the diagnosis of dementia. The need to study the specific pathophysiological significance of VEP late-component abnormalities is emphasized. (French abstract) (12 ref).

888. Vitiello, Michael V. et al. (1984). **Rapid eye movement sleep measures of Alzheimer's-type dementia patients and optimally healthy aged individuals.** *Biological Psychiatry,* 19(5), 721–734.
Examined the REM sleep of 9 mild, 9 moderate, and 9 severe dementia Ss with probable Alzheimer's disease (AD; mean ages 65.7, 70, and 73 yrs, respectively) and of 9 controls (mean age 65.6 yrs). Control and mild and moderate AD groups were screened to exclude major depression. REM latency, REM time, REM activity, and REM density were examined. Results indicate that REM sleep measures were minimally affected by mild dementia. None of the REM sleep variables successfully discriminated mild AD Ss from controls. However, REM time and REM latency were significantly affected in later stages of dementia. Total time in REM and REM latency successfully classified controls and moderate and severe AD patients. In addition, the pattern of REM density across the night was also affected by severity of dementia. Results, when compared to published REM measure findings in major depression, indicate that with proper cautions REM sleep measures may prove useful in the dif-

ferential diagnosis of dementia and depression in geriatric patient populations. (48 ref).

889. Volicer, Ladislav; Greene, Louise & Sinex, F. Marott. (1985). **Epinephrine-induced cyclic AMP production in skin fibroblasts from patients with dementia of Alzheimer type and controls.** *Neurobiology of Aging,* 6(1), 35–38.
In a search for biological markers of dementia of the Alzheimer type (DAT) that would be helpful in early diagnosis of the disease, the authors compared formation of cyclic adenosine monophosphate (AMP) in response to beta receptor stimulation in fibroblasts from 6 patients with DAT and from 3 hospitalized age-matched controls. Fibroblasts from skin biopsies were grown in culture and compared for their growth characteristics and sensitivity to epinephrine with 4 cultures from age-matched healthy individuals included in the Baltimore Longitudinal Study. The growth characteristics were similar in all 3 groups. The basal levels of cyclic AMP and the epinephrine-induced increase of cyclic AMP levels were also similar in control and DAT cells. (30 ref).

890. Weinreb, Herman J. (1985). **Fingerprint patterns in Alzheimer's disease.** *Archives of Neurology,* 42(1), 50–54.
Compared fingerprint dermatoglyphic patterns in 50 patients (aged 56–89 yrs) with senile dementia of the Alzheimer type (SDAT), 50 patient controls (aged 56–91 yrs) with other neurologic diseases, and a reference group of 5,000 British Ss (H. Cummins and C. Midlo, 1943). Results indicate that SDAT Ss evidenced an increased frequency of ulnar loops when compared with the other groups. The patterns observed in the SDAT Ss are congruent with patterns found in patients with Down's syndrome and support the associations found between these 2 diseases. (39 ref).

891. Whitehouse, Peter J. (1985). **Receptor autoradiography: Applications in neuropathology.** *Trends in Neurosciences,* 8(10), 434–437.
In neurological diseases, receptor autoradiography can be used to construct high-resolution maps of receptor distributions and to examine the relationships between specific cellular pathologies and changes in receptor densities. The advantages and limitations of this technique are summarized. Autoradiographic studies of 3 degenerative disorders—amyotrophic lateral sclerosis, Huntington's disease, and Alzheimer's disease—are reviewed.

892. Wolkowitz, Owen M.; Rubinow, David R.; Breier, Alan; Doran, Allen R. et al. (1987). **Prednisone decreases CSF somatostatin in healthy humans: Implications for neuropsychiatric illness.** *Life Sciences,* 41(16), 1929–1933.
Administration of the immunosuppressant prednisone to 9 healthy 21–41 yr olds resulted in significant reductions in cerebrospinal fluid (CSF) somatostatin-like immunoreactivity. The magnitude of these reductions was inversely related to the magnitude of prednisone-induced reductions in plasma adrenocorticotropic hormone (ACTH), suggesting a functional interaction between circulating corticosteroids, central somatostatin, and pituitary ACTH release. Implications for neuropsychiatric illnesses, including depression in Alzheimer's disease, are considered.

893. Zubenko, George S.; Cohen, Bruce M.; Reynolds, Charles F.; Boller, François et al. (1987). **Platelet membrane fluidity in Alzheimer's disease and major depression.** *American Journal of Psychiatry,* 144(7), 860–868.
Conducted double-blind fluorescence studies of platelet membrane fluidity at 37°C for 51 patients with Alzheimer-type dementia, 24 nondemented depressed patients, and 50 neurologically healthy Ss (all aged 45+ yrs). The fluidity of the hydrocarbon region of platelet membranes from the demented group, as reflected by the steady-state anisotropy of the fluorescent probe 1,6-diphenyl-1,3,5-hexatriene, was significantly greater than that for the depressed and normal

control Ss. Within the demented group, platelet membrane fluidity was significantly correlated with severity of dementia but not with duration of illness or age at onset. Demented patients with increased platelet membrane fluidity had an earlier onset, were more severely demented, and deteriorated more rapidly.

894. Zubenko, George S.; Marquis, Judith K.; Volicer, Ladislav; Direnfeld, Lorne K. et al. (1986). **Cerebrospinal fluid levels of angiotensin-converting enzyme, acetylcholinesterase, and dopamine metabolites in dementia associated with Alzheimer's disease and Parkinson's disease: A correlative study.** *Biological Psychiatry,* 21(14), 1365–1381.
Mean levels of the 2 hydrolases angiotensin-converting enzyme (ACE) and acetylcholinesterase (AChE), the dopamine metabolites dihydroxyphenylacetic acid (DOPAC) and homovanillic acid (HVA), and total protein concentration were examined in cerebrospinal fluid (CSF) samples from 13 patients (aged 48–76 yrs) with dementia of the Alzheimer's type (DAT), 10 comparably demented patients (aged 57–78 yrs) with Parkinson's disease (PD), and 15 neurologically healthy elderly controls (Cs [aged 58–86 yrs]). DAT and PD Ss exhibited a significant decrease in the mean levels of ACE activity and DOPAC per milliliter. Unlike the PD Ss, the mean HVA concentration of DAT Ss was significantly elevated. Independent of CSF protein concentration, ACE activity per milliliter exhibited a positive correlation with AChE activity per milliliter within Cs and PD Ss, whereas a significant correlation for these CSF hydrolases was not observed within the DAT group.

895. Zubenko, George S.; Wusylko, Michael; Cohen, Bruce M.; Boller, Francois et al. (1987). **Family study of platelet membrane fluidity in Alzheimer's disease.** *Science,* 238(4826), 539–542.
Investigated the relation of platelet membrane abnormality and the onset of symptoms of dementia. Ss were 23 patients with probable Alzheimer's disease (AD), 15 Ss whose AD had been confirmed by autopsy, 38 1st-degree relatives of the probands, and 34 controls. Results of fluorescence anisotropy show that platelet membrane abnormality was 3.2–11.5 times higher in relatives of probands. It is concluded that the abnormality of platelet membranes may be an inherited factor that is related to the development of AD.

GENERAL ISSUES & RESEARCH

896. ————. (1985). **Protection and advocacy for mentally ill persons act of 1985.** *Mental & Physical Disability Law Reporter,* 9(6), 466.
Compares 2 bills approved by the US Senate that address advocacy of the rights of mentally ill persons: One limits reasonable attorneys' fees for publicly funded legal aid attorneys to actual litigation costs rather than prevailing market rates and requires the exhaustion of administrative remedies "where appropriate." The other contains no such limitations and provides for the establishment of advisory boards as well as family support groups for Alzheimer's disease patients.

897. Amaducci, Luigi A.; Rocca, Walter A. & Schoenberg, Bruce S. (1986). **Origin of the distinction between Alzheimer's disease and senile dementia: How history can clarify nosology.** *Neurology,* 36(11), 1497–1499.
Discusses the history of presenile (Alzheimer's disease) and senile dementia, which reveals that the distinction was originally based on anecdotal clinical observations and that competition among universities was one of the underlying determinants. The personal opinion of E. Kraepelin played a major role. Reports based on large clinicopathologic series have shown that the pathologies of presenile and senile dementia are not qualitatively different.

898. Baker, F. M. (1986). **Legal issues affecting the older patient.** *Hospital & Community Psychiatry,* 37(11), 1091–1093.
Discusses the legal issues a psychiatrist must address when asked to establish a diagnosis, manage behavioral changes, assess capacity to refuse treatment, or make a will for a patient with a dementing illness. Specific legal issues include competency to consent to hospitalization, the legality of the living will, testimonial capacity, and guardianship and conservatorship of a patient.

899. Ball, Melvyn J. (1986). **First Canadian Symposium on the organic dementias.** Special Issue: Controversial topics on Alzheimer's disease: Intersecting crossroads. *Neurobiology of Aging,* 7(6), 591–595.
Presents an overview of highlights from the 1st Canadian Symposium on the organic dementias held at the University of Western Ontario, June 23–24, 1986. Issues addressed in 40 papers presented by researchers from Canada, the US, and the UK were grouped under 5 themes: clinical and therapeutic issues, neuropsychological challenges, cellular clues to pathogenesis, biochemical studies, and imaging of demented Ss.

900. Berg, L. et al. (1982). **Mild senile dementia of Alzheimer type: Research diagnostic criteria, recruitment, and description of a study population.** *Journal of Neurology, Neurosurgery & Psychiatry,* 45(11), 962–968.
Explored guidelines for clinical diagnostic criteria for selection of mildly impaired Ss with senile dementia of Alzheimer type (SDAT), free of other major disease. Problems of recruitment of this select population for a longitudinal study are discussed. 43 Ss with mild SDAT, 16 with questionable SDAT, and 58 healthy controls (aged 63–82 yrs) were studied over 17 mo. Diagnostic criteria for SDAT included assessment of memory, orientation, judgment and problem solving, community affairs, home and hobbies, and personal care; interviews with the S and a person close to S; and examination for physical disorders. Short term follow-up of Ss has provided preliminary support for the diagnostic criteria. (43 ref).

901. Borrie, M. J.; Crilly, R. G. & Bowring, Linda. (1987). **Age at onset and rate of Alzheimer's disease.** *Journal of the American Geriatrics Society,* 35(10), 960.
Comments on the work of F. J. Huff et al (1987) on age at onset and rate of progression of Alzheimer's disease.

902. Busby, Jan et al. (1985). **Alzheimer's disease: An annotated bibliography of recent literature.** *Journal of the American Geriatrics Society,* 33(5), 366–373.
Presents an annotated list of 92 works dealing with general knowledge, etiology, pathophysiology, diagnosis, treatment, and epidemiology of Alzheimer's disease. The list was compiled by those participating in the geriatric medicine fellowship program at the Gainesville (Florida) Veterans Administration Medical Center. These works were chosen from 400 articles on the subject published since 1981.

903. Charatan, Fred B. (1986). **An overview of geriatric psychiatry.** *New York State Journal of Medicine,* 86(12), 630–634.
Presents an overview of the field of geriatric psychiatry, including the issues of recognition of the relationship of somatic disease to mental disorder in old age, the increasing prevalence with age of organic disease of the brain, the importance of the social network, and the importance of the medical aspects of psychiatry in the treatment of elderly psychiatric patients. Also discussed are senile dementia of the Alzheimer type; depression in old age, the most common mental disorder after age 65 yrs; and age-related issues in psychotherapy, including deafness, the therapist's feelings about his/her own aging, and transference. Recommendations

for the prevention of mental disorder in old age are discussed in relation to society's attitudes toward the elderly.

904. Cronin-Golomb, Alice. (1987). **Alzheimer's disease: Advances in basic research and therapies.** *Neurochemistry International,* 11(3), 347–350.
Summarizes reports and discussions of the International Study Group on the Pharmacology of Memory Disorders Associated with Aging, January 1987, concerning basic research and therapies in regard to Alzheimer's disease (AD). Discussed were (1) clinical advances in AD, (2) neurobiology of AD, (3) phospholipid membranes, and (4) prospects for treatment. Approaches included those of genetics, neuroimaging, neuropsychology, anatomy and physiology, neurochemistry, neuropathology, and experimental animal studies.

905. Crook, Thomas H. & Miller, Nancy E. (1985). **The challenge of Alzheimer's disease.** *American Psychologist,* 40(11), 1245–1250.
Discusses, using the case of a 73-yr-old female with Alzheimer's disease, the complexity of the challenge of Alzheimer's disease (e.g., difficulty of diagnosis, treatment of the patient and his/her family) and the multi-disciplinary effort underway at the National Institute of Mental Health to meet the challenge. (3 ref).

906. Dettmann, David F. (1987). **"Alzheimer's disease: The death of the disease": Comment.** *Counseling & Values,* 31(2), 176–178.
Comments that the L. W. McBroom article on Alzheimer's disease (AD [see PA, Vol 74:28604]) gave an accurate description of the characteristics of AD. It is suggested, however, that more information could have been provided on the costs and incidence of the disease and that a discussion of typical family struggles (i.e., whether or not to institutionalize a family member with AD), the issue of diagnosis, and possible genetic factors of AD should be included.

907. Duara, Ranjan & Black, Barbara C. (1984). **Report of a statewide conference of scientific investigators of senile dementia and Alzheimer's disease sponsored by the Governor of Florida.** *Journal of Applied Gerontology,* 3(2), 206–213.
Reviews the 4 primary areas addressed at the 1st statewide meeting in Florida of scientific investigators of senile dementia and Alzheimer's disease. Topics included epidemiology, diagnosis and characteristics, treatment, and the establishment of a statewide network. Recommendations to the Governor and the Florida Committee on Aging on areas for future state involvement are discussed, including the development of a statewide information system containing a patient and resource registry, a scholarship program for dementia research, educational programs on dementing illnesses for physicians and the general public, the establishment of a statewide advisory committee, and epidemiological studies to determine the magnitude of the problem in Florida.

908. Filley, Christopher M.; Brownell, Hiram H. & Albert, Martin L. (1985). **Education provides no protection against Alzheimer's disease.** *Neurology,* 35(12), 1781–1784.
Tested the contention that educational achievement confers protection against dementia by examining the educational level and age of onset in 28 patients with Alzheimer's disease and assessing the progression of dementia over a mean period of 28 mo using both a measure of neurobehavioral status and an index of functional impairment. Findings reveal no protective effect of education in either early- or late-onset dementia. (14 ref).

909. Goldberg, Richard T. (1985). **Alzheimer's disease: From benign neglect to community living.** *Rehabilitation Literature,* 46(5–6), 122–132.
Discusses the prevalence of and research on Alzheimer's disease, which points to a basic cholinergic disruption of the basal forebrain affecting widespread areas of the cerebral

98

cortex and limbic system. Diagnosis requires a multidisciplinary team to rule out other neurological, psychological, and physical illnesses. Although no specific medical therapy can reverse the pathology, rehabilitative techniques emphasize the greatest personal freedom consistent with the patient's functional limitations. Home care with attendant community social supports is preferable to early institutionalization. Institutional care is required in the late stages. The importance of adequate attention to the patient's general health and psychological well-being is stressed. (47 ref).

910. Gubrium, Jaber F. (1987). **Structuring and destructuring the course of illness: The Alzheimer's disease experience.** *Sociology of Health & Illness,* 9(1), 1–24.
Examines the course of illness of Alzheimer's disease as a location for the assignment of developmental structure. Textual analysis and field data indicate that the stock of developmental codes for structuring the course of illness in the Alzheimer's disease experience is as varied as the manifold interests of those concerned. Structuring is practical and occasioned, realized in its variety in an ameliorative mode of communicative usage. In the tribulation mode, the course of illness is destructured. Communicative usage is discussed as a critique of developmentalism.

911. Gubrium, Jaber F. (1986). **The social preservation of mind: The Alzheimer's disease experience.** *Symbolic Interaction,* 9(1), 37–51.
Studied the activities in a small day hospital for Alzheimer's disease (AD) patients over a 4-mo period. Data from the AD experience are interpreted to extend and refine G. H. Mead's (1934) theory of mind. While Mead conceived of mind as an internal conversation, the present author argues that the disease experience shows that the reality-status of mind is more practical and radically dialogical in organization. Taken as collectively preserved, mind is circumscribed through agents by means of rule-guided articulations and closures. A medical description of the disease is followed by 4 features of the social preservation of the mind: (1) the idea of the hidden mind and the problem of realization, (2) the question of who is the mind's agent, (3) discernment and articulation rules, and (4) the organization of mental demise.

912. Heckler, Margaret M. (1985). **The fight against Alzheimer's disease.** *American Psychologist,* 40(11), 1240–1244.
Describes gains made in the US in the fight against Alzheimer's disease (AD), noting increased funding for research into its etiology and possible cure, the growth and formation of support groups for caregivers of AD patients, and investigations into alternative means of care to institutionalization such as respite care. (3 ref).

913. Huff, F. Jacob; Growdon, John H.; Corkin, Suzanne & Rosen, T. John. (1987). **Age at onset and rate of progression of Alzheimer's disease.** *Journal of the American Geriatrics Society,* 35(1), 27–30.
Evaluated age at onset, duration, and severity of dementia in 165 patients with a clinical diagnosis of Alzheimer's disease. Mean age of onset of dementia was 64.3 yrs, and 62% of the Ss were women. Rate of progression of dementia was determined in 77 Ss by repeated administration of a dementia scale. Distribution of age at onset among Ss was bimodal, with a division at about age 65 yrs. Duration of dementia at the time of initial examination was shorter, and rate of progression on a follow-up examination was more rapid in senile-onset (age 65 yrs or greater) than in presenile onset. Overlap among values for the 2 groups was observed for both variables, suggesting that age at onset is not a strong predictor of rate of progression of dementia in patients with Alzheimer's disease.

914. Huff, F. Jacob; Growdon, John H.; Corkin, Suzanne & Rosen, T. John. (1987). **"Age at onset and rate of Alzheimer's disease": Reply to Borrie, Crilly, and Bowring.** *Journal of the American Geriatrics Society,* 35(10), 961.
Replies to comments by M. J. Borrie et al (1987) on the present authors' (1987) work on age at onset and rate of progression of Alzheimer's disease. Methodological problems with the activities of daily living component of the Blessed Dementia Scale (1968) are discussed.

915. Johnson, Jean. (1985). **Nutrition as a factor of mortality in senile dementia of the Alzheimer's type.** *Psychiatric Annals,* 15(5), 323–330.
Asserts that individuals with severe senile dementia of the Alzheimer's type (SDAT) are often difficult to care for, especially in terms of ensuring adequate nutrition. Behaviors frequently observed in association with an agitated component of SDAT physically inhibit eating and decrease interest in food. Severe memory loss is also associated with forgetting to and how to eat. The link between malnutrition and immune response is addressed, and a case illustration of an 86-yr-old woman with severe organic brain syndrome is presented. Evaluation of the role of protein calorie malnutrition in the increased mortality rates of persons with SDAT is presented. (7 ref).

916. Katzman, Robert. (1987). **Alzheimer's disease: Advances and opportunities.** *Journal of the American Geriatrics Society,* 35(1), 69–73.
Discusses the prevalence and history of the investigation of Alzheimer's disease and enumerates advances in understanding of the syndrome. Three areas of progress are described: neuronal systems, neuron degeneration, and diagnostic accuracy. Future research priorities include the uses of molecular pathophysiology and molecular genetics to find the cause; cross-cultural studies to discover risk factors (e.g., peripheral markers); alternative therapies (e.g., trophic factors, brain implantation, and management of advancing disease); and initiatives in the financing of care. It is noted that Alzheimer's disease and multiple strokes presently account for three-fourths of individuals with dementia and that they are both age-dependent disorders in an era when life spans are increasing.

917. Kosik, Kenneth H. & Growdon, John H. (1982). **Aging, memory loss, and dementia.** *Psychosomatics,* 23(7), 745–751.
Discusses Alzheimer's disease (the most common cause of dementia), its diagnosis, and treatment. (10 ref).

918. Kushnir, S. L. (1982). **Reflections on Alzheimer's disease.** *Canadian Journal of Psychiatry,* 27(1), 18–22.
As longevity increases, society will face a silent epidemic of idiopathic dementias. The concept, Alzheimer's disease, reflects a cumbersome and vaguely defined cluster of signs, symptoms, and other variables that might more appropriately be labeled as the idiopathic dementias, Alzheimer-type. Diagnosis, which is made by exclusion and treatment (primarily custodial), demonstrates the complex nature and unfortunate prognosis of the problem. (French abstract) (43 ref).

919. Lehmann, Heinz E. (1986). **A call to arms for clinical research in Alzheimer's disease.** *Progress in Neuro-Psychopharmacology & Biological Psychiatry,* 10(3–5), xvii–xix.
Discusses problems in the diagnosis of Alzheimer's disease and suggests 3 tasks to be accomplished by clinical research. These include (1) the development of a method for early diagnosis of the disease, (2) the development of a new methodology for clinical drug trials in this disorder, and (3) the testing of those nootropic and other pharmacological agents that have until now produced only suggestive or equivocal results.

920. Loebel, J. Pierre. (1986). **"Understanding" in schizophrenia & Alzheimer's disease.** *American Journal of Psychiatry,* 143(7), 937.
Responds to the letter of D. E. Raskin (1985) in which he pleads for better phenomenological characterization of Alzheimer's disease. A common factor suggested in schizophrenia and Alzheimer's disease is the need to identify the psychosocial and biological contingencies of each. In his reply, Raskin agrees that only by advocating a discrimination between the disease at its neurophysiological roots and the illness, which can be exacerbated by environmental factors, can a true psychiatric approach to Alzheimer's disease be achieved. (2 ref).

921. Price, Donald L. (1986). **New perspectives on Alzheimer's disease.** *Annual Review of Neuroscience,* 9, 489–512.
New information on Alzheimer's disease (AD) is reviewed in the following areas: clinical manifestations of the disease and correlations with imaging studies; analyses of brain regions and neuronal systems affected by AD; molecular and structural pathology of affected nerve cells; and etiological factors. Significant progress has been made in refining AD diagnostic criteria and risk factors, but the roles of genetic and familial factors require further study.

922. Price, Joy A.; Price, James H.; Shanahan, Patricia M. & Desmond, Sharon M. (1986). **Elderly persons' perceptions and knowledge of Alzheimer's disease.** *Psychological Reports,* 58(2), 419–424.
148 elderly Ss (mean age 70.9 yrs) responded to an Alzheimer's disease (AD) survey consisting of 20 knowledge questions, 2 belief questions, and 1 question on sources of AD information. Only 8 of the 20 knowledge questions were correctly answered by 50% or more of the Ss. Knowledge was correlated with Ss' educational level and their having a friend or relative with AD. Sources of information on AD were TV, articles, friends, and talks. 70% did not believe they were susceptible to AD, although 84% were concerned about developing the disease.

923. Raskin, David E. (1985). **On understanding Alzheimer's disease.** *American Journal of Psychiatry,* 142(10), 1225.
Notes that, although significant advances have been made in the understanding of the schizophrenic's inner world and the meaning of schizophrenic symptomatology, there have been no similar advances in the understanding of Alzheimer's disease (AD). 100 yrs of medical experience with schizophrenia have not produced a pathological marker, while brief experience with AD has produced a pathological marker but little else. It is argued that medical professionals who have spent several years working with schizophrenics should shift their attention to patients with dementia to promote a systematic understanding of AD.

924. Ratzan, Richard M. (1986). **Communication and informed consent in clinical geriatrics.** *International Journal of Aging & Human Development,* 23(1), 17–26.
Discusses communication problems that may be involved in obtaining a valid informed consent from an elderly person, especially one with possible senile dementia of the Alzheimer's type (SDAT). Hearing loss due to normal aging or other impairments and speech and language impediments, whether as a result of stroke or SDAT, need to be addressed if the patient is to communicate effectively. Misunderstandings may arise from the use of confusing medical terms. Presbyopia, cataract, and glaucoma may make it difficult for the S to read the consent form. Recommendations for improving communication are offered.

925. Rickards, Larry D.; Zuckerman, Diana M. & West, Pamela R. (1985). **Alzheimer's disease: Current congressional response.** *American Psychologist,* 40(11), 1256–1261.
Addresses the public policy component of Alzheimer's disease (AD) by examining legislation (either proposed or passed by Congress) in the areas of research, aid and assistance to AD patients and their families, long-term care, and information dissemination. Barriers to the passage of Alzheimer's legislation in Congress are noted. (49 ref).

926. Schneck, Michael K.; Reisberg, Barry & Ferris, Steven H. (1982). **An overview of current concepts of Alzheimer's disease.** *American Journal of Psychiatry,* 139(2), 165–173.
Reviews the literature on Alzheimer's disease, the major cause of senile dementia, and presents a historical overview of senile dementia and its morbidity and mortality rates. The authors describe the clinical features of the various stages of Alzheimer's disease and discuss the differential diagnosis. Also explored are the characteristic neuropathology and neurochemical abnormalities of the disease and their etiological implications. Further information concerning neurotransmitter levels, the role of aluminum, and genetic factors is necessary. (97 ref).

927. Storandt, Martha. (1983). **Understanding senile dementia: A challenge for the future.** *International Journal of Aging & Human Development,* 16(1), 1–6.
Reviews the causes of dementia in later life. Special attention is paid to senile dementia of the Alzheimer type, its prevalence, the characteristic structural changes in the brains of persons suffering from this disorder, and the hypothesized causes of the disease. The hypothesis that Alzheimer's disease represents accelerated aging is described. Treatment issues are discussed, primarily in terms of supportive environments, differential diagnosis, and assistance to the caregiver. (6 ref).

928. Task Force on Alzheimer's Disease. (1985). **Department of Health and Human Services's Task Force on Alzheimer's disease: Report and recommendations.** *Neurobiology of Aging,* 6(1), 65–71.
Discusses 5 of the 9 areas addressed by the US Department of Health and Human Service's Task Force on Alzheimer's disease (AD) in a problem-oriented approach aimed at better defining research needs, options, and training, and service and policy issues relative to AD. The 5 areas addressed include research on epidemiology, etiology and pathogenesis, diagnosis, clinical course, and treatment. Future research directions include continuation of exploration of the cholinergic hypothesis in the development of new treatment agents for the primary cognitive impairment in AD; evaluation of the indications for, and efficacy of, psychopharmacologic agents in the treatment of secondary psychiatric symptoms and syndromes occurring concomitantly with AD; identification of naturally occurring animal diseases and the development of new experimental animal models, based on actual neuropathological findings in human populations; and development of new and more specific psychometric models that can more accurately distinguish among memory, motivation, and attention effects over time.

929. Thomas, Myfanwy & Isaac, Michael. (1987). **Alois Alzheimer: A memoir.** *Trends in Neurosciences,* 10(8), 306–307.
Presents a biographical sketch of A. Alzheimer (1907), who first established the structural basis of the most common type of presenile and senile dementia. He was able to demonstrate the neuritic plaques and neurofibrillary tangles in the brain of a demented woman 51 yrs of age. The neuropathological vs Freudian explanations of dementia and Alzheimer's disease are discussed.

930. Torack, Richard M. (1978). **The pathologic physiology of dementia—with indications for diagnosis and treatment.** *Monographien aus dem Gesamtgebiete der Psychiatrie,* 20, 155 p.

Discusses the pathologic physiology of dementia in terms of a historical overview of dementia, clinical manifestations as a determinant of dementia, treatment of senile dementia, and the epidemiology of dementia. Also discussed are current evaluations of pathologic correlates of dementia, arteriosclerotic dementia, and the nature and cause of Alzheimer's disease.

TREATMENT & COUNSELING

931. Abbott, Max W. (1986). **The Mental Health Foundation of New Zealand's primary prevention programme: 1981–1985.** *Mental Health in Australia,* 1(16), 12–21.
Provides an overview of New Zealand's Mental Health Foundation, including the foundation's activities with regard to mental health promotion, primary prevention (reactive), and primary prevention (proactive). Both reactive and proactive primary prevention activities concerned with Alzheimer's disease are described.

932. Abernethy, Darrell R. (1987). **Development of memory-enhancing agents in the treatment of Alzheimer's disease.** *Journal of the American Geriatrics Society,* 35(10), 957–958.
Describes the drug development process for therapeutic agents for senile dementia of the Alzheimer's type (SDAT) prior to the general clinical availability. It is noted that lack of specific animal models of SDAT and a limited understanding of the clinical disease in humans make selection of a therapeutic approach difficult.

933. Andrade, Luiz A. (1983). **Distúrbios de neurotransmissores e as proposições de um tratamento racional na demência senil tipo Alzheimer. / Neurotransmitter disturbances and the proposals of a rational treatment in senile dementia of the Alzheimer type.** *Neurobiologia,* 46(2), 125–140.
Senile dementia of the Alzheimer type and presenile dementia involve characteristic abnormalities such as senile plaques, neurofibrillary tangles, and a variety of neurotransmitter disturbances. An improvement in patients' cognitive functioning has not been obtained by treatments using levodopa, dopamine receptor agonists, or drugs acting on the GABAergic or serotonergic systems. Conflicting results have been obtained in studies that tested drugs, such as choline or lecithin, that act on the cholinergic system. Further research on cholinergic metabolism in dementia is recommended. (37 ref).

934. Ashford, J. Wesson et al. (1981). **Physostigmine and its effect on six patients with dementia.** *American Journal of Psychiatry,* 138(6), 829–830.
Contrary to previous reports, this study found that low doses of physostigmine did not have a beneficial effect on learning or memory in 6 Alzheimer patients as measured by 3 tests. It is concluded that physostigmine may be beneficial only if the dose is titrated individually, given in conjunction with lecithin, and administered only to Ss with mild memory impairment. (10 ref).

935. Beatty, William W.; Butters, Nelson & Janowsky, David S. (1986). **Patterns of memory failure after scopolamine treatment: Implications for cholinergic hypotheses of dementia.** *Behavioral & Neural Biology,* 45(2), 196–211.
Assessed memory on a battery of tasks in 6 healthy 20–32 yr old males who received intramuscular scopolamine (0.5 mg), glycopyrrolate (0.1–0.2 mg), or saline, once each on 3 separate occasions. The pattern of memory failure induced by scopolamine was compared to that observed on the same tasks in 15 53–79 yr olds with Alzheimer's disease (AD) and 12 29–70 yr olds with Huntington's disease (HD). In agreement with previous reports, scopolamine impaired acquisition and delayed recall of a 14-word list and disrupted retention on the Brown–Peterson distractor task, whereas the peripherally active anticholinergic glycopyrrolate was without effect. However, under scopolamine the pattern of errors differed from that seen in AD Ss. Scopolamine did not increase the number of false positive errors on delayed recognition of the word list, failed to increase the number of prior-item intrusions on the Brown–Peterson task, did not impair learning of a symbol–digit paired-associate task, and did not reduce the number of words retrieved or increase the number of words repeated on a standardized verbal fluency test. The effects of scopolamine on memory also differed from the pattern of impairments observed in demented Ss with HD. Findings question whether anticholinergic drugs adequately mimic the full range of memory impairments observed in cortical or subcortical dementias. (43 ref).

936. Beller, Suha A.; Overall, John E. & Swann, Alan C. (1985). **Efficacy of oral physostigmine in primary degenerative dementia: A double-blind study of response to different dose level.** *Psychopharmacology,* 87(2), 147–151.
Examined the efficacy of cholinergic enhancement in senile dementia of the Alzheimer type by administering oral physostigmine to 8 patients (58–83 yrs old) in a crossover trial of 3 dose levels (0.5, 1.0, and 2.0 mg) and a matching placebo. Ss met Diagnostic and Statistical Manual of Mental Disorders (DSM-III) criteria for primary degenerative dementia. Dose levels were compared in 4 consecutive 2-day trials, and each dose was administered 7 times a day. A dose-related improvement in memory as measured by objective verbal memory tests was observed. Performance was significantly better on the highest dose, 2 mg every 2 hrs, than on the lower doses. The effect was most systematically present for very short-term memory, which raises the question of whether the improvement may involve attention rather than longer term storage and retrieval. (18 ref).

937. Berman, Stephen & Rappaport, Meryl B. (1984). **Social work and Alzheimer's disease: Psychosocial management in the absence of medical cure.** *Social Work in Health Care,* 10(2), 53–70.
Notes that because Alzheimer's disease erodes and destroys an individual's personality, patients and families affected by illness have critical needs for help with its psychosocial sequelae. A model of psychosocial management is presented, which details specific interventions to help Alzheimer's patients and caregivers develop and maintain adaptations during the long course of the disease. Suggestions for counseling, living arrangements, psychosocial assessment, role of the caregiver, and methods of promoting functioning are presented for each phase of the disorder. (17 ref).

938. Blackwood, Douglas H. & Christie, Janice E. (1986). **The effects of physostigmine on memory and auditory P300 in Alzheimer-type dementia.** *Biological Psychiatry,* 21(5–6), 557–560.
12 patients (aged 54–68 yrs) with Alzheimer-type dementia were administered physostigmine (0.75 mg) to examine whether the memory improvement that resulted would be accompanied by changes in P300 latency or amplitude. There was an improvement in memory after physostigmine in 9 of the 11 Ss who completed the memory test, but there was no significant change in P300 latency or amplitude.

939. Bonder, Bette R. (1986). **Family systems and Alzheimer's disease: An approach to treatment.** *Physical & Occupational Therapy in Geriatrics,* 5(2), 13–24.
Describes family systems theory, a model which provides an explanation of the impact of senile dementia of the Alzheimer's type (SDAT) on the family as well as a framework for intervention. This approach requires a somewhat unique set of interventions on the part of the health care professional, recognizing the family as the unit for treatment, rather than the diagnosed patient. The family systems model and its application to SDAT are described.

940. Branconnier, Roland J.; Dessain, Eric C.; Cole, Jonathan O. & McNiff-Langille, Maureen E. (1984). **An analysis of dose–response of plasma choline to oral lecithin.** *Biological Psychiatry,* 19(5), 765–770.
Administered lecithin (10, 20, or 40 g/day) to 48 normal 65–85 yr olds in a placebo-controlled, double-blind, parallel-group design. A quantal dose–response analysis of the data was conducted using linear regression. Findings, which are discussed in relation to the clinical use of lecithin in treating Alzheimer's disease, indicate that reliance on contrasting arithmetic mean changes in plasma choline concentration (PCC) can lead to misinterpretation of the effective dose of lecithin required to achieve a specified PCC. (11 ref).

941. Brinkman, Samuel D. (1981). **Lecithin and memory training in Alzheimer's disease.** *Dissertation Abstracts International,* 41(8-B), 3223.

942. Brinkman, Samuel D. et al. (1982). **Lecithin and memory training in suspected Alzheimer's disease.** *Journal of Gerontology,* 37(1), 4–9.
10 patients (aged 54–73 yrs) diagnosed as having Alzheimer's disease were given 35 g/day of a 53% lecithin mixture for 2 wks in a double-blind crossover design. Ss received memory training during the lecithin condition and "placebo training" during the placebo drug condition. Repeated assessment with Buschke's Selective Reminding Procedure provided no evidence of a therapeutic lecithin effect either during the clinical trial or during follow-up. Noninvasive measurement of regional cerebral blood flow and repeated EEGs also failed to demonstrate a therapeutic effect. These latter indices reflected a decline in cerebral function over the course of the study, a finding that paralleled clinical impressions in 4 of the patients. Follow-up trials of memory training under placebo and lecithin conditions suggested that memory training may lead to some immediate improvement in list-learning ability, but the improvement was not well maintained over time. (29 ref).

943. Brinkman, Samuel D. et al. (1984). **Lithium-induced increases in red blood cell choline and memory performance in Alzheimer-type dementia.** *Biological Psychiatry,* 19(2), 157–164.
To investigate the relationship between red blood cell choline and memory in Alzheimer-type senile dementia (SDAT), lithium carbonate was administered to 14 53–81 yr old SDAT patients in doses of 400–600 mg/day for 5 wks. A battery of memory tests, including the Weschler Memory Scale—Revised, was administered at baseline and at weekly intervals. Five Ss with serum concentrations below 0.6 meq/liter developed neurotoxicity and were dropped from further analysis. For the remaining Ss, Li+ with mean serum concentrations up to 0.6 meq/liter did not alter memory scores significantly. Dramatic increases in RBC choline, however, suggest that RBC choline is not correlated with memory functioning in SDAT. (36 ref).

944. Brinkman, Samuel D. & Gershon, Samuel. (1983). **Measurement of cholinergic drug effects on memory in Alzheimer's disease.** *Neurobiology of Aging,* 4(2), 139–145.
Reviews double-blind, placebo-controlled investigations of scopolamine, physostigmine, arecoline, and tetrahydroaminoacridine in normal adults and in those having dementia of the Alzheimer type (DAT) to determine the relative sensitivity of various assessment procedures in the measurement of drug effects. Based on the limited number of possible comparisons across studies, 2 procedures appear to be useful: word list learning tasks that generate an index of intrusion errors, and visual recognition tasks. It is concluded that the lack of standardized assessments limits the ability of investigators to replicate studies, to compare relative efficacy of various drugs, or to address a number of other questions that are fundamental to the development of effective cholinergic treatments for DAT. (53 ref).

945. Bruno, Giuseppe; Mohr, Erich; Gillespie, Marjorie; Fedio, Paul et al. (1986). **Muscarinic agonist therapy of Alzheimer's disease: A clinical trial of RS-86.** *Archives of Neurology,* 43(7), 659–661.
Studied the use of 2-ethyl-8 methyl-2,8 diazospiro (4.5)-decane-1,3-dione hydrobromide (RS-86) in treating Alzheimer's disease in 3 men and 5 women (aged 55–68 yrs). Ss received up to 0.5 mg each day unless adverse effects required a reduced dose. Ss received RS-86 or a placebo for 8 days in random order with a 5-day washout period. A series of neurologic tests was given as baseline and on Day 2 and Day 7 of testing. In treated Ss there was some slight improvement in 3 tests of verbal cognitive function and in 2 tests of visuospatial function. Other tests showed no improvement or a slight decrease. All Ss had some evidence of drug-related toxic effects, namely diaphoresis. The trial did not show any consistent effect of RS-86 at this dose for an 8-day trial.

946. Burian, Ernest. (1974). **An ergot alkaloid preparation (Hydergine) in the treatment of presenile brain atrophy (Alzheimer's disease): Case report.** *Journal of the American Geriatrics Society,* 22(3), 126–128.
Administered 1 mg Hydergine 3 times/day for 90 days to 4 patients with presenile brain atrophy (Alzheimer's disease). Two Ss did not improve, 1 showed moderate improvement, and 1 S, a 62-year-old man who had become a total nursing-care problem, improved dramatically. His case is described in detail. It is concluded that the improvement and the absence of side effects justify further trials of Hydergine in presenile brain atrophy.

947. Cain, John W. (1986). **Hypertension associated with oral administration of physostigmine in a patient with Alzheimer's disease.** *American Journal of Psychiatry,* 143(7), 910–912.
Presents a case report of a 72-yr-old White woman who developed hypertensive episodes after treatment with oral physostigmine (8 mg/day), a cholinomimetic drug used in the experimental treatment of Alzheimer's disease. Although data suggest substantial memory improvement during administration, S's reaction suggests a cumulative effect of the drug. (10 ref).

948. Cardelli, Marcia B.; Russell, Mary; Bagne, Curtis A. & Pomara, Nunzio. (1985). **Chelation therapy: Unproved modality in the treatment of Alzheimer-type dementia.** *Journal of the American Geriatrics Society,* 33(8), 548–551.
Discusses the lack of effective therapeutic agents for the treatment of Alzheimer's disease (AD), which has been a contributing factor in the use by health professionals of unproved, costly, and potentially dangerous modalities, such as chelation therapy. The case histories of a 72- and a 76-yr-old woman are presented to describe the treatment of AD with chelation therapy and the lack of benefit experienced. It is concluded that until the safety and efficacy of chelating agents are demonstrated by research studies, there is no scientific rationale for their use in the treatment of AD. (25 ref).

949. Carey, Betsy & Hansen, Shannon S. (1986). **Social work groups with institutionalized Alzheimer's Disease victims.** Special Issue: Social work and Alzheimer's disease: Practice issues with victims and their families. *Journal of Gerontological Social Work,* 9(2), 15–25.
Describes groupwork experience on an Alzheimer's unit at a home for the aged. The group focused on maintaining social and mental function within the setting while discussing topics relevant to participants. It is concluded that a greater sense of belonging and togetherness developed that may be more important than the actual content of the group session. Suggestions for dealing with behavior problems, the impact of the environment, problems with evaluation, and 2 successful groups are discussed with the intent of guiding other group leaders in working with this population. (5 ref).

950. Caulfield, Malcolm & Smith, Christine. (1985). **British Pharmacological Society symposium: Alzheimer's disease—central cholinergic mechanisms.** *Neurobiology of Aging,* 6(1), 61–63.
Discusses presentations given at the Winter meeting of the British Pharmacological Society. Topics included a description of dementias, particularly Alzheimer's disease (AD); the neurochemistry of AD; animal models of the cholinergic lesion in AD; and physostigmine as a possible therapy for AD patients. The topic of the round table discussion was cholinergic synaptic function and potential therapy.

951. Christie, Janice E.; Shering, Ann; Ferguson, John & Glen, A. Iain. (1981). **Physostigmine and arecoline: Effects of intravenous infusions in Alzheimer presenile dementia.** *British Journal of Psychiatry,* 138, 46–50.
Administered physostigmine, arecoline, and saline iv over 30 min in a randomized double-blind design to 11 patients with a clinical diagnosis of Alzheimer presenile dementia. Significant improvement was seen on a picture recognition test (memory test adjusted for use with demented Ss) with physostigmine (0.375 mg) and arecoline (4 mg). A trend toward improvement was also seen with 0.25 and 0.75 mg physostigmine and 2 mg arecoline. For the majority of Ss improvement was only slight, but in 2 Ss, it was clear-cut and consistent. (29 ref).

952. Cohen, Donna; Kennedy, Gary & Eisdorfer, Carl. (1984). **Phases of change in the patient with Alzheimer's dementia: A conceptual dimension for defining health care management.** *Journal of the American Geriatrics Society,* 32(1), 11–15.
Proposes that since the progressive nature of Alzheimer's disease and related disorders of later life gradually imposes a series of significant limitations on the patient, a successful clinical management program rests on a conceptualization of changes in the patient. Postulating psychologic reactions helps professionals to understand and respond to the patient's needs and feelings at different stages of the disease. The phases discussed in the present paper provide the basis for defining treatment goals and management plans, selecting therapeutic strategies, identifying needed resources, and evolving innovative approaches to patient care. (39 ref).

953. Cohen, Gene D. (1984). **The mental health professional and the Alzheimer patient.** *Hospital & Community Psychiatry,* 35(2), 115–116, 122.
Outlines an 8-point treatment intervention-management approach that mental health professionals can use with Alzheimer's patients. The approach includes diagnosis and differential diagnosis, dealing with the unknowns of the disease, treatment of primary symptoms, treatment of concomitant physical illness causing excess disability, attention to environmental stressors or threats to the safety of the patient, support to the family, and consultation to staff working with the patient. (11 ref).

954. Coons, Dorothy H. & Weaverdyck, Shelly E. (1986). **Wesley Hall: A residential unit for persons with Alzheimer's disease and related disorders.** Special Issue: Therapeutic interventions for the person with dementia. *Physical & Occupational Therapy in Geriatrics,* 4(3), 29–53.
Describes a model residential treatment project for persons with Alzheimer's disease and related dementias. The project, Wesley Hall, is structured to maximize capacities, compensate for deficits, and foster success and self-respect on the part of residents. Interventions that have been effective in reducing such behaviors as incontinence, restlessness, and anxiety reactions are outlined. A case profile illustrates the value of designing individualized milieu intervention programs based on knowledge gained from observation and neuropsychological testing.

955. Cox, Kim G. (1985). **Milieu therapy.** Special Issue: Alzheimer's disease. *Geriatric Nursing,* 6(3), 152–154.
Describes a nursing unit whose mission is to support patients (8 men and women, aged 40–70 yrs) in the early stages of Alzheimer's disease (AZD). Patients stay from 4–6 mo; all patients have at least 1 family member participating in the program and discharge planning. The therapeutic milieu affords individuals and groups the opportunity to socially experience, explicitly recognize, and cope with the real and feared consequences of AZD. The program uses the group's sense of powerlessness paradoxically to expand emotional awareness, emotional resources, and confidence. To evaluate the effects of the milieu therapy, behavioral indicators are used as reflections of attitude change; observations collected are used to make changes in the therapeutic program.

956. Crook, Thomas. (1985). **Clinical drug trials in Alzheimer's disease.** *Annals of the New York Academy of Sciences,* 444, 428–436.
Discusses the drugs currently prescribed in the US for the treatment of Alzheimer's disease and considers a broad range of drugs recently studied or currently under study in Alzheimer's disease. Particular emphasis is placed on recent trials with cholinergic compounds, neuropeptides, and nootropic drugs. It is concluded that dramatic progress has been made recently in developing treatment strategies for Alzheimer's disease. (45 ref).

957. Crook, Thomas. (1986). **Drug effects in Alzheimer's disease.** *Clinical Gerontologist,* 5(3–4), 489–502.
Reviews the search for a miracle drug to cure, prevent, or arrest dementia. The unimpressive results wrought by such treatments as vasodilators, anticoagulants, and hyperbaric oxygenation chambers led to a rethinking of dementia and the conclusion that the neurological degeneration seen in Alzheimer's disease has characterized most cases of senile dementia. State-of-the-art antisenility medications, their utility, and side effects are discussed, including dihydroergotoxine. A cautionary note is given on the use of antipsychotics with dementia patients. Studies with some relatively experimental drugs are reviewed.

958. Cutler, Neal R. et al. (1985). **Evaluation of zimeldine in Alzheimer's disease: Cognitive and biochemical measures.** *Archives of Neurology,* 42(8), 744–748.
Conducted a placebo-controlled 23-wk study of the effects of high and low doses of zimeldine (75–175 mg or 175–275 mg) on memory in 4 49–65 yr old males with Alzheimer's disease. Ss were administered tests of reaction time (RT), learning, and delayed memory. Results suggest that alterations of serotoninergic function with zimeldine had no effect on memory function. (40 ref).

959. Cutler, Neal R. & Narang, Prem K. (1985). **Drug therapies.** Special Issue: Alzheimer's disease. *Geriatric Nursing,* 6(3), 160–163.
Describes drug therapies designed to modify some of the neurological and neurochemical deficits recently found to be associated with Alzheimer's disease (AZD). Treatments associated with AZD stages (mild, moderate, severe, and terminal) are discussed. The effects of central nervous system stimulants (amphetamines, methylphenidate, pemoline, and caffeine derivatives) and antidepressants (e.g., amitriptyline, imipramine, maprotiline) in treating pseudodementia or dementia; and vasodilators (e.g., papaverine, cyclandelate, nifedipine) to improve cerebral blood flow are discussed as therapies attempted during the mild stage of AZD. At present, the major hypotheses of AZD etiology are based on the deficiencies in the neurotransmitters and on alterations in the enzymes associated with the synthesis of glucose in the brain. Treatment strategies, therefore, are related to these alterations. The cholinergic, noradrenergic, dopaminergic/gamma-aminobutyric acid, serotonergic, and neuropeptidergic

systems are discussed in relation to drug treatment for AZD. Brain metabolism and deficiencies in the enzymes that convert glucose to acetylocoenzyme A are being explored extensively. These efforts and preliminary research with brain transplantation in rats are also discussed. (33 ref).

960. Damon, Joanne & May, Rita. (1986). **The effects of pet facilitative therapy on patients and staff in an adult day care center.** Special Issue: Therapeutic activities with the impaired elderly. *Activities, Adaptation & Aging,* 8(3–4), 117–131.
Examines adult daycare and the effect of pet facilitated intervention on individuals isolated by dementing illness. Results from 3 patients (aged 78+ yrs) with Alzheimer's disease indicate that pets can be catalysts for social behavior.

961. Davidson, Michael; Mohs, Richard C.; Hollander, Eric; Zemishlany, Ziv et al. (1987). **Lecithin and piracetam in Alzheimer's disease.** *Biological Psychiatry,* 22(1), 112–114.
10 56–72 yr old Alzheimer's disease (AD) patients were randomly administered piracetam and 1 of 3 doses of lecithin or placebo each for 1 wk. After 4 wks, an investigator blind to the drug condition selected the dose of lecithin that produced the most improvement, which was used in a replication phase. Results suggest that piracetam combined with lecithin produces only minimal improvement in some AD patients. Cholinergic dysfunction in AD is discussed.

962. Davidson, Michael; Powchik, Peter & Davis, Kenneth L. (1988). **Pisa syndrome in Alzheimer's disease.** *Biological Psychiatry,* 23(2), 213.
Presents a case of a 66-yr-old male with Alzheimer's disease who developed Pisa syndrome, a dystonic reaction, after neuroleptic treatment. The combined administration of haloperidol (6 mg/day) and amantadine (200 mg/day) improved the S's psychiatric symptoms without causing any dystonic reaction.

963. Davis, Carol M. (1986). **The role of the physical and occupational therapist in caring for the victim of Alzheimer's disease.** Special Issue: Therapeutic interventions for the person with dementia. *Physical & Occupational Therapy in Geriatrics,* 4(3), 15–28.
Briefly reviews the epidemiology and pathology associated with Alzheimer's disease and the clinical features that differentiate pseudodementia from dementia. Ways in which various forms and styles of communication can help physical and occupational therapists "break through" to Alzheimer's patients are outlined. Goals of care are also identified, along with ways of helping clients learn, handling catastrophic reactions, managing suspiciousness, understanding apathy, and communicating with depressed Alzheimer's patients.

964. Davis, Kenneth L.; Hollander, Eric; Davidson, Michael; Davis, Bonnie M. et al. (1987). **Induction of depression with oxotremorine in patients with Alzheimer's disease.** *American Journal of Psychiatry,* 144(4), 468–471.
Investigated cholinergic neurotransmission in the development of depression. Seven patients (aged 57–78 yrs) with Alzheimer's disease were given oral oxotremorine (0.25–2.0 mg), a long-acting cholinergic agonist, to assess the drug's effects on cognitive function. There were unexpected depressive reactions in 5 of the 7 Ss, 3 of whom dropped out of the study because of these side effects. Cardiovascular effects of the drug were negligible, but its effect on memory and cognition is viewed as unknown because of the small number of Ss who completed the study.

965. Davis, Kenneth L. & Mohs, Richard C. (1986). **Cholinergic drugs in Alzheimer's disease.** *New England Journal of Medicine,* 315(20), 1286–1287.

Comments on the article by W. K. Summers et al (1986) on the efficacy of cholinesterase inhibitors (e.g., tetrahydroaminoacridine) in treating patients with Alzheimer's disease. The present author hopes that the work of Summers et al will provide the impetus to the pharmaceutical industry to develop even safer and more specific cholinesterase inhibitors, as well as cholinomimetic compounds that may be capable of mitigating some of the other brain deficiencies in patients with Alzheimer's disease.

966. Davis, Kenneth L. & Mohs, Richard C. (1982). **Enhancement of memory processes in Alzheimer's disease with multiple-dose intravenous physostigmine.** *American Journal of Psychiatry,* 139(11), 1421–1424.
Administered physostigmine (.125, .25, or .50 mg, iv) or placebo over 30 min to 10 neuroleptic-free patients with Alzheimer's disease. All Ss performed better on a recognition memory task while receiving physostigmine. When placebo or the dose of physostigmine previously associated with an improvement in memory was readministered, physostigmine again enhanced performance on a recognition memory task. Results indicate that the acute augmentation of cholinergic activity in some Ss with Alzheimer's disease partially reversed the memory deficit of that disorder and provided an approach to the eventual therapy of this condition. (50 ref).

967. Davous, P. & Lamour, Y. (1985). **Bethanechol decreases reaction time in senile dementia of the Alzheimer type.** *Journal of Neurology, Neurosurgery & Psychiatry,* 48(12), 1297–1299.
In a study using a simple reaction time (RT) paradigm, 8 46–80 yr olds with senile dementia of the Alzheimer type (SDAT) were administered bethanechol (BTC [0.1 mg/kg, subcutaneously]); 8 other SDAT Ss, matched for age and level of deterioration, were administered saline. Simple RT was measured before and 15 and 30 min postinjection. Preinjection, SDAT Ss had significant longer RTs than 54 20–94 yr old nondemented controls tested in a preliminary study. A significant shortening of RTs was observed in SDAT Ss administered BTC, but not saline, 15 min postinjection. (10 ref).

968. Dawson, Pam; Kline, Karen; Wiancko, Donna C. & Wells, Donna. (1986). **Preventing excess disability in patients with Alzheimer's disease.** *Geriatric Nursing,* 7(6), 298–301.
Discusses how self-care with Alzheimer's disease patients is directed toward preventing and reversing excess disability by reinforcing the familiar and enhancing a sense of competency. Methods of nursing assessment and suggestions for intervention are described in the areas of interactional, social, and interpretive abilities.

969. Denber, Herman C. (1982). **Physostigmine in the treatment of memory disorders: A case report.** *Psychiatric Journal of the University of Ottawa,* 7(1), 8–12.
Presents a case report of a 60-yr-old male with a 4-yr history of progressive dementia with severe memory deficits. A diagnosis of Alzheimer's disease had been made, and all treatment was without success. In light of the available information, a trial with physostigmine was carried out resulting in significant improvement in his condition as evidenced by psychodiagnostic testing. The treatment was repeated a 2nd time, and after a 6-mo follow-up the improvement still was evident. (27 ref).

970. Drudge, Owen W.; Rosen, James C.; Peyser, Janis M. & Pieniadz, Jeannie. (1986). **Behavioral and emotional problems and treatment in chronically brain-impaired adults.** *Annals of Behavioral Medicine,* 8(1), 9–14.
Suggests that behavioral and emotional dysfunction is common in chronically brain-impaired adults. The factors pertaining to psychological disorder in cases of head injury, multiple sclerosis, Huntington's disease, Parkinson's disease, and Alz-

heimer's disease are discussed. Psychological disorders in these cases are capable of exacerbating adaptive dysfunction to a serious degree. Although each brain disorder poses unique problems, the most frequent psychological disorder appears to be depression. Emphasis should be placed on an integrated approach for both cognitive–emotional adaptation and behavior management, and treatment should also focus on the family.

971. Duffy, F. H.; McAnulty, G.; Albert, M.; Durwen, H. et al. (1987). **Lecithin: Absence of neurophysiologic effect in Alzheimer's disease by EEG topography.** *Neurology,* 37(6), 1015–1019.
10 patients (aged 55–76 yrs) with Alzheimer's disease (AD) participated in a 26-wk double-blind trial of lecithin (10, 15, or 20 g). EEG data were recorded at baseline, after administration of the placebo, and after administration of the drug. A direct comparison of drug and nondrug data was not significant. A comparison of differences between drug and nondrug with differences between the 2 nondrug conditions also produced no evidence of a drug treatment effect. The data confirm other reports that lecithin has no effect on spectrally analyzed EEG activity in AD.

972. Durso, R. et al. (1982). **Lysine vasopressin in Alzheimer disease.** *Neurology,* 32(6), 674–677.
Investigated the effect of lysine vasopressin on memory and cognitive deficits in Alzheimer disease in 14 Ss. In a double-blind study, 7 Ss were given 16 units of lysine vasopressin per day for 10 days and were compared with 7 Ss receiving placebo. All Ss were given a test battery before treatment, 3 days after treatment began, and twice after treatment stopped. The tests included measures of learning, memory, and perception. No significant difference in performance between the vasopressin and placebo-treated groups was found. However, significantly greater improvement in RT was seen in the vasopressin-treated group, although this effect was delayed and may have been contributed to by factors other than drug activity. (24 ref).

973. Dysken, Maurice. (1987). **A review of recent clinical trials in the treatment of Alzheimer's dementia.** *Psychiatric Annals,* 17(3), 178–191.
Reviews clinical trials that have been published over the past 5 yrs involving drugs tested for the treatment of Alzheimer's disease (AD). Knowledge about neurotransmitter deficits in the brains of AD patients and experience in the uses of pharmacological agents in animal models have suggested a variety of pharmacological treatment strategies. Cholinergic agents (e.g., lecithin) are used to restore deficient levels of brain acetylcholine in AD patients; physostigmine has been used with limited success to improve cognitive functioning. Bethanechol has resulted in some improvement in cognitive, social, and emotional functioning of AD patients. Other types of drugs have been used with varied success (e.g., opioid antagonists, ergoloid mesylates, vasopressin, lithium, and combinations of drugs).

974. Dysken, Maurice W. & Janowsky, David S. (1985). **Dose-related physostigmine-induced ventricular arrhythmia: Case report.** *Journal of Clinical Psychiatry,* 46(10), 446–447.
Describes the case of an 85-yr-old man with senile dementia of the Alzheimer's type who developed an arrhythmic effect in response to intravenous administration of 1 mg physostigmine. The observed arrhythmic effect of physostigmine is consistent with the hypothesis that central cholinergic mechanisms may regulate a variety of stress sensitive phenomena. (12 ref).

975. Eiji, Goto. (1986). **Welfare accommodations for demented old persons.** *Kyushu Neuro-psychiatry,* 32(1), 33–34.
Suggests the importance of a continuing search for a useful and meaningful life and active participation in social events by older persons in preventing senile dementia. For the care of those old persons who are demented, the following are suggested: (1) to clarify the pathological symptoms of senile dementia, especially Alzheimer's disease, (2) to participate actively in improving social awareness of senile dementia, (3) to educate and train social workers who manage geriatrics care, (4) to reevaluate the services, management, and administration of geriatric mental and health centers, and (5) to provide halfway houses for those who are recovering from diseases.

976. El Sobky, A.; El Shazly, M.; Darwish, A. K.; Davies, T. et al. (1986). **Hydergine effect on prolactin and reaction time in dementia.** *Biological Psychiatry,* 21(12), 1229–1230.
Examined whether hydergine's beneficial effect in senile dementia of the Alzheimer type (SDAT) is mediated by dopamine (DA) by studying measures of DA function serially in relation to neuropsychological parameters in 7 female SDAT patients (aged 76–87 yrs) during hydergine therapy. Findings of suppression of basal and thyrotropin-releasing hormone-induced prolactin levels indicate that hydergine has DA agonist effects.

977. Evans, John R. (1986). **Alzheimer's dementia: Some possible mechanisms related to vitamins, trace elements and minerals, suggesting a possible treatment.** *Journal of Ortho-molecular Medicine,* 1(4), 249–254.
Reviews the literature on the role of vitamins, trace elements, and minerals in the pathology of Alzheimer's dementia and discusses implications for treatment. Research evidence suggests that in some elderly people there is a diminution of transport of most vitamins, minerals, and essential trace elements at the blood–brain barrier and possibly in the gut, leading to deficiencies in brain cells. It is postulated that these deficiencies in brain cells are the primary causes of the formation of lipofuscin and neurofibrillary tangles, finally leading to cell death. Administration of vitamins and trace elements at higher than recommended intakes may halt the process at an early age, or slow down the rate of development of the disease process.

978. Fillit, Howard; Weinreb, Herman; Cholst, Ina; Luine, Victoria et al. (1986). **Observations in a preliminary open trial of estradiol therapy for senile dementia-Alzheimer's type.** *Psychoneuroendocrinology,* 11(3), 337–345.
Seven female patients with senile dementia of the Alzheimer's type (SDAT) were treated with low dosages of estradiol over a 6-wk period. Significant improvements in 3 Ss were noted on measures of attention, orientation, mood, and social interaction. These estrogen-responsive Ss were characterized by dementia associated with an affective disorder, older age at onset, and evidence of osteoporosis. Estradiol therapy thus may benefit some postmenopausal women with SDAT. The occurrence of osteoporosis in the estrogen-responsive group suggests that SDAT in some women may be associated with estrogen deficiency. However, the potential for serious side effects as a result of estrogen treatment precludes the routine clinical use of estrogen for dementia until careful clinical research trials have been performed.

979. Fisman, M. et al. (1981). **Double blind study of lecithin in patients with Alzheimer's disease.** *Canadian Journal of Psychiatry,* 26(6), 426–428.
21 61–89 yr olds with a diagnosis of Alzheimer's disease completed a double-blind trial on lecithin (25 g daily). Ss were rated on the London Psychogeriatric Rating Scale (LPRS). Equal improvement was noted in both the lecithin and placebo groups. Serum levels of lecithin measured 12–14 hrs after its administration were also not increased compared with the levels in control Ss. No significant difference was

noted on LPRS scores between the lecithin and placebo groups after 8 wks. Findings of the ineffectiveness of lecithin in patients with Alzheimer's disease are discussed in relation to the literature. (French abstract) (12 ref).

980. Fisman, Michael; Merskey, Harold & Helmes, Edward. (1981). **Double-blind trial of 2-dimethylaminoethanol in Alzheimer's disease.** *American Journal of Psychiatry,* 138(7), 970–972.
A double-blind, placebo-controlled trial of 2-dimethylaminoethanol was undertaken in 27 patients (mean age 73 yrs) with moderately severe or severe Alzheimer's disease. Of 13 Ss in the drug group, 6 were withdrawn in the 1st 5 wks of the trial because of side effects, which included drowsiness and retardation, with an increase of confusion and mild elevation of blood pressure. Results show no significant benefit from the drug treatment. (8 ref).

981. Fleischhacker, W. Wolfgang; Buchgeher, Astrid & Schubert, Harald. (1986). **Memantine in the treatment of senile dementia of the Alzheimer type.** *Progress in Neuro-Psychopharmacology & Biological Psychiatry,* 10(1), 87–93.
Studied the efficacy of the dopaminergic substance memantine in severe cases of senile dementia of the Alzheimer type using a randomized single-blind trial. 10 controls (mean age 79.6 yrs) and 10 experimental Ss (mean age 75.3 yrs) participated. Following 20 days of baseline therapy, patients received 20–30 mg of memantine per day intravenously; controls were given placebo. Ss were given measures of attention and short-term memory, psychopathology, and behavior following the baseline period. Statistical evaluation showed no significant differences between the 2 groups. Mild amelioration of sleep–wakefulness cycles and impulse and drive functions were observed clinically in both groups. Side effects (deterioration of psychopathology in 2 patients in the memantine group) disappeared after withdrawal of the substance.

982. Fovall, Penny et al. (1980). **Choline bitartrate treatment of Alzheimer-type dementias.** *Communications in Psychopharmacology,* 4(2), 141–145.
Conducted a double-blind, placebo-controlled study of the effects of choline bitartrate (CBT) on intellectual performance in 3 male and 2 female 55–77 yr old patients with early Alzheimer-type dementia. Three doses of CBT (8, 12, and 16 g) were given for 2 wks each, with a 2-wk placebo period either preceding or following the drug period. Cognitive testing (a battery of 10 tests) was conducted during a baseline period and weekly thereafter for the duration of the study. Comparison of the drug condition with placebo showed significant improvement for auditory and visual word recognition at 12 g/day of CBT. The mean plasma choline level nearly doubled from baseline to 12 g/day. Results suggest improvement in some aspects of cognitive performance during CBT treatment. (20 ref).

983. Gertz, H.-J. & Kanowski, S. (1983). **Die Therapie der senilen Demenz vom Alzheimer-Typ und der Multi-Infarkt-Demenz. / The treatment of senile dementia (Alzheimer-type) and multi-infarct dementia.** *Nervenarzt,* 54(9), 444–454.
Discusses pharmacological and nonpharmacological approaches to the treatment of senile dementia (Alzheimer type) and multi-infarct dementia. There exists no means of halting the progression of degenerative dementias, but antidepressants, neuroleptics, and tranquilizers can help reduce some symptoms of dementia. Among nonmedicative methods, milieu therapy and reality-orientation training can improve the patient's general level of activation, while behavioral treatments can effect localized behavior modifications. Judgment of the effectiveness of these methods is made difficult by the difficulty in separating the symptoms of primary brain damage from the effects of long-term institutionalization. The special significance is emphasized of advising family and caretaker personnel about these treatment possibilities, the use of outpatient therapies, and problems associated with institutionalization. (66 ref).

984. Gibeau, Janice L. (1985). **"Alzheimer's disease and long-term care: The assessment of the patient": Discussion.** *Journal of Geriatric Psychiatry,* 18(1), 27–35.
Comments on an article by B. V. Reifler and E. B. Larson (1985) that summarized issues of etiology, diagnosis, and treatment of Alzheimer's disease. It is proposed that Reifler and Larson's article suggests possible treatment methods for Alzheimer's disease. The medical profession's use of this knowledge and advocacy within the health policy sector can add to what some day may be a more predictable treatment and long-term care program for elderly people with Alzheimer's, and support for their families. (1 ref).

985. Gispen, Willem H.; Isaacson, Robert L.; Spruijt, Berry M. & de Wied, David. (1986). **Melanocortins, neural plasticity and aging.** *Progress in Neuro-Psychopharmacology & Biological Psychiatry,* 10(3–5), 415–426.
Reviews the literature to elucidate reasons for testing the efficacy of the melanocortins in providing relief from age-related brain abnormalities (e.g., Alzheimer's disease). It is concluded that peptides derived from adrenocorticotropic hormone and alpha-melanocyte-stimulating hormone exert trophic influences on peripheral and central nervous structures. Age-related brain diseases may be related to loss of neural plasticity. Melanocortins improve adaptational abilities of the nervous system.

986. González, Elizabeth R. (1984). **Drug treatment and nutrient therapy: The distinction blurs.** *New York State Journal of Medicine,* 84(9), 467–472.
Discusses the unprecedented interest in nutrition by medical investigators. Treatment of Alzheimer's disease with lecithin, unipolar depression with levotyrosine, and premenstrual syndrome with pyridoxine hydrochloride, along with other treatments, are also discussed. The current concern over the toxicity of unregulated nutrient substances is addressed. (14 ref).

987. Goodnick, P. & Gershon, S. (1984). **Chemotherapy of cognitive disorders in geriatric subjects.** *Journal of Clinical Psychiatry,* 45(5), 196–209.
Examines the neurobiology, diagnosis, and treatment of intellectual and memory impairment in the elderly. Many of the neurochemical changes associated with the aging brain, particularly lower choline acetyltransferase and higher MAO occur with greater severity in senile dementia, Alzheimer's type. These alterations correlate with neuropathologic indices (e.g., the number of senile plaques and tangles). Although many different treatment techniques have been used, most have been unsuccessful. No strong data have supported the use of stimulants, Gerovital H3, or hyperbaric oxygen. Among the vasodilators, cyclandelate and ergoloid mesylates may be of value in some but not most patients. Much recent work has focused on techniques to increase acetylcholine brain concentrations. To date, precursors such as choline seem to have limited value. Postsynaptic treatments (e.g., physostigmine) hold more hope for future benefit, if longer acting oral preparations are developed. Other compounds, such as ACTH, vasopressin, and piracetam, may have some value but need better definition and treatment indications. Recent discoveries on the influences of lecithin on membrane fluidity and receptor binding may affect the focus of future pharmacologic investigation. (140 ref).

988. Grassi, Gaddomaria. (1985). **La sindrome Parkinson-demenza: revisione critica della letteratura. / The Parkinson-dementia syndrome: A critical review of the literature.** *Rivista Sperimentale di Freniatria e Medicina Legale delle Alienazioni Mentali,* 109(5), 942–960.

Reviews the role of antiparkinsonian drugs, the clinical analysis of Parkinson's dementia, and the anatomical-pathological-biochemical aspects of this disease and of Alzheimer's disease. Iatrogenic illnesses due to drug treatment, namely anticholinergics, are discussed. The Parkinson-dementia syndrome should be considered together with the discussion about complex relations between neurotransmitters and their degeneration. (English abstract) (98 ref).

989. Grossman, Helene D.; Weiner, Audrey S.; Salamon, Michael J. & Burros, Nelson. (1986). **The milieu standard for care of dementia in a nursing home.** Special Issue: Social work and Alzheimer's disease: Practice issues with victims and their families. *Journal of Gerontological Social Work,* 9(2), 73–89.
Explores how a home for the aged developed a specialized skilled nursing facility for dementia patients and its applicability for the provision of appropriate care to demented elderly in other settings. In the developmental stage of the project, a portion of the clinical care staff and of the patients is surveyed on the question of homogeneous vs heterogeneous placement by patient function and clinical need. Development of the special care unit (SCU) requires the concurrent operation of an administrative group and a direct-care staff group. The SCU environment is viewed as an important supportive device rather than as indifferent or neutral. It is concluded that review of daily meetings notes, staff reports, and observations of patients indicate an improvement in quality of patient care and inpatient morale with the establishment of the homogeneous unit. Involvement of social workers in the developmental stages of the SCU positively affected the project. (33 ref).

990. Growdon, J. H.; Corkin, Suzanne & Huff, F. Jacob. (1985). **Clinical evaluation of compounds for the treatment of memory dysfunction.** *Annals of the New York Academy of Sciences,* 444, 437–449.
Discusses critical issues in protocol design that are specific to Alzheimer's disease in the testing of memory-enhancing drugs. These issues include the objective of the study, design and duration of the study, selection of Ss, and variables to be measured. It is pointed out that protocol design varies according to the stage of drug development. The preliminary results of an ongoing trial testing the combination of phosphatidylcholine and piracetam on 15 56–75 yr old patients with Alzheimer's disease are presented to illustrate these issues in a clinical investigation. The results of this trial highlight some of the hazards that confront clinical drug studies in Alzheimer's disease. For example, a small sample size limits any conclusions that can be drawn from the findings of a clinical drug study. (35 ref).

991. Growdon, John H.; Corkin, Suzanne; Huff, F. Jacob & Rosen, T. John. (1986). **Piracetam combined with lecithin in the treatment of Alzheimer's disease.** *Neurobiology of Aging,* 7(4), 269–276.
Administered the nootropic drug piracetam (PA), alone and in combination with phosphatidlycholine (PC), to 18 patients with Alzheimer's disease and measured the effects of treatment on a broad range of cognitive functions. PA was administered according to 3 double-blind crossover protocols and a replication study that differed in PA dose (2.4–9.9 g/day) and whether PC (18 g/day) was administered concurrently. PA was well tolerated, and there were no toxic side effects. Plasma choline levels rose significantly during PA and PC administration; monoamine metabolites in cerebrospinal fluid were unaffected by treatment. PA, either alone or in combination with PC, did not significantly affect cognition in the group as a whole, nor did it improve Ss' test performance.

992. Gustafson, L.; Edvinsson, L.; Dahlgren, N.; Hagberg, B. et al. (1987). **Intravenous physostigmine treatment of Alzheimer's disease evaluated by psychometric testing, regional cerebral blood flow (rCBF) measurement, and EEG.** *Psychopharmacology,* 93(1), 31–35.
Treated 10 patients (aged 49–71 yrs) with Alzheimer's disease with intravenous infusion of physostigmine (19.5–36.5 µg/kg) for 2 hrs. The acute effects on cognitive function, regional cerebral blood flow, and EEG were compared to placebo (isotonic glucose) using a double-blind cross-over design. Physostigmine caused a limited improvement of psychomotor performance and EEG and an increase of blood flow in the most severely affected cortical areas, predominantly in an early phase of Alzheimer's disease.

993. Habbema, J. Dik & Dippel, Diederik W. (1986). **Survivors-only bias in estimating survival in Alzheimer's disease and vascular dementias.** *Neurology,* 36(7), 1009.
Comments on the paper by L. L. Barclay et al (1985) on survival in Alzheimer's disease, suggesting that they reported overoptimistic life-expectancy figures.

994. Hall, Geri; Kirschling, M. Virginia & Todd, Susan. (1986). **Sheltered freedom: An Alzheimer's unit in an ICF.** *Geriatric Nursing,* 7(3), 132–137.
Describes the development, operation, and evaluation of an Alzheimer's disease (AD) unit at an 89-bed intermediate care facility (ICF). The special unit was developed to improve the quality of life for AD patients by decreasing their stressful encounters with physically frail but alert residents. The unit care plans are designed to accommodate the special needs of residents with progressively diminishing intellectual capacity and tolerance for multiple stimuli and change and with increasing susceptibility to fatigue. In-service training and support for staff promote high quality care for unit residents. Evaluation of the unit after 3 mo of operation showed that the unit had a calming effect on residents, increased their social interactions, and decreased their need for medication.

995. Hamerman, David; Dubler, Nancy N.; Kennedy, Gary J. & Masdeu, Joseph. (1986). **Decision making in response to an elderly woman with dementia who refused surgical repair of her fractured hip.** *Journal of the American Geriatrics Society,* 34(3), 234–239.
Presents the case of a 79-yr-old woman with Alzheimer's disease whose refusal of surgical care for a fractured hip was honored and who thereafter remained chairbound. The authors discuss the physical, psychological, and legal implications of the case and conclude that an interdisciplinary geriatric team conference with an advocate identified for the patient should have been held. If the group had concurred on the indications for intervention, reference to the court would have been appropriate. The authors recommend that an interdisciplinary approach is appropriate for geriatric patients with severe dementia. The inability of the patient to weigh options and the medical and psychosocial consequences of respecting his/her statements must be considered. (29 ref).

996. Hayter, Jean. (1974). **Patients who have Alzheimer's disease.** *American Journal of Nursing,* 74(8), 1460–1463.
Describes the treatment of patients with Alzheimer's disease, a chronic neuropsychiatric disorder of unknown etiology characterized by impairment of intellectual ability. Occurrence of the disease and possible theoretical explanations of its source are reviewed. Symptoms result from destruction of neurons in the cerebral cortex, particularly those of the frontal, parietal, and temporal lobes. Characteristic symptoms include memory loss, time disorientation, and lack of spontaneity. Since there is no known cure for this illness, it is suggested that nursing care should focus on making the patient and his family as comfortable and satisfied as possible. Gentleness is viewed as the best possible approach in this relationship between pa-

tient and nurse, since the patient often is unable to communicate or to let the nurse know that he understands language.

997. Helgeson, Elsbeth M. & Willis, Scott C. (1986). **Handbook of group activities for impaired older adults.** *Activities, Adaptation & Aging,* 9(2), 107.
Presents a description of activities conducted at a daycare and day treatment facility for patients with Alzheimer's disease and related disorders. These activities are designed to provide a foundation for a daily program that becomes therapy for participants and respite for their families. They seek to enable clients to obtain human interaction and to achieve a sense of self-worth. Each activity is rated with symbols according to its principal therapeutic value; the activities are also categorized according to their potential to facilitate emotional expression, enhance problem-solving skills, stimulate sensory systems, and encourage interaction. Guidelines for leading groups with impaired adults and tailoring activities to meet the needs of particular groups are also presented.

998. Herrmann, N.; Sadavoy, J. & Steingart, A. (1987). **"Use of THA in treatment of Alzheimer-like dementia: Pilot study in twelve patients": Comment.** *New England Journal of Medicine,* 316(25), 1603–1604.
Suggests that the results of a study by W. K. Summers et al (1986) of the use of oral tetrahydroaminoacridine in treating senile dementia of the Alzheimer's type were biased by choice of outcome variables, use of improved diagnostic techniques, and use of lecithin by some Ss.

999. Hollander, Eric; Davidson, Michael; Mohs, Richard C.; Horvath, Thomas B. et al. (1987). **RS 86 in the treatment of Alzheimer's disease: Cognitive and biological effects.** *Biological Psychiatry,* 22(9), 1067–1078.
12 patients with Alzheimer's disease completed a double-blind crossover study comparing oral RS 86, a long-acting and specific muscarinic agonist, with placebo. Cognitive and noncognitive effects were assessed using a rating scale developed by W. G. Rosen et al (1984). RS 86 was found to improve test scores consistently (both cognitive and noncognitive subscales) in 7 Ss, with a clinically obvious improvement in only 2 Ss. RS 86 produced a significant increase in peak nocturnal cortisol levels, correlated with improvement on testing. Biological findings suggest that RS 86 was effective only to the extent that it enhanced central cholinergic activity.

1000. Hollister, Leo E. (1986). **Drug therapy of Alzheimer's disease: Realistic or not?** *Progress in Neuro-Psychopharmacology & Biological Psychiatry,* 10(3–5), 439–446.
Discusses problems in evaluating drug therapy of Alzheimer's disease (AD). It is suggested that treatment approaches with drugs have been either symptomatic or specific. Treatments are discussed that include stimulants, cerebral vasodilators, drugs that increase brain metabolism, drugs with special actions, enhancement of neurotransmission, and neuropeptides. It is concluded that it is reasonable to try to treat AD with drugs even though a definite rationale for such treatment is not established.

1001. Hoss, Mary K. (1986). **Recreation activities and an examination of the effects of activity programming on persons with Alzheimer's Disease.** *Dissertation Abstracts International,* 47(6-B), 2399.

1002. Hu, Teh-wei; Huang, Lien-fu & Cartwright, William S. (1986). **Evaluation of the costs of caring for the senile demented elderly: A pilot study.** *Gerontologist,* 26(2), 158–163.
Evaluated economic costs for 25 nursing home patients (average age 82.08 yrs) and 19 elderly individuals (average age 78.17 yrs) with senile dementia (Alzheimer's or multi-infarct) living in their own homes through a household survey. Using time records compiled by nurses or family members over a 2-

wk period, the costs incurred annually in caring for an elderly person with senile dementia at home were estimated to average $11,735; in a nursing home, the cost was estimated to be $22,458.

1003. Hughes, Donna Y. (1987). **Alzheimer's disease and psychiatric nursing: Treating the depression.** *Perspectives in Psychiatric Care,* 24(1), 5–8.
Discusses efforts by a staff of experienced psychiatric nurses at the National Institutes of Health to deal with depression observed in some patients with Alzheimer's disease (AD) participating in research on AD. The approach included the involvement of a multidisciplinary team, which provided a therapeutic milieu with a weekly structure of activities and meetings and group psychotherapy to help patients and family members develop coping strategies.

1004. Hyman, Bradley T.; Eslinger, Paul J. & Damasio, Antonio R. (1985). **Effect of naltrexone on senile dementia of the Alzheimer type.** *Journal of Neurology, Neurosurgery & Psychiatry,* 48(11), 1169–1171.
Performed a double-blind crossover trial of naltrexone, an orally active long-acting opiate antagonist, in 17 Alzheimer-type dementia patients (57–81 yrs old). Ss received 100 mg/day of naltrexone HCl orally or placebo each week for 6 wks. None showed any improvement in assessments of day-to-day living skills or on a battery of neuropsychological tests. In the dosage used, naltrexone appears not to be useful in Alzheimer-type dementia. (17 ref).

1005. Janowsky, David S. et al. (1985). **Effects of physostigmine on pulse, blood pressure, and serum epinephrine levels.** *American Journal of Psychiatry,* 142(6), 738–740.
Explored the cardiovascular and sympathetic amine-releasing effect in 14 patients (aged 25–52 yrs) of the centrally active cholinesterase inhibitor physostigmine. Ss, who had been diagnosed with affective disorder, were pretreated with methscopolamine and received .022 mg/kg (up to 2.0 mg) of physostigmine salicylate, iv, 30 min later. The physostigmine infusion caused significant and often profound increases in the Ss' epinephrine levels, pulse rates, and blood pressure. These cardiovascular effects may have clinical importance for the experimental use of physostigmine in the treatment of elderly Ss with Alzheimer's disease. (12 ref).

1006. Jenike, Michael A. (1986). **"Caution urged in using MAOIs with the elderly": Dr. Jenike replies.** *American Journal of Psychiatry,* 143(1), 119.
Responds to cautions offered by C. Salzman (1986) regarding the use of monoamine oxidase inhibitors (MAOIs) with depressed patients with degenerative dementia (Alzheimer's disease)—treatment recommended by the present author (1985)—and contends that, though care should be taken, patients with more severe dementia should not be excluded from a trial of an MAOI. (5 ref).

1007. Jenike, Michael A. (1985). **Monoamine oxidase inhibitors as treatment for depressed patients with primary degenerative dementia (Alzheimer's disease).** *American Journal of Psychiatry,* 142(6), 763–764.
Reports 2 case histories of a 73-yr-old woman and a 68-yr-old man with disabling depression who failed to respond to standard antidepressants but improved with an MAO inhibitor. It is noted that the cholinergic system is involved in Alzheimer's symptoms and that demented patients have high MAO levels. (10 ref).

1008. Jenike, Michael A.; Albert, Marilyn S.; Heller, Hope; LoCastro, Susan et al. (1986). **Combination therapy with lecithin and ergoloid mesylates for Alzheimer's disease.** *Journal of Clinical Psychiatry,* 47(5), 249–251.

Conducted a 10-wk placebo-controlled double-blind crossover protocol of combination therapy with 20 gm lecithin and 6 mg ergoloid mesylates with 7 patients (aged 55–74 yrs) with presenile and senile dementia, Alzheimer's type. Ss' abilities to detect spatial arrangements, to recognize faces, and to identify new words on a delayed recognition span test were not significantly improved. Dementia Rating Scale scores before treatment were not significantly different from those after treatment.

1009. Jenkie, Michael A. (1986). **Alzheimer's disease: Clinical care and management.** *Psychosomatics,* 27(6), 407–416.
Suggests that the diagnosis of Alzheimer's disease is best made by evaluating the overall course of the illness and by ruling out other causes of dementia, some of which are potentially treatable. Management of the Alzheimer patient necessitates that the physician assist family members and be familiar with use of psychotropics and cognition-enhancing drugs. Concomitant depression, psychosis, anxiety, or behavioral problems are generally responsive to medication. Means of managing behaviors such as suspiciousness and emotional overresponse are described, and consultation with the family is discussed in terms of optimizing home care of the patient.

1010. Johnson, Leayn H. (1987). **The effects of an educational program on anxiety, locus of control, and knowledge in nurses' aides caring for Alzheimer's patients in nursing homes.** *Dissertation Abstracts International,* 48(2-B), 581.

1011. Jorm, A. F. (1986). **The dissemination of research findings: Some limitations revealed when attempting a meta-analysis.** *Australian & New Zealand Journal of Psychiatry,* 20(3), 384–385.
A meta-analysis of the literature on drug treatments for Alzheimer's disease, conducted by the author (1986), revealed the following limitations in the dissemination of research findings: (1) multiple publication of findings, (2) failure to report basic descriptive statistics, and (3) failure to respond to written requests for additional information on the research. Possible reasons for these problems and remedies for them are discussed.

1012. Jorm, Anthony F. (1986). **Effects of cholinergic enhancement therapies on memory function in Alzheimer's disease: A meta-analysis of the literature.** *Australian & New Zealand Journal of Psychiatry,* 20(2), 237–240.
Reports that a quantitative analysis of the literature on cholinergic enhancement of memory function in Alzheimer's disease showed that such therapies have an effect if dosages are individualized. Treatments that combine a precursor with an anticholinesterase appear to be the most promising for clinically useful results, although the number of studies that have evaluated this combination treatment is small.

1013. Kirwin, Patricia M. (1986). **Adult day care: An integrated model.** Special Issue: Social work and Alzheimer's disease: Practice issues with victims and their families. *Journal of Gerontological Social Work,* 9(2), 59–71.
Suggests that for frail elders and those afflicted with Alzheimer's disease, adult daycare is a maturing service option linking clients and their caregivers with formal community supports. Integrating 2 programs for the aging, such as an adult daycare program and a senior center, increases participant service options while decreasing service cost. Those who benefit most from this service include families and caregivers who get respite from the continuous pressures of full-time care; frail elders who need social contact in a highly supervised setting; current senior center members who have become more dependent; and the well spouse who is not able to leave the frail mate unattended to participate in senior center activities. Basic program services include socialization, health service, nutrition counseling and education, transportation, family support groups, and staff needs and training. Difficulties in integrating daycare in a senior center are described. An annotated bibliography is provided for 24 publications related to adult daycare.

1014. Knopman, David S. & Hartman, Marilyn. (1986). **Cognitive effects of high-dose naltrexone in patients with probable Alzheimer's disease.** *Journal of Neurology, Neurosurgery & Psychiatry,* 49(11), 1321–1322.
Assessed the cognitive effects of chronic administration of the narcotic antagonist, naltrexone (50–300 mg/kg, orally), in 10 probable Alzheimer's disease patients (aged 67–73 yrs). Improvements on measures of total word recall suggest a beneficial effect of naltrexone on aspects of episodic memory not found in other studies (e.g., B. T. Hyman et al; 1986).

1015. Kopelman, Michael. (1987). **"Use of THA in treatment of Alzheimer-like dementia: Pilot study in twelve patients": Comment.** *New England Journal of Medicine,* 316(25), 1604.
Notes problems with S assignment to blinded and nonblinded phases in a study by W. K. Summers et al (1986) on the use of oral tetrahydroaminoacridine in treating senile dementia of the Alzheimer's type.

1016. Kopelman, Michael D. (1985). **Multiple memory deficits in Alzheimer-type dementia: Implications for pharmacotherapy.** *Psychological Medicine,* 15(3), 527–541.
Compared primary and secondary memory in 16 56–75 yr old patients with Alzheimer's disease (AD), 16 38–66 yr old Korsakoff patients, and 16 38–73 yr old healthy controls, using the Digit Span subscale of the Wechsler Adult Intelligence Scale (WAIS), the Wechsler Memory Scale, and measures of short- and long-term forgetting. Results show that AD Ss had deficits in both primary and secondary memory. Previous pharmacological studies have suggested that there is no impairment of primary and marked impairment of secondary memory on the basis of cholinergic depletion. The present findings of primary memory deficits are unlikely to be accounted for in terms of cholinergic depletion but provide a possible explanation for the disappointing results of trials of cholinergic replacement therapy in AD Ss. The pattern of deficit in secondary memory is consistent with that expected from cholinergic depletion. (10 ref).

1017. Kral, V. A. (1983). **The relationship between senile dementia (Alzheimer type) and depression.** *Canadian Journal of Psychiatry,* 28(4), 304–306.
Describes the symptomatology and treatment of the various types of depressions found in Alzheimer patients and discusses some of the theoretical problems that are posed. (French abstract) (12 ref).

1018. Kurlychek, Robert T. (1983). **Use of a digital alarm chronograph as a memory aid in early dementia.** *Clinical Gerontologist,* 1(3), 93–94.
Describes a digital alarm chronograph that serves as a cue for brain-damaged persons to consult their datebook. A 64-yr-old man with a diagnosis of early Alzheimer's disease was able to remember to consult his schedule of programs while wearing a watch that was set to chime every hour. S became able to attend his scheduled programs without being directed, and he regained some lost self-confidence.

1019. Kurz, A.; Rüster, P.; Romero, B. & Zimmer, R. (1986). **Cholinerge Behandlungsstrategien bei der Alzheimerschen Krankheit. / Cholinergic treatment strategies in Alzheimer's disease.** *Nervenarzt,* 57(10), 558–569.
Discusses cholinergic treatment strategies for Alzheimer's disease, since neurochemical, neuropathological, and pharmacological investigations show that this form of senile dementia involves a dysfunction of the cholinergic neurotransmitter system. A cholinergic deficit has become an important factor in the design of pharmacological treatments for Alzheimer

patients. An overview is presented of 78 therapy studies, published between 1978 and 1984, that involved Ss treated with different cholinergic medications. Special cognitive and mnesic performance tests showed only minor improvements in a few Ss.

1020. Kushnir, Seymour L.; Ratner, Jack T. & Gregoire, Pierre A. (1987). **Multiple nutrients in the treatment of Alzheimer's disease.** *Journal of the American Geriatrics Society,* 35(5), 476–477.
Reports that the treatment of 8 patients who met Diagnostic and Statistical Manual of Mental Disorders (DSM-III) criteria for primary degenerative dementia with daily doses of lecithin, tryptophan, and tyrosine, the nutrient precursors of acetylcholine, serotonin, and dopamine/noradrenaline, resulted in 3 of the patients being more relaxed, alert, and socially involved. Assessment with the Brief Psychiatric Rating Scale revealed significant improvement in all 8 patients.

1021. Lesko, L. J.; Fiore, D.; Leslie, J.; Narang, P. K. et al. (1986). **Estimation of protein binding of zimelidine and norzimelidine using cerebrospinal fluid and ultrafiltration.** *Research Communications in Psychology, Psychiatry & Behavior,* 11(2–3), 95–111.
Steady-state concentrations of the bicyclic antidepressant zimelidine (ZIM) and its active metabolite norzimelidine were measured in the cerebrospinal fluid (CSF) and serum of 5 males (aged 51–76 yrs) with Alzheimer's disease. Results suggest that the CSF/serum ratio of bicyclic antidepressants cannot be accurately predicted from in vitro measurements of an unbound fraction. Findings on the biochemical and cognitive effects of ZIM are discussed in terms of attempts to correlate serum drug concentration with clinical response.

1022. Little, Adrienne; Levy, Raymond; Chuaqui-Kidd, Paz & Hand, David. (1985). **A double-blind, placebo controlled trial of high-dose lecithin in Alzheimer's disease.** *Journal of Neurology, Neurosurgery & Psychiatry,* 48(8), 736–742.
51 Ss with senile dementia of the Alzheimer type were given either 20–25 g/day purified soya lecithin (containing 90% phosphatidyl plus lysophosphatidyl choline) or placebo for 6 mo and were followed up for at least a further 6 mo. Plasma choline levels were monitored throughout treatment. No differences were found between the placebo group and the lecithin group, but there was improvement in a subgroup of relatively poor lecithin compliers. These were older and had intermediate levels of plasma choline. It is suggested that there may be an optimal dose of lecithin in Alzheimer's disease that the poor compliers received by chance. (57 ref).

1023. Mace, Nancy. (1986). **Home and community services for Alzheimer's disease.** Special Issue: Therapeutic interventions for the person with dementia. *Physical & Occupational Therapy in Geriatrics,* 4(3), 5–13.
Discusses the need for therapeutic home and community programs—including day care, recreation programs in nursing homes, home help, and outpatient services—for Alzheimer's patients and their families. Methods of service delivery are described. Four principles of patient care are outlined: Conduct a complete and thorough assessment; treat all concurrent illnesses; treat disabling symptoms; and make the patient's environment work for him/her. A supportive environment recognizes the patient's limited ability to tolerate stress and helps the patient withdraw when demands or noise and confusion become too much. The need for a continuum of care is also emphasized, from short-term respite care for families to residential care and hospice programs. Implications for quality assurance and information dissemination are noted.

1024. Mace, Nancy L. (1987). **Principles of activities for persons with dementia.** *Physical & Occupational Therapy in Geriatrics,* 5(3), 13–27.

Asserts that the experience of day care and residential care programs that serve people with dementing illnesses such as Alzheimer's disease has been that a program of planned activities is a vital part of therapy. Activity programs can give meaning to one's life, reestablish valued interpersonal roles, confirm dignity and enable pleasure in the face of illness, and support experiences of success. Participants in such programs often show improved social functioning; evidence of increased life satisfaction; and a decrease of some disturbed behaviors, even with severe cognitive deficits. Activities are most effective when they seek to support remaining strengths and are supportive of the specific deficits that people with dementing illnesses experience. Potentially useful activities and tasks are discussed.

1025. Margolin, Richard A. & Ban, Thomas A. (1986). **Neuroimaging and psychopharmacology in the diagnosis and treatment of dementia.** *Progress in Neuro-Psychopharmacology & Biological Psychiatry,* 10(3–5), 493–500.
Reviews contributions of noninvasive brain imaging technologies to the diagnosis of organic dementias, with special reference to Alzheimer's disease. These techniques include computed tomography, magnetic resonance imaging, and positron emission tomography. Biochemical hypotheses with possible relevance to the pathogenesis of Alzheimer's disease are presented, and their therapeutic implications are discussed. Included among the hypotheses are interference with protein synthesis, acetylcholine deficiency, and aluminum deposition. The status of pharmacotherapy of Alzheimer's disease is outlined.

1026. Martin, Eileen M. (1987). **Intraventricular bethanechol infusion for Alzheimer disease.** *Dissertation Abstracts International,* 47(9-B), 3964.

1027. McBroom, Lynn W. (1987). **Alzheimer's disease: The death of the disease.** *Counseling & Values,* 31(2), 165–173.
Describes the behavioral and physical symptoms of Alzheimer's disease and offers specific suggestions for care of patients with the disease so that counselors can use this information to provide family members and others dealing with Alzheimer's patients with knowledge and practical advice about dealing with the changes occurring in the patient.

1028. Miller, Terry P.; Davies, Helen D.; Yesavage, Jerome A. & Tinklenberg, Jared R. (1984). **Presenile dementia associated with elevated aluminum and zinc levels: A case report.** *Clinical Gerontologist,* 2(3), 55–59.
Reports a failure of an attempted treatment of a 43-yr-old male patient with progressive dementia associated with markedly elevated serum, urine, and CSF levels of aluminum with the aluminum chelating agent tetracycline (1,000 mg) for 3 mo. Implications are discussed in terms of the role of aluminum in Alzheimer's disease. (2 ref).

1029. Mohs, Richard C. et al. (1985). **Oral physostigmine treatment of patients with Alzheimer's disease.** *American Journal of Psychiatry,* 142(1), 28–33.
Administered 0, .5, 1, 1.5, and 2 mg of oral physostigmine to 8 male and 4 female 52–76 yr old Alzheimer's patients every 2 hrs for 3–5 days in an evaluation of the effects of oral physostigmine on Alzheimer's disease. Ss' symptoms after each dose were assessed with the Alzheimer's Disease Assessment Scale. Placebo and the dose associated with the least severe symptoms were then readministered for 3–5 days each in the 2nd phase of the study. Of the 10 Ss who completed the study, 3 showed clinically significant improvement on the highest physostigmine dose in both phases, 4 more were marginally improved in both phases, and 3 had inconsistent responses to physostigmine. Cortisol measures obtained during the 2nd phase suggested that Ss whose symptoms im-

proved on physostigmine were those in whom oral physostigmine enhanced central cholinergic activity. (55 ref).

1030. Mohs, Richard C. et al. (1985). **Clinical studies of the cholinergic deficit in Alzheimer's disease: II. Psychopharmacologic studies.** *Journal of the American Geriatrics Society,* 33(11), 749–757.
Intravenous physostigmine (.125–.5 mg) significantly and reliably enhanced memory in 13 of 16 patients (aged 53–75 yrs) with definite or probable Alzheimer's disease or senile dementia of the Alzheimer type (AD/SDAT), but the dose producing the improvement varied among Ss. Oral physostigmine (.5–2 mg/2 hrs) decreased overall symptom severity in a reliable way in 7 of 12 AD/SDAT patients (aged 52–76 yrs). The extent of improvement was correlated with the increase in mean cortisol secretion produced by physostigmine, suggesting that the drug improved behavior and cognition only to the extent that it had a specific central cholinomimetic effect. There was no significant association between response to physostigmine and results of a dexamethasone suppression test, and physostigmine had no effect on growth hormone secretion. (62 ref).

1031. Mohs, Richard C. & Davis, Kenneth L. (1982). **A signal detectability analysis of the effect of physostigmine on memory in patients with Alzheimer's disease.** *Neurobiology of Aging,* 3(2), 105–110.
10 50–68 yr old patients with clinically diagnosed Alzheimer's disease were given tests of recognition memory (the Memory and Information Test and the Dementia Rating Scale) while receiving placebo or physostigmine given iv over 30 min. Doses of 0.0, 0.125, 0.25, and 0.5 mg were given in random order on 4 separate days. All Ss had their best performance following one of the doses of physostigmine rather than saline, although dose–response curves varied from one S to another. The dose associated with the best performance in each S was compared with saline in a replication study. The total number of correct responses on the recognition memory task was significantly greater following physostigmine than following saline. To determine whether this improvement in performance was a result of an increase in the amount of information stored in memory or was secondary to a change in the Ss' criteria for saying that they recognized an item, the results were subjected to a signal detectability analysis. Studied items and new items were more discriminable following physostigmine, as evidenced by an increase in d', and the criteria for saying which items had been studied also changed following physostigmine, as evidenced by an increase in C. The increase in d' indicated that physostigmine enhanced storage of information in memory, while the change in C was consistent with the view that patients altered their decision criteria to maximize the number of correct responses in both conditions. (43 ref).

1032. Narang, Prem K. & Cutler, Neal R. (1986). **Pharmacotherapy in Alzheimer's disease: Basis and rationale.** *Progress in Neuro-Psychopharmacology & Biological Psychiatry,* 10(3–5), 519–531.
Suggests that research has revealed behavioral symptoms in Alzheimer's disease associated with underlying biochemical changes in the cholinergic, dopaminergic/gamma-aminobutyric acid (GABA)ergic, noradrenergic, serotoninergic, neurochemical, and neuropeptidergic systems. Pharmacological strategies involving manipulation of these systems as a means of relieving Alzheimer's disease symptoms are reviewed from several perspectives (e.g., those involving transmitter substitution, enzyme inhibition, direct specific receptor stimulation).

1033. Newhouse, Paul A. et al. (1986). **Intravenous nicotine in a patient with Alzheimer's disease.** *American Journal of Psychiatry,* 143(11), 1494–1495.
Investigated the effects of intravenous nicotine (≤0.5 μg/kg/minute) on cognitive and psychological functioning in a 57-yr-old male nonsmoker with progressive degenerative dementia and in 20 nonsmokers (aged 21–62 yrs) given doses up to 0.70 μg/kg/minute. Results suggest that the potential threshold for achieving improved cognitive functioning may be lower in Alzheimer patients than in young normal Ss. (5 ref).

1034. O'Donnell, Vincent M. (1982). **Neurochemical correlates of memory function in Korsakoff's syndrome and Alzheimer's disease.** *Dissertation Abstracts International,* 42(8-B), 3434.

1035. Palmer, Mary H. (1983). **Alzheimer's disease and critical care: Interactions, implications, interventions.** *Journal of Gerontological Nursing,* 9(2), 86–90, 116.
Contends that a knowledge of Alzheimer's disease (AD) and its progression helps the critical care unit (CCU) nurse implement anticipatory and preventive interactions to promote the quality of life and maintain the cognitive functions of the patient. Careful planning, open communication, and awareness of one's own feelings regarding aging and chronic dementing disorders will minimize trauma to both the nursing staff routine and to the client while providing superior care tailored to the many challenging needs AD poses. A case study of a 56-yr-old AD female is presented to illustrate the needs of a patient in a CCU. (39 ref).

1036. Paschke, Mary J. (1984). **Day care within a community mental health center.** *Physical & Occupational Therapy in Geriatrics,* 3(4), 67–70.
Describes a day-care program conducted by a community mental health center for at-risk and frail elderly persons. The social day-care program was an outgrowth of the center's psychiatric day program and offered support groups for Alzheimer's patients, depressed patients, and those with significant physical impairments. Two major goals of the program were to provide an alternative to institutionalization and to sustain the skills that the elderly needed for daily independent living. (2 ref).

1037. Peabody, Cecilia A. et al. (1985). **Desglycinamide-9-arginine-8-vasopressin (DGAVP, organon 5667) in patients with dementia.** *Neurobiology of Aging,* 6(2), 95–100.
Investigated the effects of DGAVP (Organon 5667) on learning and memory in a double-blind parallel group study with 17 demented Ss. Nine Ss met Diagnostic and Statistical Manual of Mental Disorders (DSM-III) criteria for primary degenerative dementia (Alzheimer's disease) with insidious onset prior to age 65 yrs; the other 8 Ss met DSM-III criteria for dementia associated with alcoholism. Ss were given either DGAVP (92 μg intranasally 3 times/day) or an identical placebo for 1 wk after having received 1 wk of placebo. The DGAVP group had a statistically significant improvement on the list learning of low-imagery words; however, it is argued that this finding needs to be replicated before any definite conclusions can be drawn. There were no other appreciable behavioral effects of this DGAVP regimen, and there was no evidence of any DGAVP-related adverse effects, except for possible weight gain. (37 ref).

1038. Peabody, Cecilia A.; Deblois, Thomas E. & Tinklenberg, Jared R. (1986). **Thyrotropin-releasing hormone (TRH) and Alzheimer's disease.** *American Journal of Psychiatry,* 143(2), 262–263.
To examine whether thryotropin-releasing hormone (TRH) would have beneficial effects in treating Alzheimer's disease (AD), 4 AD patients participated in a double-blind study. Neither a 300- or a 500-μg injection of TRH exerted positive behavioral effects in Ss, as measured by a neuropsychological battery. (5 ref).

111

1039. Peabody, Cecilia A.; Davies, Helen D.; Berger, Philip A. & Tinklenberg, Jared R. (1986). **Desamino-D-arginine-vasopressin (DDAVP) in Alzheimer's disease.** *Neurobiology of Aging,* 7(4), 301–303.
14 Alzheimer Ss participated in a parallel group study of DDAVP. All Ss received 1 wk of single-blind placebo. Then, on a double-blind basis, the active group received DDAVP intranasally in doses starting at 30 µg/day and increasing over a 3-wk period to 180 µg/day. Using a repeated measures analysis of variance (ANOVA), 3 of 31 measures were significant for DDAVP treatment: the Hamilton Rating Scale for Depression and the Affect and Interpersonal subscales of the Sandoz Clinical Assessment Geriatric Scale.

1040. Peabody, Cecilia A.; Warner, M. Dhyanne; Whiteford, Harvey A. & Hollister, Leo E. (1987). **Neuroleptics and the elderly.** *Journal of the American Geriatrics Society,* 35(3), 233–238.
Presents the case of a 63-yr-old patient with Alzheimer's disease treated with temazepan (15 mg at bedtime and every 6 hrs as needed for agitation). The present authors discuss the case in terms of changes in kinetics of drugs in the elderly, indications for use, side effects (e.g., tardive dyskinesia), extrapyramidal reactions, orthostatic hypotension, anticholinergic side effects, sedation, cardiac toxicity, choice of neuroleptics, and drug interactions.

1041. Peppard, Nancy R. (1986). **Special nursing home units for residents with primary degenerative dementia: Alzheimer's Disease.** Special Issue: Social work and Alzheimer's disease: Practice issues with victims and their families. *Journal of Gerontological Social Work,* 9(2), 5–13.
Describes a special nursing home unit for Alzheimer's disease patients designed to provide proper care for the patients while remaining supportive of family and staff. A design was formulated to create a wholistic environment that would allow behavior management techniques appropriate to individual and group needs and abilities. Admission criteria include a complete neurological assessment by a neurologist with a diagnosis of Alzheimer's disease or a related irreversible dementia. Daily activities are designed to be appropriate to the level of each resident participant. To achieve specialization, training, and modification of traditional roles, staff work only in the special unit. Training is conducted at 3 levels and includes everyone who interacts on the unit. Family members are encouraged to spend as much time as they desire on the unit. Based on the evolution of this program, it is suggested that specific training and support result in high quality, wholistic patient care; development of effective behavioral management techniques; and increased job satisfaction for staff, resulting in lower turnover. (10 ref).

1042. Pirozzolo, Francis J.; Baskin, David S.; Swihart, Andrew A. & Appel, Stanley H. (1987). **Oral tetrahydroaminoacridine in the treatment of senile dementia, Alzheimer's type.** *New England Journal of Medicine,* 316(25), 1603.
Identifies methodological problems in a study by W. K. Summers et al (1986) on the use of oral tetrahydroaminoacridine in the treatment of senile dementia of the Alzheimer's type.

1043. Pomara, Nunzio et al. (1985). **Multiple, single-dose naltrexone administrations fail to affect overall cognitive functioning and plasma cortisol in individuals with probable Alzheimer's disease.** *Neurobiology of Aging,* 6(3), 233–236.
Conducted a double-blind placebo-controlled study with 9 Ss (mean age 66.4 yrs) with probable Alzheimer's disease to assess the effects of varying doses of naltrexone (0, 25, 50, and 100 mg) on cognitive functioning and on plasma cortisol. Naltrexone improved performance in only 1 of the 6 psychometric tasks employed (the Token Test). However, enhancement of Token Test performance was limited to the 25-mg naltrexone dose and was mainly the result of an improve-ment on the part of the 2 most severely impaired Ss. In contrast to previous reports of elevations of plasma cortisol following administration of opiate antagonists to younger, nondemented Ss, naltrexone failed to produce any significant increase in plasma cortisol. (24 ref).

1044. Pomara, Nunzio et al. (1983). **Failure of single-dose lecithin to alter aspects of central cholinergic activity in Alzheimer's disease.** *Journal of Clinical Psychiatry,* 44(8), 293–295.
Assessed the effect of a single dose (15 g/70 kg) of lecithin (95% phosphatidylcholine) on several measures of central cholinergic activity (memory, cortisol, prolactin, pulse, and blood pressure) in 6 Ss (aged 62–82 yrs) with Alzheimer's disease. In contrast to the reported effects of physostigmine, a cholinesterase inhibitor, lecithin had no effect on these parameters despite significant increases in plasma and erythrocyte choline. (14 ref).

1045. Pomara, Nunzio et al. (1983). **Elevation of RBC glycine and choline levels in geriatric patients treated with lithium.** *American Journal of Psychiatry,* 140(7), 911–913.
Investigated the effect of Li on red blood cell (RBC) glycine and choline and on cognitive functioning in persons with Alzheimer's disease. During 6 wks of Li treatment, the RBC glycine and choline levels of 5 cognitively impaired geriatric Ss (4 with Alzheimer's disease) without affective disorders increased significantly and correlated with RBC and plasma Li levels. Ss' cognitive processes did not improve. (10 ref).

1046. Pomara, Nunzio et al. (1984). **Combined Piracetam and cholinergic precursor treatment for primary degenerative dementia.** *IRCS Medical Science: Psychology & Psychiatry,* 12(5–6), 388–389.
Reports on a double-blind study of the effects of a piracetam/lecithin combination in treating 9 55–75 yr old patients with Alzheimer's disease. One-way ANOVAs of scores on a computerized psychometric assessment battery (e.g., selective reminding and RT tasks) showed no significant differences among the combination treatment, piracetam alone, or placebo treatment. When directly compared with the piracetam-alone condition, the combination treatment decreased Sperling task (G. Sperling, 1963) scores and increased Ss' reliance on short-term retrieval in the selective reminding task. (10 ref).

1047. Pomara, Nunzio; Bagne, Curtis A.; Stanley, Michael & Yarbrough, George G. (1986). **Prospective strategies for cholinergic interventions in Alzheimer's disease.** *Progress in Neuro-Psychopharmacology & Biological Psychiatry,* 10(3–5), 553–569.
Suggests that the cholinergic hypothesis of memory dysfunction, which has guided proposals for treating symptoms of Alzheimer's disease (AD), is in need of revision. Two assumptions of the cholinergic hypothesis are examined: the beliefs that cholinoceptive neurons would function normally with adequate stimulation and that AD is characterized by generalized cholinergic hypoactivity. Evidence for cortisol hypersecretion, abnormal dexamethasone suppression, and occurrence of depressive symptoms and sleep abnormalities in AD patients is more consistent with regional cholinergic hyperactivity than generalized hypoactivity. It is suggested that cholinoceptive neurons could be hypersensitive or subsensitive or have unaltered responsivity, and these options have different treatment implications.

1048. Rabinowitz, Ellen. (1986). **Day care and Alzheimer's disease: A weekend program in New York City.** Special Issue: Therapeutic interventions for the person with dementia. *Physical & Occupational Therapy in Geriatrics,* 4(3), 95–103.

112

Notes that relatively few daycare programs have been established exclusively for individuals with Alzheimer's disease. A New York City program that operates on Saturdays is described; it is staffed entirely by occupational therapy personnel. A description of the program is presented, including intake procedures, clinical characteristics of participants, physical environment, staffing patterns, and activities that have been found to be successful with mildly to moderately demented individuals.

1049. Rabins, Peter V. (1986). **Establishing Alzheimer's disease units in nursing homes: Pros and cons.** *Hospital & Community Psychiatry,* 37(2), 120–121.
Discusses favorable and unfavorable aspects of maintaining specialized units for patients with dementia, suggesting that more experience should be gained before these units become widespread and that nursing homes now planning Alzheimer's disease units should consider their negative and positive aspects when designing them. (9 ref).

1050. Rabins, Peter V. & Mace, Nancy L. (1986). **Some ethical issues in dementia care.** *Clinical Gerontologist,* 5(3–4), 503–512.
Discusses the fact that since dementia makes an individual less capable of making his/her own decisions, the caregiver must usurp autonomy and perhaps even limit the patient's freedom. Related issues are the professional commitment to beneficence and nonmaleficence as well as the legal principle of incompetency. Four cases (Ss aged 63–78 yrs) illustrate the ethical dilemmas posed by dementia, death, and disability. It is advised that dementia, in and of itself, does not necessarily entail mental incompetence. The expressed wishes of the patient should be considered. Family issues are also reviewed.

1051. Rai, G. S. (1986). **Chelation therapy in dementia.** *Journal of the American Geriatrics Society,* 34(5), 413.
Expands on the danger of zinc loss due to administration of ethylenediaminetetraacetic acid, as noted by M. B. Cardelli et al (1985). It is suggested that Cardelli et al fail to expand on the danger of this procedure for patients with Alzheimer-type dementia.

1052. Randels, Patricia M. et al. (1984). **Lithium and lecithin treatment in Alzheimer's disease: A pilot study.** *Hillside Journal of Clinical Psychiatry,* 6(2), 139–147.
10 males (aged 47–70 yrs) who met DSM-III criteria for primary degenerative dementia received oral administrations of lithium carbonate to maintain serum lithium levels between 0.6–1.0 mEq/l for 4 wks. Lecithin granules were concurrently administered for 2 wks. Of the 6 Ss who completed the regimen (4 Ss dropped out because of toxic effects and an intervening illness), 2 showed behavioral improvement; none showed improvement on measures of cognitive functioning (e.g., Mini-Mental State Examination). Possible mechanisms of action are discussed. (28 ref).

1053. Randels, Patricia M.; Marco, Luis A.; Hanspal, N. S. & Robinson, Bessie. (1984). **Possible lithium-induced extrapyramidal effects in Alzheimer's disease.** *Hillside Journal of Clinical Psychiatry,* 6(1), 117–121.
Documents 2 cases—a 60-yr-old man with primary degenerative dementia (PDD) and a 47-yr-old man with Alzheimer's disease—who, following lithium treatment for less than a week, developed severe extrapyramidal symptomatology. It is emphasized that, in the presence of organic mental disorder, even brief treatment with lithium may induce severe extrapyramidal signs. Furthermore, toxicity to lithium may occur even though serum lithium levels are at therapeutic levels. Following termination of lithium, symptoms subsided quickly in the PDD patient (5 days) but more slowly in the Alzheimer's patient (16 days). (10 ref).

1054. Reifler, Burton V. & Larson, Eric B. (1985). **Alzheimer's disease and long-term care: The assessment of the patient.** *Journal of Geriatric Psychiatry,* 18(1), 9–26.
Reviews work on Alzheimer's disease, especially as it relates to long-term care. Models for accurate assessments, both for patients with dedicated families and for those who are isolated, are described. It is argued that depression and medical illness are more likely to aggravate Alzheimer's than to imitate it. (25 ref).

1055. Reifler, Burton V.; Larson, Eric B.; Teri, Linda & Poulsen, Marilyn. (1986). **Dementia of the Alzheimer's Type and depression.** Second International Congress on Psychogeriatric Medicine (1985, Umea, Sweden). *Journal of the American Geriatrics Society,* 34(12), 855–859.
Retrospectively reviewed the medical records of 131 dementia of the Alzheimer's type (DAT) Ss (aged 60+ yrs), 41 of whom also had a major affective disorder. Of those DAT plus depression Ss whose records reflected treatment (usually with a tricyclic antidepressant), 85% showed clear evidence of improvement in mood, vegetative signs, or activities of daily living. Analysis of change in cognitive function (measured by the Mini-Mental State Examination) and 5 global measures failed to reveal any differences between the depressed and nondepressed groups after a mean interval of 17 mo.

1056. Reisberg, Barry; Borenstein, Jeffrey; Salob, Stacy P.; Ferris, Steven H. et al. (1987). **Behavioral symptoms in Alzheimer's disease: Phenomenology and treatment.** *Journal of Clinical Psychiatry,* 48(5, Suppl), 9–15.
Examined the incidence, nature, and treatment of behavioral symptoms in patients with Alzheimer's disease by conducting a chart review of 57 patients (aged 55–93 yrs). Results show that 33 Ss had significant behavioral symptomatology (most commonly delusions, nonspecific agitation, and diurnal rhythm disturbances). 27 were treated with thioridazine (10–250 mg/day), 15 of whom were judged to have a positive response (mean maximum dose 55 mg/day). Information regarding the characteristic phenomenology of the behavioral symptoms studied was used to design a clinical rating instrument (appended) that may be useful in prospective studies of behavioral symptoms as well as in pharmacologic trials.

1057. Renvoize, E. B.; Kent, J. & Klar, H. M. (1987). **Delusional infestation and dementia: A case report.** *British Journal of Psychiatry,* 150, 403–405.
Reports the case of an 82-yr-old woman with delusional infestation and senile dementia of the Alzheimer type. The S's symptoms of infestation ceased with pimozide (8 mg daily) given for 5 wks and did not recur during follow-up over 9 mo. The importance of organic factors in patients with this disorder is emphasized.

1058. Reyes, Patricio F.; Dwyer, Boyd A.; Schwartzman, Robert J. & Sacchetti, Thomas. (1987). **Mental status changes induced by eye drops in dementia of the Alzheimer type.** *Journal of Neurology, Neurosurgery & Psychiatry,* 50(1), 113–115.
Reports 3 cases in which elderly patients (aged 72, 76, and 77 yrs) developed central nervous system (CNS) manifestations following pilocarpine administration and were subsequently found to have dementia of the Alzheimer type. Pilocarpine, a cholinomimetic agent, is a commonly prescribed eyedrop for middle aged and elderly patients.

1059. Risse, Steven C. & Barnes, Robert. (1986). **Pharmacologic treatment of agitation associated with dementia.** *Journal of the American Geriatrics Society,* 34(5), 368–376.
Reviews studies conducted over the past 30 yrs that have investigated the efficacy of psychotropic medications in controlling behavioral disturbances in elderly demented patients. The review, which emphasizes double-blind, placebo-controlled studies, discusses research having to do with neuroleptics, benzodiazepines, lithium, propranolol, carbamazepine,

alcohol, and other drugs used by clinicians. It is suggested that more studies are needed to evaluate the effectiveness of pharmacologic agents in specific types of dementia, particularly Alzheimer's disease.

1060. Risse, Steven C.; Lampe, Thomas H. & Cubberley, Lyndel. (1987). **Very low-dose neuroleptic treatment in two patients with agitation associated with Alzheimer's disease.** *Journal of Clinical Psychiatry*, 48(5), 207–208.
Presents the cases of 2 agitated male patients (aged 59 and 82 yrs) with Alzheimer's disease who either failed to respond or worsened with conventional low-dose neuroleptic and other pharmacologic treatment. Both demonstrated sustained improvement with very low-dose neuroleptics, one with haloperidol (0.125 mg) and the other with thioridazine (5 mg). Clinical, pharmacokinetic, and pharmacodynamic factors that may have accounted for this response are discussed.

1061. Rogers, Joan C. (1986). **Occupational therapy services for Alzheimer's disease and related disorders.** *American Journal of Occupational Therapy*, 40(12), 822–824.
Describes the uses of occupational therapy assessment and intervention in the management of irreversible dementing illnesses such as Alzheimer's disease. Assessment may aid in differential diagnosis and the evaluation of medical treatments, provides a baseline for assessing intervention, and suggests appropriate interventions. Interventions, such as environmental structuring and patterning of social interactions, are designed to maintain functional capacity, promote participation in activities, and ease caregiving activities.

1062. Rose, Robert P. & Moulthrop, Mark A. (1986). **Differential responsivity of verbal and visual recognition memory to physostigmine and ACTH.** *Biological Psychiatry*, 21(5–6), 538–542.
Describes the case of a 79-yr-old White woman admitted with a 4-yr history of progressively worsening confusion and memory problems and a presumed etiology of Alzheimer's disease. The S showed good nonmnemonic cognitive functions. Drug trials with 3 doses of physostigmine (0.125, 0.25, and 0.50 mg) and 2 doses of adrenocorticotropic hormone (ACTH [15 and 30 mg]) showed that different aspects of the S's memory had distinctive dose responses for both drugs.

1063. Rosse, Richard B.; Allen, Andree & Lux, Warren E. (1986). **Baclofen treatment in a patient with tardive dystonia.** *Journal of Clinical Psychiatry*, 47(9), 474–475.
Describes the treatment of a 70-yr-old female with a clinical diagnosis of Alzheimer's disease who developed tardive dystonia after 8 wks of haloperidol therapy and experienced complete remission of her dystonia while taking baclofen (60 mg/day).

1064. Sahakian, Barbara; Joyce, Eileen & Lishman, W. A. (1987). **Cholinergic effects on constructional abilities and on mnemonic processes: A case report.** *Psychological Medicine*, 17(2), 329–333.
Assessed the effects of physostigmine (0.4 mg) on test performance of a 58-yr-old female patient with multiple cognitive deficits. Scores on learning and memory tests and tests of visuospatial and constructional ability were improved by physostigmine, while lecithin only improved learning and memory scores. Results support enhancement of learning/memory by physostigmine in studies of patients with dementia of the Alzheimer's type.

1065. Salzman, Carl. (1986). **Caution urged in using MAOIs with the elderly.** *American Journal of Psychiatry*, 143(1), 118–119.

Comments on recommendations made by M. A. Jenike (1985) concerning the use of monoamine oxidase inhibitors (MAOIs) as treatment for depressed patients with primary degenerative dementia (Alzheimer's disease) and cautions that, since MAOIs increase agitation and confusion, MAOI treatment should be used only with elderly patients with mild dementia. (3 ref).

1066. Samorajski, T.; Vroulis, G. A. & Smith, R. C. (1985). **Piracetam plus lecithin trials in senile dementia of the Alzheimer type.** *Annals of the New York Academy of Sciences*, 444, 478–481.
Examined the neuropsychological effects of long-term treatment with a combination of lecithin and piracetam in 11 patients (mean age 67.1 yrs) with senile dementia of the Alzheimer type. Ss participated in a 6-mo double-blind, placebo-controlled crossover study. Neuropsychological evaluations showed that 8 of the 11 Ss improved more during the medication phase than during the placebo phase. (6 ref).

1067. Schafer, Susan C. (1985). **Modifying the environment.** Special Issue: Alzheimer's disease. *Geriatric Nursing*, 6(3), 157–159.
Discusses a nursing program for diagnostic evaluation that supports the Alzheimer patient. This is done by individualizing the patient's care and daily activities to simulate his/her home life. The nurse adapts the physical and psychosocial surroundings to the patient rather than asking the patient to adapt to the unit's routine. In this way, the patient's behaviors become the criteria for unit functioning. Staff–patient and patient–patient interactions are structured to maximize patient independence. Aspects of the program (encouraging patient's control, modifying stimuli, individualizing the schedule, and modifying the internal environment) are discussed. It is concluded that creating the environment in which Alzheimer's disease patients feel safe and comfortable can strengthen their incentive to continue using whatever capacities they have for as long as possible. (3 ref).

1068. Schwartz, Arthur S. & Kohlstaedt, Elizabeth V. (1986). **Physostigmine effects in Alzheimer's disease: Relationship to dementia severity.** *Life Sciences*, 38(11), 1021–1028.
11 demented patients (aged 61–83 yrs) were administered physostigmine (.004, .009, and .013 mg/kg, intramuscularly) and placebo, double-blind, in Phase 1. The most effective dose (in terms of Ss showing the best memory score) was repeated during Phase 2. Five Ss improved their verbal memory scores in Phases 1 and 2; these 5 responders were significantly more demented than the 6 nonresponders. Drug-induced increases in memory scores were significantly correlated with illness severity. The association between physostigmine effect and degree of dementia suggests that the severe cases may have more permeable blood–brain barriers and that drug availability to the brain is an important factor in evaluating treatment of senile dementia of the Alzheimer type with cholinergic substances.

1069. Serby, Michael. (1986). **Neuroleptic malignant syndrome in Alzheimer's disease.** *Journal of the American Geriatrics Society*, 34(12), 895–896.
Describes a case of neuroleptic malignant syndrome (NMS) in a 65-yr-old man with Alzheimer's disease (AD), suggesting that clinicians should be alert to early signs of NMS in geriatric Ss, especially in those with AD.

1070. Serby, Michael; Resnick, Richard; Jordan, Barbara; Adler, John et al. (1986). **Naltrexone and Alzheimer's disease.** *Progress in Neuro-Psychopharmacology & Biological Psychiatry*, 10(3–5), 587–590.

Administered naltrexone (5–100 mg/day), an oral opiate antagonist, to 9 patients with Alzheimer's-type dementia. Two Ss demonstrated apparent cognitive enhancement on 100 mg daily and were then tested in a double-blind crossover period. Only 1 of these Ss improved during active naltrexone administration.

1071. Small, Gary W.; Spar, J. Edward & Plotkin, Daniel A. (1987). **"Use of THA in treatment of Alzheimer-like dementia: Pilot study in twelve patients": Comment.** *New England Journal of Medicine,* 316(25), 1604.
Discusses the methodological shortcomings in a study by W. K. Summers et al (1986) on the use of oral tetrahydroaminoacridine in treating senile dementia of the Alzheimer's type.

1072. Soininen, H. et al. (1985). **Treatment of Alzheimer's disease with a synthetic ACTH 4–9 analog.** *Neurology,* 35(9), 1348–1351.
Administered the synthetic adrenocorticotropic hormone 4–9 analog, Org 2766, or placebo to 77 patients with Alzheimer's disease for 6 mo in a double-blind study. The 39 Ss in the treatment group had a mean age of 71.8 yrs; those in the control group (38 Ss) had a mean age of 74.6 yrs. Four Ss in the placebo group were dropped from the study. Org 2766 was tolerated well but no significant effect was found in terms of rating scales or cognitive functions. (17 ref).

1073. Sourander, Leif B.; Portin, Raija; Mölsä, Pekka; Lahdes, Anne et al. (1987). **Senile dementia of the Alzheimer type treated with aniracetam: A new nootropic agent.** *Psychopharmacology,* 91(1), 90–95.
44 patients with senile dementia of the Alzheimer type were randomly allocated into double-blind treatment with either 1 g aniracetam (RO 13-5057) or placebo daily for 3 mo. Neurological examinations were made before and after treatment, and psychometric tests were performed before and after 1 and 3 mo treatment. Treatment was interrupted due to occurrence of confusion in 4 cases in the aniracetam group and in 1 case in the placebo group. During treatment, an improvement was seen in several cognitive tests, especially those associated with memory, but this improvement occurred in the placebo as well. In clinical evaluation, no difference was seen in efficacy between the 2 treatment groups.

1074. Spar, James E. (1984). **Psychopharmacology of Alzheimer's disease.** *Psychiatric Annals,* 14(3), 186–189.
Inconclusive or negative results have generally been obtained with experimental agents for the treatment of Alzheimer's disease such as pentylenetetrazol, methylphenidate, and desferioxamine. Data from a study by the author and colleagues with 10 Alzheimer's patients also show no significant improvement on the WAIS and Mini-Mental State Examination as the result of naloxone (1 mg/kg, iv) treatment. However, conventional psychopharmacological agents such as tricyclic antidepressants, neuroleptics, and benzodiazepines can be used to control the complications of the basic disease process. (29 ref).

1075. Steele, Cynthia; Lucas, Mary J. & Tune, Larry. (1986). **Haloperidol versus thioridazine in the treatment of behavioral symptoms in senile dementia of the Alzheimer's type: Preliminary findings.** *Journal of Clinical Psychiatry,* 47(6), 310–312.
To compare the efficacy and side effects of haloperidol (HAL) and thioridazine (THZ) in the management of behavioral symptoms of senile dementia of the Alzheimer's type, 16 patients (mean age 76 yrs; duration of illness 2–9 yrs) were studied in an open crossover design study. Following 2-wk drug washout, Ss were assigned to either HAL (1, 2, and 5 mg/day for 2 wks) or THZ (25, 50, and 75 mg/day for 2 wks). Six Ss completed the crossover design, 1 received only HAL, and 9 received only THZ. Both drugs were effective in man-

aging target behaviors, including hostility, uncooperativeness, bothersomeness, emotional lability, and irritability. Complaints of fatigue and extrapyramidal side effects were greater with HAL than with THZ. Neither compound produced significant impairments in cognition as assessed by the Mini-Mental State Examination score or caused orthostatic hypertension.

1076. Steffes, Robert & Thralow, Joan. (1985). **Do uniform colors keep patients awake?** *Journal of Gerontological Nursing,* 11(7), 6–9.
Investigated the correlation between the color of nursing staff uniforms and the amount of nighttime disturbed behavior of patients housed in a closed ward for the cognitively impaired. 25 34–86 yr old males participated in the study. Ss' diagnoses included Alzheimer's Disease, cerebral vascular accidents, alcoholism, organic dementia, schizophrenia, and Huntington's chorea. During the 4-wk test period, the nursing staff wore dark brown or white uniforms at random. Prior to the study each S was evaluated to determine blindness, color blindness, depth perception, and general visual acuity. Results indicate that in Ss whose vision was unimpaired, nursing uniform color made no apparent difference. However, in older Ss with impaired vision and with a somewhat confused or agitated mental state, nurses in white uniforms took on a ghostlike appearance in semidarkened rooms. This gave rise to an increase in disturbed behavior just after nursing rounds were made. (5 ref).

1077. Steiger, William A. et al. (1985). **Effects of naloxone in treatment of senile dementia.** *Journal of the American Geriatrics Society,* 33(2), 155.
Reports on a randomized controlled clinical trial using a double-blind crossover design that assessed the efficacy of naloxone (10 mg/wk for 4 wks) in treating 16 patients with early to moderate stages of Alzheimer's disease. No positive effects on cognitive function were observed, based on caregivers' reports and scores on a cognitive rating scale. (2 ref).

1078. Summers, William K. (1987). **Fee-for-service research on THA: An explanation.** *New England Journal of Medicine,* 316(25), 1605–1606.
Discusses the present author and colleagues' (1986) fee-for-service research on the use of tetrahydroaminoacridine in treating senile dementia of the Alzheimer's type.

1079. Summers, William K.; Majovski, Lawrence V.; Marsh, Gary M.; Tachiki, Kenneth et al. (1987). **"Use of THA in treatment of Alzheimer-like dementia: Pilot study in twelve patients": Reply.** *New England Journal of Medicine,* 316(25), 1605.
Replies to comments by F. J. Pirozzolo et al (1987), N. Herrmann et al (1987), G. W. Small et al (1987), M. Kopelman (1987), and P. N. Tariot and E. D. Caine (1987) on the present authors' (1986) study of the use of oral tetrahydroaminoacridine in treating senile dementia of the Alzheimer's type.

1080. Summers, William K.; Majovski, Lawrence V.; Marsh, Gary M.; Tachiki, Kenneth et al. (1986). **Oral tetrahydroaminoacridine in long-term treatment of senile dementia, Alzheimer type.** *New England Journal of Medicine,* 315(20), 1241–1245.
Investigated the effects of oral tetrahydroaminoacridine (THA), using 17 patients (mean age 70.65 yrs) in the middle and late stages of suspected Alzheimer's disease. In Phase 1, 25–200 mg of THA was administered over a period of 7–10 days. Results show significant improvement compared with pretreatment status on global assessment. During Phase 2, the optimal drug dose and placebo were randomly assigned. Among the 14 Ss completing Phase 2, THA produced significantly better results than placebo on the global assessment and other tests. 12 Ss have entered Phase 3, which involves

long-term administration of oral THA. The average duration of treatment in these Ss at present is 12.6 mo; symptomatic improvements have occurred. It is suggested that THA may be temporarily useful in the long-term palliative treatment of Alzheimer's disease.

1081. Summers, William K.; Viesselman, John O.; Marsh, Gary M. & Candelora, Kent. (1981). **Use of THA in treatment of Alzheimer-like dementia: Pilot study in twelve patients.** *Biological Psychiatry,* 16(2), 145–153.
Administered the centrally acting anticholinesterase THA (1, 2,3,4 tetrahydro-5-aminoacridine; 0.25–1.5 mg/kg, iv) to 12 unselected cases (aged 42–85 yrs) of Alzheimer-like senile dementia. Significant improvement in memory testing occurred in 6 Ss; 9 improved in clinical staging. Analysis of results with respect to staging of dementia revealed that the degree of improvement was inversely related to the severity of dementia. (21 ref).

1082. Sunderland, Trey et al. (1985). **Scopolamine challenges in Alzheimer's disease.** *Psychopharmacology,* 87(2), 247–249.
Designed a challenge paradigm to test the functional sensitivity to anticholinergic agents in Alzheimer's disease. 10 patients (42–73 yrs old) with dementia of the Alzheimer type were serially administered 3 intravenous doses (0.1, 0.25, and 0.5 mg) of the centrally active anticholinergic drug scopolamine and placebo. Testing was carried out in a placebo-controlled, double-blind fashion to measure cognitive, physiologic, and behavioral changes. Cognitive testing assessed vigilance, new learning, and knowledge memory. Ss showed a marked, dose-related behavioral and cognitive sensitivity to temporary cholinergic blockade. It is suggested that scopolamine testing may serve as an index of the status of central cholinergic functional integrity, and may ultimately prove useful as a diagnostic or staging test in the evaluation of the cholinergic system in dementia. (13 ref).

1083. Sunderland, Trey; Tariot, Pierre N.; Cohen, Robert M.; Weingartner, Herbert et al. (1987). **Anticholinergic sensitivity in patients with dementia of the Alzheimer type and age-matched controls: A dose-response study.** *Archives of General Psychiatry,* 44(5), 418–426.
Tested dose–response relationships in 10 normal elderly controls (mean age 61.3 yrs) and 10 patients (mean age 58.8 yrs) with dementia of the Alzheimer type (DAT) to examine whether the sensitivity to central cholinergic blockade is primarily a function of age or due to the disease process itself. Following a series of baseline tests over 30 min, Ss received 1 of 3 scopolamine doses (0.1, 0.25, or 0.5 mg, intravenously) or placebo in a double-blind, pseudorandomized fashion. The dependent variables included a cognitive battery used to assess drug effects on vigilance, category retrieval, selective reminding, and continuous performance. Ss with DAT showed significant impairment in most cognitive tasks and behavioral measures at lower doses of scopolamine than the controls and relatively more impairment at higher doses.

1084. Sunderland, Trey; Tariot, Pierre N.; Weingartner, Herbert; Murphy, Dennis L. et al. (1986). **Pharmacologic modelling of Alzheimer's disease.** *Progress in Neuro-Psychopharmacology & Biological Psychiatry,* 10(3–5), 599–610.
Suggests that evidence of a central role for the cholinergic system in normal human memory function and disorders such as Alzheimer's disease (AD) has grown tremendously. Anticholinergic and noncholinergic agents have been found to create transient memory impairments in young adults that mimic the changes associated with normal aging or amnesia. The rationale for using scopolamine (a centrally active anticholinergic agent) as a pharmacologic probe of memory function is reviewed, using data from studies in animals and humans. The cognitive functioning of 10 normal elderly controls (aged 42–72 yrs) given scopolamine was compared to the baseline functioning of patients with Alzheimer's disease. The use of scopolamine as a modeling agent for dementia is discussed.

1085. Tariot, Pierre N. et al. (1986). **Naloxone and Alzheimer's disease: Cognitive and behavioral effects of a range of doses.** *Archives of General Psychiatry,* 43(8), 727–732.
12 42–72 yr old Ss with a clinical diagnosis of dementia of the Alzheimer type (DAT) participated in 3 test days (separated by at least 72 hrs) consisting of 2 sequential infusions (5 sec and 2 min, 60 min apart) of (a) placebo and placebo, (b) naloxone hydrochloride (NAL [5 µg/kg—test dose and 0.1 mg/kg—low dose]), and (c) NAL (5 µg/kg—test dose and 2 mg/kg—high dose). Both observer ratings and self-ratings of physical and psychological/behavioral signs and symptoms were obtained at intervals throughout the day. Cognitive assessment consisted of tasks previously shown to be sensitive to DAT or chosen for the potential for demonstrating improvement. Results show that neither low- nor high-dose NAL facilitated performance on measures of cognitive function. Behavioral changes after low-dose NAL therapy were noted: moderate restlessness, irritability, hostility, and mild drowsiness associated with moderate dysphoria. After the high dose, Ss experienced more persistent drowsiness associated with milder restlessness and irritability without hostility or dysphoria. (39 ref).

1086. Tariot, Pierre N.; Cohen, Robert M.; Sunderland, Trey; Newhouse, Paul A. et al. (1987). **l-Deprenyl in Alzheimer's disease: Preliminary evidence for behavioral change with monoamine oxidase B inhibition.** *Archives of General Psychiatry,* 44(5), 427–433.
Conducted a double-blind, placebo-controlled serial study of levodeprenyl (LDP) in dementia of the Alzheimer's type, using 17 hospitalized patients fulfilling Diagnostic and Statistical Manual of Mental Disorders (DSM-III) criteria for primary degenerative dementia and criteria for probable Alzheimer's disease. A 2nd group of 9 patients who did not receive medication was also studied. The medication Ss were administered LDP (10 mg/day for 21 days and 40 mg/day for 22 days). The lower dose of LDP resulted in significant changes in observer ratings of behavior in the 17 Ss. Significant and dose-dependent changes in the hemodynamic state as well as in neurotransmitter metabolites in the cerebrospinal fluid (CSF), consistent with monoamine oxidase inhibition, were also observed.

1087. Tariot, Pierre N. & Caine, Eric D. (1987). **"Use of THA in treatment of Alzheimer-like dementia: Pilot study in twelve patients": Comment.** *New England Journal of Medicine,* 316(25), 1604–1605.
Outlines unanswered questions resulting from a study by W. K. Summers et al (1986) on the use of oral tetrahydroaminoacridine in treating senile dementia of the Alzheimer's type.

1088. Tariot, Pierre N.; Sunderland, Trey; Murphy, Dennis L.; Cohen, Martin R. et al. (1986). **Design and interpretation of opiate antagonist trials in dementia.** *Progress in Neuro-Psychopharmacology & Biological Psychiatry,* 10(3–5), 611–626.
Outlines some possible rationales for the study of endogenous opiate systems in dementia of the Alzheimer type (DAT) and reviews pharmacologic and clinical considerations in the design and interpretation of a multidose naloxone trial in 12 Ss with DAT. These considerations include the nature and timing of observations made, as well as the importance of considering the differential effects of varying doses of naloxone. Naloxone had no clinical or cognitive benefits for Ss but did have behavioral effects that varied with dosage.

116

1089. Tariot, Pierre N.; Sunderland, Trey; Weingartner, Herbert; Murphy, D. L. et al. (1987). **Cognitive effects of l-deprenyl in Alzheimer's disease.** *Psychopharmacology,* 91(4), 489–495.
Studied the effects of levodeprenyl (LD), a monoamine oxidase (MAO) inhibitor, on several types of cognitive function in 17 patients (aged 42–72 yrs) with dementia of the Alzheimer type (DAT). Two doses of LD (10 and 40 mg/day) and placebo were compared in a double-blind, serial treatment design. Episodic learning and memory, knowledge memory, attention, recognition, and performance on a continuous performance task were assessed at baseline and under these drug and placebo conditions. Significant improvement was noted in performance on an episodic memory and learning task requiring complex information processing and sustained conscious effort during treatment with LD (10 mg/day). Knowledge memory, intrusions, and other cognitive functions relevant to DAT were not altered by LD at either dose.

1090. Tennant, Forest S. (1987). **Preliminary observations on naltrexone for treatment of Alzheimer's type dementia.** *Journal of the American Geriatrics Society,* 35(4), 369–370.
Reports preliminary results of the use of naltrexone (50 mg/day for 6 wks) with 9 50–84 yr olds who met criteria for probable senile dementia of the Alzheimer type (SDAT). Three were studied on a placebo-controlled, double-blind, crossover basis. Findings suggest that naltrexone may ameliorate symptoms of SDAT in some patients.

1091. Teri, Linda & Reifler, Burton V. (1986). **Sexual issues of patients with Alzheimer's disease.** Special Issue: The physician's guide to sexual counseling. *Medical Aspects of Human Sexuality,* 20, 86–91.
Discusses sexual functioning and problems of patients with Alzheimer's disease. Problems range from diminished interest in sex to inappropriate activity due to confusion. The patient's spouse faces problems in that the disease-related changes in the patient may impair the healthy spouse's enjoyment of or desire for sex; stress and fatigue generated by emotional trauma and pressures of daily activities may greatly reduce his/her motivation and energy for sexual activity; and feelings of loss, despair, grief, and depression cause further negative reactions and effects on sexuality. Management strategies, including medication, can help make the situation more tolerable.

1092. Thal, Leon J.; Masur, David M.; Sharpless, Nansie S.; Fuld, Paula A. et al. (1986). **Acute and chronic effects of oral physostigmine and lecithin in Alzheimer's disease.** *Progress in Neuro-Psychopharmacology & Biological Psychiatry,* 10(3–5), 627–636.
16 Alzheimer patients were treated with lecithin and gradually increasing doses (3–16 mg/day) of oral physostigmine. 10 Ss showed improvement in total recall, retrieval from long-term storage, and decrease in intrusions. During a replication study, all 10 Ss again responded. During long-term (4–20 mo) treatment of 5 Ss, most continued drug response initially but then lost responsiveness to physostigmine, and their dementia progressed. Physostigmine treatment appeared to improve memory with or without concomitant lecithin therapy. The degree of memory improvement correlated with increasing cerebrospinal fluid (CSF) cholinesterase inhibition.

1093. Thornton, Joe E.; Davies, Helen D. & Tinklenberg, Jared R. (1986). **Alzheimer's disease syndrome.** *Journal of Psychosocial Nursing & Mental Health Services,* 24(5), 16–22.
Suggests that effective treatment of Alzheimer's disease (AD) requires linkage of research, clinical service, and social support. Many of the symptoms associated with AD are treatable with either antipsychotic or anticholinergic medication or behavioral management. Instructions for caregivers (e.g., nurses) are presented, the neuropathology of AD is outlined,

and the impact of AD on family dynamics is discussed. AD support groups are also described.

1094. Toseland, Ronald W.; Derico, Anthony & Owen, Mary L. (1984). **Alzheimer's disease and related disorders: Assessment and intervention.** *Health & Social Work,* 9(3), 212–226.
Presents an overview of organic brain syndromes, describes effective assessment techniques, and discusses methods of intervention successful in providing support to both patients and caregivers. The case of a 76-yr-old female who became progressively confused is presented to illustrate applications of these techniques. Benefits associated with allowing social workers earlier interventions in these cases are discussed.

1095. Turkel, Henry & Nusbaum, Ilse. (1986). **Down syndrome and Alzheimer's disease contrasted.** *Journal of Orthomolecular Medicine,* 1(4), 219–229.
Discusses the association between Down's syndrome (DS) and Alzheimer's disease (AD), and describes orthomolecular treatment of DS patients with the Turkel U-series (H. Turkel). Reports in the lay and professional press have linked DS and AD because of comparable structural and chemical alterations of the brain and dermatoglyphic similarities. Several reports have stated that all adults with DS above the age of 35 yrs will develop AD. However, these predictions are not supported by an international, 3-yr study by J. B. Wyngaarden (1986) or by clinical observations at the Turkel Clinic for DS. The Turkel U-series of orthomolecular therapy for DS patients has proven to be effective in delaying or preventing the age-related decline in IQ scores and possibly in accelerating the myelination process, thereby reducing early onset of AD in DS patients.

1096. Turnbull, Ian M.; McGeer, P. L.; Beattie, L.; Calne, D. et al. (1985). **Stimulation of the basal nucleus of Meynert in senile dementia of Alzheimer's type: A preliminary report.** Ninth Meeting of the World Society for Stereotactic and Functional Neurosurgery (1985, Toronto, Canada). *Applied Neurophysiology,* 48(1–6), 216–221.
Tested the hypothesis that electrical stimulation of the basal nuclei would bring about clinical improvement and increase cortical glucose metabolic activity in senile dementia of Alzheimer's type (SDAT). An electrode was implanted into the left basal nucleus of a 74-yr-old man with SDAT. Repetitive cycles of stimulation for 9 mo had no definite effect on memory or cognition, but a follow-up positron emission tomography scan showed that cortical glucose metabolic activity was preserved in the ipsilateral temporal and parietal lobes while it declined elsewhere in the cortex.

1097. Verebey, Karl G. & Mulé, Salvatore J. (1986). **Naltrexone (Trexan): A review of hepatotoxicity issues.** Proceedings of the 47th Annual Scientific Meeting of the Committee on Problems of Drug Dependence: Problems of drug dependence, 1985 (1985, Baltimore, Maryland). *National Institute on Drug Abuse: Research Monograph Series,* 67, 73–81.
A literature review on studies that investigated the hepatotoxicity of naltrexone (NT) indicates that opiate agonists rather than antagonists are responsible for the elevation of hepatic enzymes. The literature is not clear whether the enzyme elevations after opiate agonists are the result of hepatocellular damage or temporary enzyme leakage into the circulation. Some studies indicate that tolerance develops to hepatic enzyme elevations following chronic treatment with opiate agonists. The major indictment of NT are studies on the obese and the elderly suffering from Alzheimer's disease. It is suggested that the alteration in hepatic enzymes in these abnormal models may be due to predisposition aggravated by an agonist metabolite of NT.

117

1098. Vitaliano, Peter P. et al. (1985). **The Ways of Coping Checklist: Revision and psychometric properties.** *Multivariate Behavioral Research,* 20(1), 3–26.
Examined the psychometric properties of the original 7 factored scales derived by C. Aldwin et al (1980) from S. Folkman and R. S. Lazarus's (1980) Ways of Coping Checklist (WCCL) vs a revised set of scales. Four psychometric properties were examined, including the reproducibility of the factor structure of the original scales, the internal consistency reliabilities and intercorrelations of the original and revised scales, the construct and concurrent validity of the scales, and their relationships to demographic factors. These properties were studied on 3 distressed samples: 83 psychiatric outpatients (mean age 32.5 yrs), 62 spouses (mean age 65.8 yrs) of patients with Alzheimer's disease, and 425 medical students (mean age 25.8 yrs) The revised scales were consistently more reliable and shared substantially less variance than the original scales across all samples. In terms of construct validity, depression was positively related to the revised Wishful Thinking scale and negatively related to the revised Problem-Focused scale consistently across samples. Anxiety was also related to these scales and was positively related to the Seeks Social Support scale across samples. The Mixed Scale was the only original scale that was consistently related to depression and anxiety across the 3 samples. Validity was indicated by the fact that medical students in group therapy had significantly higher original and revised scale scores than students not participating in such groups. Both sets of scales were generally free of demographic biases. (34 ref).

1099. Vitaliano, Peter P.; Maiuro, Roland D.; Russo, Joan & Becker, Joseph. (1987). **Raw versus relative scores in the assessment of coping strategies.** *Journal of Behavioral Medicine,* 10(1), 1–18.
Compared 2 approaches to the analysis and interpretation of coping efforts, using 145 psychiatric outpatients (mean age 32.5 yrs), 66 spouses of patients with senile dementia of the Alzheimer's type (mean age 65.8 yrs), and 185 1st- and 2nd-yr medical students (mean age 25.8 yrs). Raw scores (frequency of efforts) vs relative scores (percentage of efforts) were compared. It was hypothesized that, conditional on the source of and appraisal of a stressor, problem-focused coping should be inversely related and wishful thinking should be positively related to depression when relative scores were used, but raw problem-focused scores would be less clearly related to depression in such a way. Given the maladaptive status of the psychiatric outpatients, it was hypothesized that they would report more emotion-focused strategies and less problem-focused coping than the nonclinical samples and that these differences would be better observed using relative rather than raw scores. The hypotheses were generally supported.

1100. Volicer, Ladislav. (1986). **Need for hospice approach to treatment of patients with advanced progressive dementia.** *Journal of the American Geriatrics Society,* 34(9), 655–658.
Discusses cases of "mercy killing" in which the victim had progressive dementia of the Alzheimer type and argues that most cases of mercy killing are due to inappropriate use of medical technology and lack of consensus concerning ethical and legal acceptability of limited medical care for patients in a vegetative state or with advanced dementia. Issues with regard to life-shortening decisions during a terminal illness, misuse of medical technology, passive euthanasia, and court decisions having to do with discontinuation of treatment with terminal patients are discussed. Finally, it is contended that all decisions to limit treatment should take place before an emergency occurs.

1101. Vroulis, George et al. (1982). **Reduction of cholesterol risk factors by lecithin in patients with Alzheimer's disease.** *American Journal of Psychiatry,* 139(12), 1633–1634.

10 patients (aged 50–76 yrs) with Alzheimer's dementia had significantly lower cholesterol risk ratios after 2–3 mo of treatment with lecithin (53% phosphatidylcholine). No significant effect of lecithin on learning and memory was noted. (10 ref).

1102. Wald, Judith. (1984). **The graphic representation of regression in an Alzheimer's disease patient.** *Arts in Psychotherapy,* 11(3), 165–175.
Presents the case of a 58-yr-old woman who had been diagnosed as having Alzheimer-type dementia and had received treatment for 2 yrs in a neurological day treatment program. Through the S's artwork, her severe regression and intrapsychic reactions to the degenerative effects of this neuropathological disease, which usually causes death within 5 yrs of diagnosis, were followed. (9 ref).

1103. Wald, Judith. (1983). **Alzheimer's disease and the role of art therapy in its treatment.** *American Journal of Art Therapy,* 22(2), 57–64.
Discusses the course of Alzheimer's disease, the use of art expressions in diagnosing and evaluating dementia, and the value of art therapy in treatment. Art therapy is a process of physical and emotional involvement on the part of the patient and provides a tangible product in which the patient can take pride. Precautions related to the functional deficits of Alzheimer's patients are noted, and examples of therapy sessions are presented. (4 ref).

1104. Walsh, Arthur C. (1987). **Treatment of senile dementia of Alzheimer type by a psychiatric-anticoagulant regimen.** *Journal of Orthomolecular Medicine,* 2(3), 188–190.
Suggests that many patients diagnosed as having senile dementia of the Alzheimer type also have a circulatory deficiency of the brain, which can be improved by adding anticoagulant therapy to the standard psychiatric treatment. This is illustrated by the case history of a 56-yr-old male patient.

1105. Weaverdyck, Shelly E. (1987). **A cognitive intervention protocol for dementia: Its derivation from and application to a neuropsychological case study of Alzheimer's disease.** *Dissertation Abstracts International,* 48(2-B), 576.

1106. Weiss, Brian L. (1987). **Failure of nalmefene and estrogen to improve memory in Alzheimer's disease.** *American Journal of Psychiatry,* 144(3), 386–387.
Reports a study in which estradiol and nalmefene failed to enhance memory in 4 postmenopausal women with moderate dementia of the Alzheimer type. A reversible deterioration occurred in 1 of the 4 Ss.

1107. Welden, Sherman. (1986). **Behavioral and contextual interventions for Deficit-Type I and Type II Dementias (Alzheimer's Disease).** *Clinical Gerontologist,* 6(1), 35–43.
Contends that there are 2 distinct populations subsumed under the diagnosis Alzheimer's disease, referred to here as Deficit I and II dementias. Deficit I dementias respond to an environmental design in which interventions are physiological. Deficit II populations respond to an environment of simpler and more meaningful constituents, lowering the level of present stimulation to allow the environment to become more in keeping with earlier and familiar levels of controllable functioning. Examples of 3 Alzheimer patients are given to illustrate the 2 different types of dementias and the interventions used.

1108. Welden, Sherman & Yesavage, Jerome A. (1982). **Behavioral improvement with relaxation training in senile dementia.** *Clinical Gerontologist,* 1(1), 45–49.

Investigated the effectiveness of intensive relaxation training in 48 52–93 yr old White inpatients with diagnoses of senile dementia of the Alzheimer's type or multi-infarct dementia. Results indicate that relaxation training may be an effective aid in the management of behavioral problems in demented elderly patients. (16 ref).

1109. Wesnes, Keith; Simpson, Pauline M. & Kidd, Alexander. (1987). **The use of a scopolamine model to study the nootropic effects of tenilsetam (CAS 997) in man.** *Medical Science Research: Psychology & Psychiatry,* 15(17–20), 1063–1064.
Tested cognitive function in 18 male undergraduates administered tenilsetam after receiving scopolamine hydrobromide or saline. Subjective mood rating scales were completed, as was an automated cognitive test battery (e.g., tasks on verbal recall, verbal recognition, choice reaction, logical reasoning). Tenilsetam improved cognitive performance both under normal conditions and in antagonism to mental deficiencies induced by scopolamine, suggesting that the drug may prove useful in treating age-associated cognitive declines, including those associated with Alzheimer's disease.

1110. Whitford, G. Mervyn. (1986). **Alzheimer's disease and serotonin: A review.** *Neuropsychobiology,* 15(3–4), 133–142.
Reviews data from postmortem brain, cerebrospinal fluid (CSF), and 5-hydroxytryptamine (5-HT) synapse and platelet uptake studies indicating serious impairment of the serotonergic system in patients with Alzheimer's disease (AD). The link between decreased levels of the 5-HT metabolite, 5-hydroxyindoleacetic acid and aggressive behavior—which may further complicate management of AD patients—is discussed. It is noted that results of treatment with levotryptophan, aimed at influencing the 5-HT deficit, have proved generally disappointing. Present intensive research indicates that no single form of chemotherapy is likely to be effective in treating AD. Thus, a multitherapy approach to treatment of the many neurotransmitter abnormalities involved is likely.

1111. Wiancko, Donna C.; Crinklaw, Linda D. & Mora, Cathy D. (1986). **Nurses can learn from wives of impaired spouses.** *Journal of Gerontological Nursing,* 12(11), 28–33.
Describes issues raised in a 7-wk support group for wives of institutionalized men with either Alzheimer's disease or dementia and chronic physical disease. Discussion themes included the universality or uniqueness of experiences, patient advocacy, visiting, communication with health-care providers, and patient care issues. It is concluded that such discussions offer much value for nursing practice, especially awareness of issues the family encounters in having an institutionalized, cognitively impaired member.

1112. Wilson, Catherine A. (1986). **Society for Drug Research Symposium: Senile dementia of the Alzheimer type.** Society for Drug Research Symposium: Senile dementia of the Alzheimer type (1985, London, England). *Neurobiology of Aging,* 7(3), 219–222.
Reviews recent studies concerned with senile dementia of the Alzheimer type (SDAT). Studies considered include those investigating anatomical and biochemical changes in Alzheimer's disease and clinical symptoms and treatment. It is suggested that current treatment is solely symptomatic and rarely distinguishes between the types of dementias. Current pharmacological research into possible treatments for SDAT appears mainly to be concentrating on overcoming the deficits in the cholinergic system, and much work has been done on the effect of cholinergic agents on cognitive and behavioral activity.

1113. Winogrond, Iris R.; Fisk, Albert A.; Kirsling, Robert A. & Keyes, Barbara. (1987). **The relationship of caregiver burden and morale to Alzheimer's disease patient function in therapeutic setting.** *Gerontologist,* 27(3), 336–339.
Examined caregiver stress and Alzheimer's disease patient function at the time of initial entry in a day hospital program and again at 6 mo, using 18 patients (aged 59–84 yrs) and 18 caregivers (9 spouses, 5 children, 3 siblings, and a friend). Results show a significant decline in patient cognitive function with no increase in behavior problems. Significant changes also occurred over time in the relationship between patients' functioning and caregivers' perceptions of stress, suggesting an improvement in coping. Findings indicate that a therapeutic program for patients and their caregivers may slow behavior deterioration in patients and promote enhanced coping in caregivers.

1114. Winslade, William J.; Lyon, Martha A.; Levine, Martin L. & Mills, Mark J. (1984). **Making medical decisions for the Alzheimer's patient: Paternalism and advocacy.** *Psychiatric Annals,* 14(3), 206–208.
Discusses decision procedures that the clinician should consider in attempting to serve the interests and to protect the rights of patients with Alzheimer's disease. The importance of accurate diagnosis and consideration of the capacities and limitations of the particular patient are stressed. Five decision procedures are outlined that rely on medical authority, family decision makers, court order, patient advocates, and durable power of attorney. (4 ref).

1115. Wolkowitz, Owen M.; Tinklenberg, Jared R. & Weingartner, Herbert. (1985). **A psychopharmacological perspective of cognitive functions: II. Specific pharmacologic agents.** *Neuropsychobiology,* 14(3), 133–156.
Reviews human and animal studies on the effects of specific drugs and neurotransmitter systems on cognitive functions. Drug treatments considered include acetylcholine, catecholamines, benzodiazepines, gamma-aminobutyric acid (GABA), serotonin, stimulants, vasodilators, vasopressin, oxytocin, adrenocorticotropic hormone, corticosteroids, and opioids. The effects of each drug are considered with respect to memory, arousal, attention, and sensory thresholds. Implications for the treatment of disorders such as senile dementia of the Alzheimer type, depression, amnesia, and Cushing's syndrome are noted. A taxonomy of the pharmacology of memory is presented that highlights the value of viewing memory as consisting of several differentiated processes. (7 p ref).

1116. Yarbrough, George G. & Pomara, Nunzio. (1985). **The therapeutic potential of thyrotropin releasing hormone (TRH) in Alzheimer's disease (AD).** *Progress in Neuro-Psychopharmacology & Biological Psychiatry,* 9(3), 285–289.
Reviews the literature on the use of TRH in the management of Alzheimer's patients. Topics considered include the dysfunction of cholinergic systems in AD, principles of cholinergic treatment strategies, and the pharmacotherapeutic effects of TRH in AD and in amyotrophic lateral sclerosis. It is suggested that while limited success with the TRH strategy has been achieved to date, the evidence does document unique facilitative interactions of this peptide with cholinergic neurons. (31 ref).

1117. Zachary, Ruth A. (1984). **Day care within an institution.** *Physical & Occupational Therapy in Geriatrics,* 3(4), 61–67.
Discusses the purposes of day-care for Alzheimer's patients and describes a program conducted in an institutional setting. Separating Alzheimer's residents and others with similar characteristics is a key to success, as is keeping families informed. Specific examples of activities (e.g., arts and crafts, dancing, remotivation, sensory stimulation, and word games) are included.

TREATMENT & COUNSELING

Family Relations & Caregiving

1118. Albert, Marilyn S. (1984). **Dementia and family dynamics: Discussion.** Scientific meeting of the Boston Society for Gerontologic Psychiatry: Family issues in geriatric psychiatry (1983, Boston, Massachusetts). *Journal of Geriatric Psychiatry,* 17(1), 57–60.
Responds to the paper by G. Niederehe and E. Frugé (1984), which reviewed clinical research on the family dynamics involved in tending to a family member with dementia (Alzheimer's disease). The present author elaborates on an issue briefly discussed in the paper: the degree to which professional intervention can or should be involved in studying the families of demented patients and the degree to which the absence of intervention may produce misleading conclusions. It is noted that families often misunderstand the psychiatric changes associated with the disease. It is not uncommon for family members to look for an environmental cause for depressive symptomatology.

1119. Aronson, Miriam K.; Levin, Gilbert & Lipkowitz, Rochelle. (1984). **A community-based family/patient group program for Alzheimer's disease.** *Gerontologist,* 24(4), 339–342.
Describes an Alzheimer's family/patient group program that consists of simultaneous family and patient groups meeting for 1.5 hrs/wk at a gerontology center. Members are outpatients with dementia and their primary caregivers. The family group helps members cope with declining family organization, provides a support network, and encourages the expressing of feelings, learning new activities, and making decisions and new adaptations. The patient group provides activities for socialization at an appropriate functional level. Although services are provided free, the approximate cost is $1,500/patient/year. (9 ref).

1120. Bråne, Görel. (1986). **Normal aging and dementia disorders: Coping and crisis in the family.** *Progress in Neuro-Psychopharmacology & Biological Psychiatry,* 10(3–5), 287–295.
Interviewed the relatives of 28 Alzheimer's disease (AD)/senile dementia of Alzheimer type (SDAT) patients (aged 43–75 yrs) admitted to a geropsychiatric ward and the relatives of 28 AD/SDAT patients (aged 65–88 yrs) cared for in long-stay wards. 26 individuals (aged 85 yrs or older) who lived at home served as a control group and were interviewed about formal and informal help, and their mental functions were rated. It is concluded that the very old individuals, even those who were very healthy, needed much support. All families of patients with dementia disorders needed support to some degree, including either group therapy or individual psychotherapy. It is suggested that adequate formal help from society and psychological support to the primary caregivers probably delays institutionalization.

1121. Brink, T. L. (1983). **Paranoia in Alzheimer's patients: Prevalence and impact on caretakers.** *International Journal of Behavioral Geriatrics,* 1(4), 53–55.
Studied the incidence of paranoia, uncooperativeness, and verbal abusiveness in Alzheimer's patients, as reported by their caretaking family members ($N = 39$), and measured the level of depression in the caretakers. Results show that 38% of the patients were described as frequently paranoid, 36% as frequently uncooperative, and 13% as frequently verbally abusive. Although the average depression score for the caretakers was in the mildly depressed range, the range of scores was quite large and there was no correlation between caretaker depression and the patient's behavior: paranoid, uncooperative, or verbally abusive. (7 ref).

1122. Chenoweth, Barbara & Spencer, Beth. (1986). **Dementia: The experience of family caregivers.** *Gerontologist,* 26(3), 267–272.
Surveyed 289 caregivers of family members with dementia of the Alzheimer's type for their experiences with early symptoms, obtaining a diagnosis, home care, and institutionalization. Over half were spouses, and half were aged 50–70 yrs. Results show that at each stage in the process of providing care there were new and different stresses that could be ameliorated by appropriate professional assistance.

1123. Cole, Laura; Griffin, Karla & Ruiz, Barbara. (1986). **A comprehensive approach to working with families of Alzheimer's patients.** Special Issue: Social work and Alzheimer's disease: Practice issues with victims and their families. *Journal of Gerontological Social Work,* 9(2), 27–39.
Suggests that families who care for patients with Alzheimer's disease face severe psychosocial problems. A comprehensive approach for social work practice with such families is presented. The use of both clinical and social interventions is recommended to assist families in managing daily activities, alleviating stress, planning for long-term care, and coping with the emotional sequelae of the disease. Information-giving, teaching, and advocacy are stressed as a way of providing families with the tools they need to cope with the problems of caring for someone with a chronic, degenerative condition. A case study is presented of a 65-yr-old woman whose 68-yr-old husband has Alzheimer's disease and whose social worker recommends clinical, social and family supports to alleviate the S's stresses related to caring for her husband. (6 ref).

1124. Colerick, Elizabeth J. & George, Linda K. (1986). **Predictors of institutionalization among caregivers of patients with Alzheimer's disease.** *Journal of the American Geriatrics Society,* 34(7), 493–498.
Examined why some families continue to shoulder the burden of care for a relative with Alzheimer's disease, often beyond healthful limits, while others relinquish care to professionals. 209 caregivers of Alzheimer's patients were surveyed in 1983 and again 1 yr later. Four dimensions of caregiver well-being were assessed: physical health, mental health, participation in social and recreational activities, and perceived economic status. Using logistic regression techniques, caregiver characteristics and caregiver well-being, rather than patient characteristics, emerged as important predictors of placement decisions. Results suggest that practitioners, in evaluating the family's need for institutionalization, must move beyond duration of illness and current cognitive functioning to aspects of the caregiver support system.

1125. Coppel, David B.; Burton, Catherine; Becker, Joseph & Fiore, Joan. (1985). **Relationships of cognitions associated with coping reactions to depression in spousal caregivers of Alzheimer's disease patients.** *Cognitive Therapy & Research,* 9(3), 253–266.
Examined (1) attributions (globality and stability) related to the reformulated learned-helplessness model of depression by L. Y. Abramson et al (1978) and the attributes, self-evaluations, and expectancies concerning coping reactions (degree of upset, success, satisfaction, control in future, future coping success) postulated by C. B. Wortman and L. Dintzer (1978) for their respective relations to severity and prevalence of diagnosable depression in spouse caregivers of Alzheimer's disease (AD) patients. Attribution-related cognitions of 68 37–85 yr old spouses of 21 institutionalized and 47 at-home patients were obtained. An unpredictable upsetting behavior by the AD patient and significant life change experienced by the caregiver as a result of spouse's AD provided the situational contexts for semi-structured interview. Results indicate that only globality was related to depression related to the AD patient's unpredictable behavior; both globality and stability were related to depression for S's life-change situation. The pattern of the other depressogenic coping cognitions was also different for the 2 contexts: While ratings of upset and lack of current and future control were related to depression related to the AD patient's behavior, ratings of

poor current and future coping, lack of coping success, and coping dissatisfaction were related to depression resulting from S's life-change context. (19 ref).

1126. Creasey, Gary L. (1988). **Alzheimer's disease: Effects on child and family life.** *Dissertation Abstracts International,* 48(8-B), 2474.

1127. Cutler, Loraine. (1985). **Counseling caregivers.** *Generations,* 10(1), 53–57.
Reviews the problems and stresses faced by caregivers and discusses the counseling of caregivers. Assessment and treatment planning, education, support, family role, and intrapsychic issues are addressed using case studies.

1128. Davies, Helen; Priddy, J. Michael & Tinklenberg, Jared R. (1986). **Support groups for male caregivers of Alzheimer's patients.** *Clinical Gerontologist,* 5(3–4), 385–395.
Describes a pilot intervention for male caregivers that consisted of short-term support groups. Recruitment, format, and group cohesion are discussed. Some of the themes emerging in the group were caregiver pride, the decision for institutionalization, and needs for validation, information, networks, and physical care.

1129. Dundon, Margaret M. (1987). **Distress and coping among caregivers of victims of Alzheimer's disease and related disorders.** *Dissertation Abstracts International,* 48(2-A), 339.

1130. Dunkle, Ruth E. & Nevin, Michael. (1987). **Stress of the caregiver: Effective management of dementia patients in hospital and community settings.** *Journal of Sociology & Social Welfare,* 14(1), 73–84.
Explored management problems among elders with dementia and their medical and family caregivers. 25 patients (mean age 78 yrs) with Alzheimer's type dementia, multi-infarct dementia, simple dementia, or organic brain syndrome were interviewed, as were professional health care personnel and family members. Findings indicate that professional assessment facilitates home caregiving but had little bearing on successful coping by the caregiver. Variability of coping was related to the strategy employed.

1131. Fabisewski, Kathy J. & Howell, Mary C. (1986). **A model for family meetings in the long term care of Alzheimer's Disease.** Special Issue: Social work and Alzheimer's disease: Practice issues with victims and their families. *Journal of Gerontological Social Work,* 9(2), 113–117.
Describes a model for routine, periodic family conferences for families of Alzheimer's disease patients. The conferences, which include the long-term care multidisciplinary treatment team, promote assessment of family structure and needs, teach about the course of the disease as well as possible causes and the probable prognosis, and provide assistance in the process of making decisions about modes of care. Families participate in the planning and provision of treatment regimens and are assisted in developing guidelines for medical intervention in the event of life-threatening illness. Family members are encouraged to recognize and name their feelings of grief, anticipatory mourning, anger, and sadness. It is suggested that this model facilitates the establishment of trust between family members and the treatment team and assists the treatment team in understanding and meeting the needs of the family. (5 ref).

1132. Famighetti, Robert A. (1986). **Understanding the family coping with Alzheimer's disease: An application of theory to intervention.** *Clinical Gerontologist,* 5(3–4), 363–384.
Discusses the crisis families face with progressive mental deterioration of a member in terms of a multiple-crisis syndrome and H. McCubbin and J. M. Patterson's (unpublished paper) Double ABC-X crisis model and family development theory. It is suggested that families, like individuals, go through stages, adjusting to both epigenetic needs and unan-

ticipated crises. How the crisis affects the family depends on the crisis, how the family sees it, and what the family does about it. Family coping in phases—precrisis, diagnosis, exhaustion, consolidation, adjustment—is charted.

1133. Fiore, Joan; Becker, Joseph & Coppel, David B. (1983). **Social network interactions: A buffer or a stress.** *American Journal of Community Psychology,* 11(4), 423–439.
44 45–85 yr old caregivers of spouses with a diagnosis of Alzheimer's disease provided a stressed population considered at high risk for depression. Unlike more typical unidirectional measures of perceived social support quality, ratings were elicited separately as to how helpful as well as how upsetting each network member was in 5 support categories. Correlations between perceived network "upset" and depression (Beck Depression Inventory) were highly significant, while in no case did perceived "helpfulness" relate to depression. Stepwise multiple regression analyses revealed that the set of 5 support category upset ratings predicted depression better than did helpful/upset ratios, which in turn predicted depression better than the helpfulness ratings as a group. Implications for the conceptualization of social support and its measurement are discussed. (51 ref).

1134. Fiore, Joan; Coppel, David B.; Becker, Joseph & Cox, Gary B. (1986). **Social support as a multifaceted concept: Examination of important dimensions for adjustment.** *American Journal of Community Psychology,* 14(1), 93–111.
Investigated the relationship between 4 operationalizations of the social support concept network (contact frequency; satisfaction with support, including 9 dimensions; perceived availability of support; and use of support), 2 measures of psychological adjustment, and 1 measure of physical adjustment. Ss were 68 45–85 yr old, highly stressed caregivers to spouses with Alzheimer's disease. Results indicate that of the operationalizations, satisfaction with support was the only significant predictor of depression and general psychopathology. The set of 4 support variables showed the strongest relationship to depression level, next strongest to general psychopathology, and least to physical health. (51 ref).

1135. George, Linda K. & Gwyther, Lisa P. (1986). **Caregiver well-being: A multidimensional examination of family caregivers of demented adults.** *Gerontologist,* 26(3), 253–259.
Examined the well-being of 510 family caregivers of older memory-impaired adults in 4 dimensions (physical health, mental health, financial resources, and social participation). Most of the Ss were middle-aged or older. Results indicate that, relative to random community samples, caregivers were most likely to experience problems with mental health and social participation. Characteristics of the caregiving situation were more closely associated with caregiver well-being than were illness characteristics of the patients.

1136. Glosser, Guila & Wexler, Debra. (1985). **Participants' evaluation of educational/support groups for families of patients with Alzheimer's disease and other dementias.** *Gerontologist,* 25(3), 232–236.
Examined the effectiveness of educational/support groups for relatives of patients with Alzheimer's disease and other dementias. 54 participants of 7 8-wk educational/support groups evaluated the helpfulness of various aspects of their group experience. Evaluations were generally very positive. The supportive aspects of the group and the information provided about medical and behavioral management of the patient were most highly rated. Resolution of intrafamilial conflict and information pertaining to specific legal, financial, and social problems were evaluated as somewhat less helpful. It is suggested that these problems may require more individualized interventions. Findings also indicate the limitations of a formal group as the sole support for isolated family caregivers and imply that interventions in the natural social network of

caregivers are important adjuncts to educational/support groups. Difficulties related to the termination of the program are considered. (13 ref).

1137. Gwyther, Lisa P. & Matteson, Mary A. (1983). **Care for the caregivers.** *Journal of Gerontological Nursing*, 9(2), 92–95, 110.
The Alzheimer's disease patient and family caregivers need sustained, long-term, comprehensive, appropriate, and acceptive services during the specific stages of the illness. Nurses and social workers should be available to provide continuity or a "superstructure" for the caregiver throughout the illness and bereavement. Professional and self-help groups can supplement and complement one another in providing this continuity and superstructure. This is a therapeutic and preventive activity that can positively affect the long-term care needs of a rapidly growing segment of the population. (10 ref).

1138. Haley, William E.; Brown, S. Lane & Levine, Ellen G. (1987). **Experimental evaluation of the effectiveness of group intervention for dementia caregivers.** *Gerontologist*, 27(3), 376–382.
Tested the hypothesis that support-group participation by caregivers of elderly dementia patients would lead to decreased depression, increased life satisfaction, and increased social activity. 54 family caregivers assigned to 1 of 2 types of support groups completed pregroup, postgroup, and follow-up assessments. A waiting list condition was also used. Ss completed the Beck Depression Inventory, interview assessments of their impaired relatives' degree of disability, measures of any changes in caregiver coping responses, and a follow-up questionnaire indicating their satisfaction with the groups. Results indicate that although caregivers rated the groups as quite helpful, group participation did not lead to improvements on measures of depression, life satisfaction, social support, or coping variables. Methodological issues in assessing the efficacy of caregiver groups are discussed.

1139. Hemshorn, Agnes. (1985). **They call it Alzheimer's disease.** *Journal of Gerontological Nursing*, 11(1), 36–38.
Presents the experiences of a spouse whose husband developed an inability to follow conversations, restlessness, insecurity, and inappropriate behavior that was diagnosed after a brain scan as a type of Alzheimer's disease. When she could no longer care for him at home, he was placed in a nursing home. After 9 mo of difficulty, he became more subdued. The difficulties in adjustment for both husband and wife are discussed.

1140. Henderson, Dana H. (1986). **Presentation of information via video tape to increase knowledge and reduce stress in family caretakers of Alzheimer patients.** *Dissertation Abstracts International*, 47(5-B), 2139.

1141. Hepburn, Kenneth & Wasow, Mona. (1986). **Support groups for family caregivers of dementia victims: Questions, directions, and future research.** *New Directions for Mental Health Services*, 29, 83–92.
Discusses the concept and goals of support groups in general and some models of groups for the caregivers of Alzheimer's and dementia patients. Four existing models of group leadership are identified, along with 4 major foci of the groups. The former include professionally led groups, peer-led groups, professional/peer coleader groups, and leaderless groups; the latter include education, support, and provision of a safe place for venting feelings and ideas. Three alternative models are outlined: one based on the Alcoholics Anonymous program, another revolving around recreational activities, and a seminar model allowing discussion of current knowledge of a given disorder. Concerns in the establishment and conduct of support groups are considered (e.g., sexuality, preparation for

the death of the patient, divorce, the right to death). Public policy and research issues are also addressed. (9 ref).

1142. Humphry, Derek. (1986). **Mercy denied to Roswell Gilbert.** *Euthanasia Review*, 1(1), 13–19.
Discusses the controversy precipitated by the 25-yr prison sentence with no parole received by a 76-yr-old man, Roswell Gilbert, for shooting his wife who was suffering from Alzheimer's disease. Details of the case are described. Questions regarding the resources spent on the sick and elderly and the timeliness of lawful voluntary euthanasia are raised.

1143. Jenkins, Terry S. (1983). **Alzheimer's Disease: Perceptions of stress burden, social support, and help orientation.** *Dissertation Abstracts International*, 44(5-B), 1617.

1144. Jenkins, Terry S.; Parham, Iris A. & Jenkins, Larry R. (1985). **Alzheimer's disease: Caregivers' perceptions of burden.** Special Issue: Aging and mental health. *Journal of Applied Gerontology*, 4(2), 40–57.
Examined factors contributing to the burden of 120 primary caregivers (aged 25–87 yrs) of Alzheimer's disease patients. The relationship between burden and other relevant variables including stress responses, help orientation, social support, and predisease caregiver–patient relationship was assessed. Analyses indicate that burden was uncorrelated overall with level of dementia. However, there were significant differences in level of burden reported by Ss caring for patients in varying stages of the disease. While burden was negatively correlated with the predisease caregiver–patient relationship, burden was positively correlated with stress response and support-group impact. Level of dementia, burden, and support group attendance exhibited significant increases at a retest 9 mo later, and caregivers reported a decrease in help beliefs consistent with the medical model. (45 ref).

1145. Kahan, Jason; Kemp, Bryan; Staples, Fred R. & Brummel-Smith, Kenneth. (1985). **Decreasing the burden in families caring for a relative with a dementing illness: A controlled study.** *Journal of the American Geriatrics Society*, 33(10), 664–670.
Investigated the efficacy of a specifically designed group support program for relatives of patients with Alzheimer's disease and related disorders. The group program included educational/supportive activities and used basic principles of the cognitive-behavioral approach. 22 Ss participated in an 8-session program, while 18 control Ss received no treatment. Ss were 16–77 yrs old. Measures of family burden, levels of depression, and knowledge of dementia were obtained. Results indicate that group program Ss showed a significant decrease in total family burden, whereas control Ss showed a significant increase. Experimental Ss also showed reduction in depression levels and demonstrated a significantly greater improvement than control Ss on knowledge of dementia. Findings suggest that a relatively short but intensive support experience can have a positive effect in reducing some of the burden and depression associated with the care of a demented relative. (22 ref).

1146. Kahan, Jason S. (1984). **The effects of a group support program on decreasing feelings of burden and depression in relatives of patients with Alzheimer's disease and other dementing illnesses.** *Dissertation Abstracts International*, 45(3-A), 963–964.

1147. Kiecolt-Glaser, Janice K.; Glaser, Ronald; Shuttleworth, Edwin C.; Dyer, Carol S. et al. (1987). **Chronic stress and immunity in family caregivers of Alzheimer's disease victims.** *Psychosomatic Medicine*, 49(5), 523–535.
34 family caregivers of Alzheimer's disease (AD) patients were more distressed than 34 comparison Ss without similar responsibilities. Greater impairment in the AD victim was associated with greater distress and loneliness in caregivers. Caregivers had significantly lower percentages of total T lym-

phocytes and helper T lymphocytes than did comparison Ss, as well as significantly lower helper–suppressor cell ratios; caregivers also had significantly higher antibody titers to Epstein-Barr virus than did comparison Ss. Finally, caregivers showed greater depression, lower life satisfaction, and fewer social contacts than controls.

1148. LaBarge, Emily. (1981). **Counseling patients with senile dementia of the Alzheimer type and their families.** *Personnel & Guidance Journal,* 60(3), 139–143.
In senile dementia of the Alzheimer type, there is an overabundance of plaques and neurofibrillary tangles of the cortex; that is, the structure of the brain cells is altered and cognitive functioning is impaired. The author discusses counseling patterns for treatment and the stresses encountered by the family. It is suggested that educated family members can help alleviate stress for the patient, provide a structured milieu, and monitor changes in the patient's activities so care can be properly maintained. (25 ref).

1149. Lundervold, Duane & Lewin, Lewis M. (1987). **Effects of in-home respite care on caregivers of family members with Alzheimer's disease.** *Journal of Clinical & Experimental Gerontology,* 9(3), 201–214.
Investigated the effects of short-term, in-home respite care on 3 caregivers of family members with Alzheimer's disease, and an additional caregiver who served as a no-treatment control. The effects of 4–6 hrs of respite care each week on measures of caregiver health, depression, stress, and burden were evaluated over a period of up to 6 mo. Results indicate that the respite care did not result in clinically significant changes in depression, stress, or burden compared with no-respite conditions. Perceived health improved somewhat with the implementation of respite services. Measures of social support indicated no change in the frequency, type, or persons providing support.

1150. Mayhew, Patricia A. (1986). **The coping process in family-member caregivers of patients with Alzheimer's disease and related disorders.** *Dissertation Abstracts International,* 47(5-B), 1930.

1151. McNew, Judith A. (1987). **Alzheimer's Disease: Conceptualizing caregiver competence and practice implications.** *Journal of Applied Social Sciences,* 11(2), 167–190.
Contends that Alzheimer's disease (AD) has been identified as a major problem, not only for the patient, but for the primary caregiver as well. In attempting to develop a theoretical understanding of the impact of AD on caregivers, 3 major components emerged as contributing to caregiver competence: (1) A transactional component, environmental support, explains how competence is affected by the ability to enhance and adapt to environments; (2) a personal capacity component, interpersonal effectiveness, explains how interpersonal relationships affect competence; and (3) a cognitive component, perceived personal control, directs attention to how individual perceptions affect competence. Based on this conceptualization, suggestions for practice with the AD caregiver are presented.

1152. Miller, Baila. (1987). **Gender and control among spouses of the cognitively impaired: A research note.** *Gerontologist,* 27(4), 447–453.
Explored perceptions of caring for cognitively impaired spouses in interviews of 15 elderly spouses. Male and female spouses differed in the way they perceived dimensions of control as reflected in interpretation of the disease process, assumption of authority, control over the environment, and use of social support. Case examples are presented of elderly male and female spouses caring for mates with dementia and Alzheimer's disease, respectively. Findings suggest a high reliance on previous patterns of sex-role behavior. It is noted that the women stressed nurturance and relationship, whereas the men focused on authority and taking charge.

1153. Mobily, Kenneth E. & Hoeft, Thea M. (1985). **The family's dilemma: Alzheimer's disease.** *Activities, Adaptation & Aging,* 6(4), 63–71.
Notes that researchers have found increasing evidence to support the contention that Alzheimer's disease is the single leading cause of dementia in the elderly, although onset can occur at younger ages. Principles for enhancing the quality of life for the client and caregiver alike through leisure activities are presented. Such activities should make use of intact sensory channels as far as possible; they should also aim at maximizing the quality of life without impairing stability. Recreation should be a medium through which a family and client can facilitate positive affective experiences, communication, and successful utilization of remaining abilities. It is concluded that, by simplifying activities employing regular physical activity and using leisure counseling techniques, the practitioner can improve the lot of the Alzheimer's disease victim and his/her family. (11 ref).

1154. Montgomery, Dorothy R. & Still, Joyce A. (1985). **Alzheimer's disease: A select bibliography relating to the families of victims of this disease.** *Activities, Adaptation & Aging,* 6(4), 73–79.
Presents a bibliographic collection of over 100 materials written for the general public that may be of interest and assistance to families of Alzheimer patients or to others interested in the disease from a medical standpoint. Books and journal articles are included.

1155. Morycz, Richard K. (1983). **Family burden and outpatients with Alzheimer's disease.** *Dissertation Abstracts International,* 43(10-A), 3420.

1156. Morycz, Richard K. (1985). **Caregiving strain and the desire to institutionalize family members with Alzheimer's disease: Possible predictors and model development.** *Research on Aging,* 7(3), 329–361.
Determined whether the strain experienced by caregivers of relatives with Alzheimer's disease is strongly related to the desire of families to institutionalize their older members. Data were collected from structured interviews and a telephone follow-up survey of 80 families caring for Alzheimer patients (average patient age 78 yrs; average caregiver age 55 yrs). Extent of family burden, stressors such as functional deficits and incapacities of the patient, environmental factors, family strain, and vigilance/disruptiveness were assessed. The desire of a caregiver to institutionalize a patient with Alzheimer's disease was found to be greater when the caregiver experienced increased strain or burden, when a patient was widowed, when more physical labor was involved in caregiving tasks, and when the patient lived alone. Intensity of family strain (or felt stress) could be best predicted by the availability to the caregiver of social support: less support implied more strain. However, for male caregiving groups and for all Black caregivers, strain did not play a significant role in predicting the desire to institutionalize. (4 p ref).

1157. Morycz, Richard K.; Malloy, Julie; Bozich, Maryann & Martz, Pamela. (1987). **Racial differences in family burden: Clinical implications for social work.** 37th Annual Meeting of the Gerontological Society of America (1984, San Antonio, Texas). *Journal of Gerontological Social Work,* 10(1–2), 133–154.
Examined the clinical implications for social work practice of the differential impact of caregiving strain according to race. Data were drawn from a study of 95 Black and 715 White patients (mean ages 75 and 76 yrs, respectively) in a community-based geriatric assessment center. Measures included the Mini-Mental State Examination and the OARS Multidimensional Functional Assessment Questionnaire. There was a dif-

ference within the interaction of race and the care for an elderly person with Alzheimer's disease. A classification schema is suggested of specific interventions for different caregiving groups and subgroups, based on both race and relationship. This schema encompasses cognitive guidance, emotional support, socialization, tangible assistance, and self-disclosure.

1158. Nathan, Peggy K. (1986). **Helping wives of Alzheimer's patients through group therapy.** *Social Work with Groups,* 9(2), 73–81.
Examined, 1 yr after the group began, the treatment of 17 women (aged 49–74 yrs) members whose husbands were institutionalized with Alzheimer's disease. Ss had experienced negative changes in functioning, self-esteem, life satisfaction, and physical health, and increases in anxiety, depression, and guilt. Treatment involved working through guilt and anxiety associated with the disease and developing self-esteem and identity. It is concluded that group support was effective in alleviating the suffering of spouses of those with dementia.

1159. Oliver, Rose & Bock, Frances A. (1985). **Alleviating the distress of caregivers of Alzheimer's disease patients: A rational-emotive therapy model.** *Clinical Gerontologist,* 3(4), 17–34.
Argues that caring for a person with senile dementia of the Alzheimer type places a large emotional burden on the caregiver. Common responses of caregivers include denial, anger, guilt, self-pity, and depression. These negative emotions exacerbate the difficulties of caring for the patient and constrict the caregiver's ability to develop appropriate coping skills for his/her own life. Rational-emotive therapy (RET) specifies the maladaptive cognitions that elicit and sustain maladaptive emotions and behaviors and provides a model for cognitive, affective, and behavioral change. Excerpts from RET sessions are presented to illustrate the process. (18 ref).

1160. Ory, Marcia G. et al. (1985). **Families, informal supports, and Alzheimer's disease: Current research and future agendas.** *Research on Aging,* 7(4), 623–644.
Reviews the knowledge on how families and other social supports affect and are affected by Alzheimer's disease (AD) and related disorders and suggests a future research agenda. Topics discussed include availability of family members to care for AD patients, caregivers' perceptions of and responses to AD symptoms, the influence of familial factors on the onset and/or exacerbation of AD symptoms, and the burden of AD on caregivers. (4 p ref).

1161. Pagel, Mark & Becker, Joseph. (1987). **Depressive thinking and depression: Relations with personality and social resources.** *Journal of Personality & Social Psychology,* 52(5), 1043–1052.
We studied depression, depressive cognitions, social supports, and self-esteem in a sample of 68 spouse-caregivers of patients with Alzheimer's Disease in an attempt to identify possible buffering mechanisms of the latter 2 variables. Specifically, we hypothesized that the well-known relation of depressive cognitions to depression would vary as a function of satisfaction with social supports and with level of self-esteem. Hierarchical multiple regression analyses conducted to predict depression revealed significant and independent main effects for depressive cognitions, social supports, and self-esteem, with depressive cognitions associated with higher depression and the other 2 variables associated with reduced depression. In addition, the relation of depressive cognitions with depression varied substantially depending on the level of social supports; caregivers with high levels of depressive cognitions had high levels of depression only if social supports were low. Self-esteem and depressive cognitions showed a similar interaction, but it failed to reach significance. Analyses to determine whether self-esteem and social supports were directly associated with lower depressive cognitive activity yielded a main effect for self-esteem only.

1162. Pagel, Mark D.; Becker, Joseph & Coppel, David B. (1985). **Loss of control, self-blame, and depression: An investigation of spouse caregivers of Alzheimer's disease patients.** *Journal of Abnormal Psychology,* 94(2), 169–182.
Tested several predictions derived from the reformulated learned helplessness (RLH) depression model developed by L. Y. Abramson et al (1978) and from recent critiques of that model, in a longitudinal study of spouses caring for a husband or wife with Alzheimer's disease. During initial interviews, 68 caregivers (aged 37–85 yrs) rated the uncontrollability of important upsetting events related to their spouse's disease and were scored on an index of internal–external causal attribution (CATN) for those events. In addition, at both the initial and follow-up interviews ($n = 38$) about 10 mo later, caregivers were rated for depression, anxiety, and hostility. Results indicate that the indices of loss of control and CATN were more consistently related to depression than to anxiety or hostility, although hostility was related to CATNs. Correlations of the loss of control and CATN variables with depression remained significant after controlling for a measure of the spouse's objective disability. In hierarchical regression analyses, perceived loss of control and its interaction with CATN significantly predicted follow-up depression after controlling for initial depression. The interaction showed that loss of control combined with an internal attribution predicted higher depression than did either one alone. The importance of including specific uncontrollable events when studying the RLH model is emphasized. (36 ref).

1163. Pagel, Mark D.; Erdly, William W. & Becker, Joseph. (1987). **Social networks: We get by with (and in spite of) a little help from our friends.** *Journal of Personality & Social Psychology,* 53(4), 793–804.
Investigated both the helpful or positive and the upsetting or negative aspects of social networks in a longitudinal study of spouses caring for a husband or wife with Alzheimer's disease, a progressive senile dementia. Measures of helpful and upsetting aspects of the care givers' networks, derived from interviews and daily interaction ratings, were studied for their relations with overall network satisfaction and depression at an initial interview period ($n =68$) and at a follow-up period about 10 months later ($n = 38$). Results from hierarchical multiple regression analyses, in which care givers' age and sex and measure of the spouses' health status were controlled, showed that the care givers' degree of upset with their networks was strongly associated with lower network satisfaction and increased depression at both time periods. Helpful aspects bore little or no direct relation to either depression or network satisfaction. Helpful aspects of the network did, however, interact with network upset in predicting network satisfaction, and depression (combined probabilities test, $p < .05$). Longitudinal predictions of follow-up depression, after age, sex, care givers' health status, and initial depression levels were controlled, showed that changes in upsetting aspects of one's network were predictive of changes in depression over time. We interpreted these results within an attributional framework that emphasizes the salience of upsetting events within a social network.

1164. Pallett, Phyllis J. (1987). **Determinants and effects of stress experienced by caregiving spouses of patients with Alzheimer's dementia.** *Dissertation Abstracts International,* 47(8-B), 3297.

1165. Pollack, Mona M. (1985). **The general well-being of caregivers of older persons with dementing illnesses.** *Dissertation Abstracts International,* 45(10-B), 3204–3205.

1166. Powell, Lenore S. (1985). **Alzheimer's disease: A practical, psychological approach.** Special Issue: Health needs of women as they age. *Women & Health,* 10(2–3), 53–62.
Discusses Alzheimer's Disease (AD) and provides suggestions to help both the Alzheimer patient and the caregiver. AD is a

crippling, organic brain disorder that causes the loss of recent memory, intellectual deterioration, unpredictable behavioral changes, and personality deterioration. The etiology and phases of AD are described and it is suggested that the disease has 2 victims, the AD patient and the caregiver. Caregivers often experience shame, embarrassment, denial, frustration, anger, depression, and guilt as they care for an AD patient. It is concluded that those who deal with AD must recognize that both the patient and the caregiver are victims and that adequate treatment is needed for both. Help should be offered in practical terms, enlisting as wide a support network as possible. (15 ref).

1167. Pratt, Clara C.; Schmall, Vicki L.; Wright, Scott & Cleland, Marilyn. (1985). **Burden and coping strategies of caregivers to Alzheimer's patients.** Special Issue: The family and health care. *Family Relations: Journal of Applied Family & Child Studies,* 34(1), 27–33.
Examined coping strategies used by 240 caregivers (mean age 61.3 yrs) of Alzheimer's disease patients and the relationship of those strategies to the caregivers' subjective sense of burden. Ss completed a battery of instruments, including a caregiver burden scale and a scale that assessed coping strategies. Data show that differences in burden scores were not significantly affected by caregivers' age, sex, income, education, or patient residence (i.e., community dwellings, institutions). However, burden scores were significantly related to caregivers' health status. Burden scores were not significantly related to presence of confidant or support group membership. Three internal coping strategies (confidence in problem solving, reframing the problem, passivity) and 2 external coping strategies (spiritual support and extended family) were significantly related to caregiver burden scores. (25 ref).

1168. Pratt, Clara C.; Schmall, Vicki L. & Wright, Scott. (1986). **Family caregivers and dementia.** *Social Casework,* 67(2), 119–124.
Presents an overview of senile dementia, including Alzheimer's disease, and discusses the role of family caregiving for dementia patients. 240 family caregivers (mean age 61.3 yrs) completed a caregiver burden scale and a family coping strategies instrument. Results show, in part, that S morale scores were significantly negatively correlated to S burden. Burden scores were significantly higher among Ss who reported the patient's mental status to be poor. Ss who reported that their emotional relationship with the patient before caregiving had not been close had significantly higher burden scores compared with Ss who reported previously close relationships.

1169. Pratt, Clara C.; Wright, Scott & Schmall, Vicki. (1987). **Burden, coping and health status: A comparison of family caregivers to community dwelling and institutionalized Alzheimer's patients.** Special Issue: Gerontological social work with families: A guide to practice issues and service delivery. *Journal of Gerontological Social Work,* 10(1–2), 99–112.
Investigated caregiver health, burden, and coping strategies of 240 family caregivers (mean age 61.3 yrs) to institutionalized and community-dwelling Alzheimer's disease patients. Questionnaire data indicated that patient residence was significantly related to caregiver health status, sources of burden, and the efficacy of various strategies for reducing burden. However, total burden did not significantly differ between caregivers to community-dwelling or institutionalized patients, indicating that family caregivers do not necessarily rebound from the strains of caregiving once daily responsibilities are removed. Implications for intervention with family caregivers are discussed.

1170. Rabins, Peter V. (1984). **Management of dementia in the family context.** *Psychosomatics,* 25(5), 369–375.
Examines the impact of the cognitive, emotional, and behavioral concomitants of Alzheimer's disease and other demen-

tias on the family and examines interventions for these families. In addition to role changes necessitated in the course of the illness, the family will experience a variety of emotions that may be conceptualized as chronic grieving and that share the attributes of acute grief reactions: denial, sadness and depression, anger and frustration, guilt, and hopelessness. Recommendations are presented for providing advice, reassurance, and support to these families. Emphasis is on education and psychotherapeutic intervention and potential use of respite services, community agencies, self-help groups, and other professionals. (12 ref).

1171. Reisman, Bernard. (1986). **Adjusting to a residential facility for older persons: A child's perspective.** Special Issue: Social work and Alzheimer's disease: Practice issues with victims and their families. *Journal of Gerontological Social Work,* 9(2), 91–100.
Describes the present author's personal experience of helping his father, an Alzheimer's disease patient, adjust to full-time placement in a nursing home. Specific steps taken to facilitate the adjustment are described, including reassuring the patient, finding an appropriate care facility, and communicating with staff.

1172. Rusk, Carla L. (1986). **Alzheimer's Disease: Effects on the family.** *Dissertation Abstracts International,* 47(5-B), 2144.

1173. Sands, Dan. (1984). **Use of the Burden Interview in an adult day care setting.** Special Issue: Dementia assessment. *Clinical Gerontologist,* 3(2), 37–38.
Describes the use of the "burden" interview as part of the intake procedure used by a daycare center operating a support program for families of patients with Alzheimer's disease. The interview was found to have predictive validity with regard to families in which the patient was female. (2 ref).

1174. Schmidt, Gregory L. & Keyes, Barbara. (1985). **Group psychotherapy with family caregivers of demented patients.** *Gerontologist,* 25(4), 347–350.
The authors' experience with a support group for caregivers of relatives with Alzheimer's disease led to the identification of a group defense against individual expression of painful emotions. An active psychotherapeutic approach was employed to confront this defense with no overall detriment to the group and apparent benefit to some individual members. The dynamics of the transition from support group to therapy group are outlined. The role of the leaders in group therapy with family caregivers is seen as a critical one—they must make an initial offer to the group that encourages emotional expression but that does not prevent members from receiving the benefits of the supportive and educational components of the group experience. (9 ref).

1175. Scott, Jean P.; Roberto, Karen A. & Hutton, J. Thomas. (1986). **Families of Alzheimer's victims: Family support to the caregivers.** *Journal of the American Geriatrics Society,* 34(5), 348–354.
Examined the instrumental and social-emotional support provided by families to the primary caregivers of Alzheimer's patients. Ratings of instrumental assistance, social-emotional support, adequacy of support, and coping effectiveness were made by trained raters from transcribed interviews with 23 primary caregivers of Alzheimer's patients and a 2nd family member. While the major caregiving tasks were performed by the primary caregiver, the types of assistance from family that seemed most appreciated were visits and having persons stay with the patient so that the caregiver could take a trip, rest, run errands, or get out of the house for social activities. The majority of caregivers felt a high degree of support from their families and reported low levels of emotional upset resulting from family support efforts. Data confirmed the hypothesis

that family support was positively associated with the caregiver's coping effectiveness.

1176. Shibbal-Champagne, Sue & Lipinska-Stachow, D. M. (1986). **Alzheimer's Educational/Support group: Considerations for success—awareness of family tasks, pre-planning, and active professional facilitation.** Special Issue: Social work and Alzheimer's disease: Practice issues with victims and their families. *Journal of Gerontological Social Work,* 9(2), 41–48.
Describes the formation of educational/support groups to assist families of Alzheimer's disease patients in learning more about the disease, community resources, and effective coping strategies. In addition, the groups provide an opportunity to share emotional reactions and develop a network with others experiencing a common issue. A set of requirements facilitate group cohesion, attendance, and participation. It is concluded that awareness of family tasks, pre-planning, time-limited sessions, and professional facilitation were elements in releasing the supportive potential of the group members and increasing their adaptive capacities. (10 ref).

1177. Simank, Margaret H. & Strickland, Kenny J. (1986). **Assisting families in coping with Alzheimer's disease and other related dementias with the establishment of a mutual support group.** Special Issue: Social work and Alzheimer's disease: Practice issues with victims and their families. *Journal of Gerontological Social Work,* 9(2), 49–58.
Suggests that Alzheimer's disease is a family disease in the sense that the caregiver (usually a spouse, child, or sibling) is involved in a progressively more active role as caregiver to a person who does not get better but who deteriorates mentally and physically. The progression of the family's emotions over the course of the patient's dementia is described. It is suggested that mutual support groups led by social workers offer relatives information, referral to existing resources in the community, and a setting where they can feel acceptance, can share the emotional burden, and can receive support and empathy from those who have experienced the same kind of grief and loss. (7 ref).

1178. Simonton, Linda J. (1987). **Assessing caregiver information needs: A brief questionnaire.** Special Issue: Gerontological social work with families: A guide to practice issues and service delivery. *Journal of Gerontological Social Work,* 10(1–2), 177–180.
Suggests that the type of information needed by caregivers of Alzheimer's disease patients varies, depending on the stage of the caregiver's emotional acceptance of the illness and on the patient's condition. A brief questionnaire is presented for identifying caregiver information needs.

1179. Spence, Donald L. & Miller, Dulcy B. (1986). **Family respite for the elderly Alzheimer's patient.** Special Issue: Social work and Alzheimer's disease: Practice issues with victims and their families. *Journal of Gerontological Social Work,* 9(2), 101–112.
Describes a respite care program designed to provide temporary relief for families caring for a relative with Alzheimer's disease or a related disorder at home. The program provides an apartment or space in a nursing home for the patient and a caregiver on a short-term basis. The short-term placement is limited, compared to long-term nursing home placement, in making the patient feel part of the nursing home family. However, in providing the alternatives of an apartment or the nursing home setting, the program can develop a range of services specific to the clients. Criteria for judging the effectiveness of such a program are discussed. (16 ref).

1180. Steuer, Joanne L. & Clark, Elisabeth O. (1982). **Family support groups within a research project on dementia.** *Clinical Gerontologist,* 1(1), 87–95.

Reports on the effectiveness of 3 support groups for caregivers of patients with senile dementia who were participating in a larger study of Alzheimer's disease. One group participated in structural, open-ended sessions, while the other 2 groups participated in closed, time-limited sessions. The most cohesive and supportive group was unstructured and time limited. It also consisted of caregivers whose relationships to the patients were similar (i.e., spouses). (16 ref).

1181. Teusink, J. Paul & Mahler, Susan. (1984). **Helping families cope with Alzheimer's disease.** *Hospital & Community Psychiatry,* 35(2), 152–156.
Describes what appears to be an intense 5-stage reaction process that many families of patients with Alzheimer's disease undergo and how mental health professionals can help during each stage. The 5 stages are the following: denial, overinvolvement, anger, guilt, and acceptance. Family members also appear to face several specific problems when coping with the onset and progression of the disease, including role reversal, reactivated interpersonal problems, lack of understanding about the illness, fears about heredity, and shopping for cures. It is suggested that mental health professionals must provide families with education about the disease and with supportive guidance, so that family members will successfully work through their reactions and be able to mourn their loved one, make necessary decisions for his/her care, and reestablish family equilibrium. (10 ref).

1182. Tsemberis, Sam L. (1985). **Social networks of older people with early and moderate Alzheimer's disease.** *Dissertation Abstracts International,* 46(3-B), 1003.

1183. Ware, Lorene A. & Carper, Mark. (1982). **Living with Alzheimer disease patients: Family stresses and coping mechanisms.** *Psychotherapy: Theory, Research & Practice,* 19(4), 472–481.
Provides basic information on Alzheimer disease and its common manifestations. Critical diagnostic and therapeutic issues involved in the treatment of patients with Alzheimer disease and their families are discussed, including recognizing the difference between depression (pseudodementia) and Alzheimer disease; appropriate treatment based on diagnosis; psychotherapeutic intervention with the spouse and/or family; and using neuropsychological test data in clearly defining the patient's cognitive strengths and weaknesses, and use of this information for maximally beneficial management. The history, neuropsychological test profile, and tactics for therapeutic intervention of a "typical" case of Alzheimer disease are also presented. (14 ref).

1184. Wasow, Mona. (1986). **Support groups for family caregivers of patients with Alzheimer's disease.** *Social Work,* 31(2), 93–97.
The author discusses the assumptions, dilemmas, and questions related to Alzheimer's disease (AD) and support groups for AD based on her experience as a co-leader of a support group for family caregivers of AD patients, conversations with other facilitators of AD support groups, and a literature review. Dilemmas related to therapy vs support provision, focusing, coping expectation, group composition, and cultural values are explored. It is suggested that, while it is clear that educational information about the disease and its treatment and emotional support are important elements of a successful support group, methods of dealing with group and individual resistances to coping with strong negative feelings are less clear. It is concluded that the most important issue to be addressed by support groups is the recognition that caregivers have different needs and coping mechanisms that require a flexible approach to support provision and a wide variety of support-group models.

1185. Williams-Schroeder, Mary L. (1984). **Meeting the needs of the Alzheimer's caregiver.** *Physical & Occupational Therapy in Geriatrics,* 3(4), 33–38.
Describes the educational, emotional, physical, social, and professional needs of caregivers for Alzheimer's patients. Suggestions for dealing with the stress that this disorder causes among staff and among families of patients are presented. It is contended that caregiving leaves physical, emotional, and financial marks on those involved and that many people in the society are not able to comprehend the magnitude of the problems caused by dementia. (8 ref).

1186. Wood, Joan B. (1987). **Coping with the absence of perceived control: Ethnic and cultural issues in family caregiving for patients with Alzheimer's disease.** *Dissertation Abstracts International,* 48(5-B), 1551.

1187. Wright, Scott D. (1986). **The relationship of personal and social resources on coping and individual well-being in caregivers of dementia patients.** *Dissertation Abstracts International,* 47(3-A), 1078.

1188. Wright, Scott D.; Lund, Dale A.; Pett, Marjorie A. & Caserta, Michael S. (1987). **The assessment of support group experiences by caregivers of dementia patients.** *Clinical Gerontologist,* 6(4), 35–59.
Investigated the assessment of support groups established to help caregivers for dementia patients by studying questionnaire responses of 646 caregivers (mean age 60.4 yrs) who had attended at least 1 support group meeting. 73% of the Ss were female, 95% were White, and 86.6% were married. Results show that the group factors of universality, group cohesiveness, and imparting of knowledge were positive features of support groups; content of meetings, logistics, and emotions/feelings were negative features.

Section II. Citations to Recently Published Journal Articles

This section includes the most recent citations from the journal literature on Alzheimer's disease, retrieved from the PsycALERT database, and arranged alphabetically by author. When abstracting and full indexing are completed, the records will appear in *Psychological Abstracts* and the PsycINFO database.

1189. Abalan, Francois. (1988). **Alzheimer's disease: The nutritional hypothesis.** *Journal of Orthomolecular Medicine,* 3(1), 13–17.

1190. Amaducci, L. & Lippi, A. (1988). **Risk factors and genetic background for Alzheimer's disease.** Proceedings of the 27th Scandinavian Congress of Neurology (1988, Kuopio, Finland). *Acta Neurologica Scandinavica,* 77(116, Suppl), 13–18.

1191. Bartus, Raymond T. & Dean, Reginald L. (1988). **Lack of efficacy of clonidine on memory in aged cebus monkeys.** *Neurobiology of Aging,* 9(4), 409–411.

1192. Beatty, William W.; Salmon, David P.; Butters, Nelson; Heindel, William C. et al. (1988). **Retrograde amnesia in patients with Alzheimer's disease or Huntington's disease.** *Neurobiology of Aging,* 9(2), 181–186.

1193. Beck, Cornelia; Heacock, Patricia; Mercer, Susan; Thatcher, Rozanne et al. (1988). **The impact of cognitive skills remediation training on persons with Alzheimer's disease or mixed dementia.** *Journal of Geriatric Psychiatry,* 21(1), 73–88.

1194. Becker, James T.; Huff, F. Jacob; Nebes, Robert D.; Holland, Audrey L. et al. (1988). **Neuropsychological function in Alzheimer's disease: Pattern of impairment and rates of progression.** *Archives of Neurology,* 45(3), 263–268.

1195. Becker, Joseph & Morrissey, Elizabeth. (1988). **Difficulties assessing depressive-like reactions to chronic severe external stress as exemplified by spouse caregivers of Alzheimer patients.** *Psychology & Aging,* 3(3), 300–306.

1196. Becker, R.; Giacobini, E.; Elble, R.; McIlhany, M. et al. (1988). **Potential pharmacotherapy of Alzheimer disease: A comparison of various forms of physostigmine administration.** Proceedings of the 27th Scandinavian Congress of Neurology (1988, Kuopio, Finland). *Acta Neurologica Scandinavica,* 77(116, Suppl), 19–32.

1197. Benson, D. Frank. (1988). **PET/dementia: An update.** *Neurobiology of Aging,* 9(1), 87–88.

1198. Berrettini, Wade H.; Kaye, Walter H.; Sunderland, Trey; May, Conrad et al. (1988). **Galanin immunoreactivity in human CSF: Studies in eating disorders and Alzheimer's disease.** *Neuropsychobiology,* 19(2), 64–68.

1199. Berry, Ira R. & Borkan, Lionel. (1988). **Advances in Alzheimer's disease: A report.** *Journal of Orthomolecular Medicine,* 3(2), 68–76.

1200. Bigler, Erin D. (1987). **The clinical significance of cerebral atrophy in dementia.** *Archives of Clinical Neuropsychology,* 2(2), 177–190.

1201. Blass, John P.; Gleason, Patricia; Brush, Dorothea; DiPonte, Pompeo et al. (1988). **Thiamine and Alzheimer's disease: A pilot study.** *Archives of Neurology,* 45(8), 833–835.

1202. Botwinick, Jack; Storandt, Martha; Berg, Leonard & Boland, Susan. (1988). **Senile dementia of the Alzheimer type: Subject attrition and testability in research.** *Archives of Neurology,* 45(5), 493–496.

1203. Butters, Nelson; Salmon, David P.; Cullum, C. Munro; Cairns, Patricia et al. (1988). **Differentiation of amnesic and demented patients with the Wechsler Memory Scale—Revised.** Special Issue: Initial validity studies of the new Wechsler Memory Scale—Revised. *Clinical Neuropsychologist,* 2(2), 133–148.

1204. Campbell, Scott S.; Kripke, Daniel F.; Gillin, J. Christian & Hrubovcak, J. C. (1988). **Exposure to light in healthy elderly subjects and Alzheimer's patients.** *Physiology & Behavior,* 42(2), 141–144.

1205. Chipperfield, Barbara; Smith, Timothy A. & Moyes, Isabel C. (1987). **Plasma cholinesterase activities in dementias, depressions and schizophrenia.** *International Journal of Geriatric Psychiatry,* 2(4), 247–254.

1206. Christie, J. E.; Kean, D. M.; Douglas, R. H.; Engleman, H. M. et al. (1988). **Magnetic resonance imaging in pre-senile dementia of the Alzheimer-type, multi-infarct dementia and Korsakoff's syndrome.** *Psychological Medicine,* 18(2), 319–329.

1207. Cleary, T. Anne; Clamon, Cheryl; Price, Marjorie & Shullaw, Gail. (1988). **A reduced stimulation unit: Effects on patients with Alzheimer's disease and related disorders.** *Gerontologist,* 28(4), 511–514.

1208. Cohen, Donna & Eisdorfer, Carl. (1988). **Depression in family members caring for a relative with Alzheimer's disease.** *Journal of the American Geriatrics Society,* 36(10), 885–889.

1209. Coyle, Joseph T.; Oster-Granite, Mary L.; Reeves, Roger H. & Gearhart, John D. (1988). **Down syndrome, Alzheimer's disease and the tristomy 16 mouse.** *Trends in Neurosciences,* 11(9), 390–394.

1210. Cronin-Golomb, Alice. (1988). **Alzheimer's disease: Advances in basic research and therapies.** *Neuropsychologia,* 26(1), 187–193.

1211. Crystal, Howard A.; Wolfson, Leslie I. & Ewing, Stephanie. (1988). **Visual hallucinations as the first symptom of Alzheimer's disease.** *American Journal of Psychiatry,* 145(10), 1318.

1212. Cummings, J. L.; Darkins, A.; Mendez, M.; Hill, M. A. et al. (1988). **Alzheimer's disease and Parkinson's disease: Comparison of speech and language alterations.** *Neurology,* 38(5), 680–684.

1213. Cutler, Neal R. (1988). **Cognitive and brain imaging measures of Alzheimer's disease.** *Neurobiology of Aging,* 9(1), 90–92.

1214. Cutler, Neal R. & Narang, Prem K. (1988). **Alzheimer's disease, dementia and Down syndrome: An evaluation using positron emission tomography (PET).** Special Issue: Neuroradiology: Applications in neurology and neurosurgery. *Journal of Mind & Behavior,* 9(3), 351–366.

129

1215. Danielsson, Erik; Eckernäs, Sven-Åke; Westlind-Danielsson, Anita; Nordström, Öie et al. (1988). **VIP-sensitive adenylate cyclase, guanylate cyclase, muscarinic receptors, choline acetyltransferase and acetylcholinesterase, in brain tissue afflicted by Alzheimer's disease/senile dementia of the Alzheimer type.** *Neurobiology of Aging,* 9(2), 153–162.

1216. Dannenbaum, Stephen E.; Parkinson, Stanley R. & Inman, Vaughan W. (1988). **Short-term forgetting: Comparisons between patients with dementia of the Alzheimer type, depressed, and normal elderly.** *Cognitive Neuropsychology,* 5(2), 213–233.

1217. Davidson, Michael; Bastiaens, Leo; Davis, Bonnie M.; Shah, Mahendra B. et al. (1988). **Endocrine changes in Alzheimer's disease.** *Neurologic Clinics,* 6(1), 149–157.

1218. Davidson, Michael; Davis, Bonnie M.; Bastiaens, Leo; Macaluso, Joseph et al. (1988). **Growth hormone response to edrophonium in patients with Alzheimer's disease and normal control subjects.** *American Journal of Psychiatry,* 145(8), 1007–1009.

1219. Davidson, Michael; Zemishlany, Zvi; Mohs, Richard C.; Horvath, Thomas B. et al. (1988). **4-Aminopyridine in the treatment of Alzheimer's disease.** *Biological Psychiatry,* 23(5), 485–490.

1220. Davies, D. C. & Hardy, J. A. (1988). **Blood brain barrier in ageing and Alzheimer's disease.** *Neurobiology of Aging,* 9(1), 46–48.

1221. Davies, Peter. (1988). **Neurochemical studies: An update on Alzheimer's disease.** *Journal of Clinical Psychiatry,* 49(5, Suppl), 23–28.

1222. Davis, Kenneth L.; Davidson, Michael; Yang, Ren-kui; Davis, Bonnie M. et al. (1988). **CSF somatostatin in Alzheimer's disease, depressed patients, and control subjects.** *Biological Psychiatry,* 24(6), 710–712.

1223. Davous, P.; Roudier, M.; Piketty, M. L.; Abramowitz, C. et al. (1988). **Pharmacological modulation of cortisol secretion and dexamethasone suppression in Alzheimer's disease.** *Biological Psychiatry,* 23(1), 13–24.

1224. Degrell, István & Niklasson, Frank. (1988). **Purine metabolites in the CSF in presenile and senile dementia of Alzheimer type, and in multi infarct dementia.** *Archives of Gerontology & Geriatrics,* 7(2), 173–178.

1225. de Leon, M. J.; George, A. E.; Marcus, D. L. & Miller, J. D. (1988). **Positron emission tomography with the deoxyglucose technique and the diagnosis of Alzheimer's disease.** *Neurobiology of Aging,* 9(1), 88–90.

1226. Devanand, D. P.; Sackeim, Harold A. & Mayeux, Richard. (1988). **Psychosis, behavioral disturbances, and the use of neuroleptics in dementia.** *Comprehensive Psychiatry,* 29(4), 387–401.

1227. Dick, Malcolm B.; Kean, Mary-Louise & Sands, Dan. (1988). **The preselection effect on the recall facilitation of motor movements in Alzheimer-type dementia.** *Journals of Gerontology,* 43(5), P127–P135.

1228. Dieckmann, Lisa; Zarit, Steven H.; Zarit, Judy M. & Gatz, Margaret. (1988). **The Alzheimer's Disease Knowledge test.** *Gerontologist,* 28(3), 402–407.

1229. Emery, Olga B. (1988). **The deficit of thought in senile dementia Alzheimer's type.** 27th Annual Meeting Group-Without-A-Name International Psychiatric Research Society (1985, Toronto, Canada). *Psychiatric Journal of the University of Ottawa,* 13(1), 3–8.

1230. Erkinjuntti, T.; Haltia, M.; Palo, J. & Sulkava, R. (1988). **Accuracy of the clinical diagnosis of vascular dementia: A prospective clinical and post-mortem neuropathological study.** *Journal of Neurology, Neurosurgery & Psychiatry,* 51(8), 1037–1044.

1231. Erkinjuntti, Timo; Larsen, T.; Sulkava, R.; Ketonen, L. et al. (1988). **EEG in the differential diagnosis between Alzheimer's disease and vascular dementia.** *Acta Neurologica Scandinavica,* 77(1), 36–43.

1232. Ferrier, I. Nicol; Pascual, Juanita; Charlton, Bruce G.; Wright, Carolyn et al. (1988). **Cortisol, ACTH, and dexamethasone concentrations in a psychogeriatric population.** *Biological Psychiatry,* 23(3), 252–260.

1233. Filinson, Rachel. (1988). **A model for church-based services for frail elderly persons and their families.** *Gerontologist,* 28(4), 483–486.

1234. Fisman, Michael; Inaba, Ted; Kalow, Werner; Fox, Hannah et al. (1988). **Oxazepam as a probe of hepatic metabolism in patients with Alzheimer's disease.** 10th Annual Meeting of the Canadian College of Neuro-psychopharmacology: Perspectives in Canadian neuro-psychopharmacology (1987, Ottawa, Canada). *Progress in Neuro-Psychopharmacology & Biological Psychiatry,* 12(2–3), 255–261.

1235. French, Carolyn J. (1986). **The development of special services for victims and families burdened by Alzheimer's disease.** *Pride Institute Journal of Long Term Home Health Care,* 5(3), 19–27.

1236. Friedland, Robert P.; Horwitz, Barry & Koss, Elisabeth. (1988). **Measurement of disease progression in Alzheimer's disease.** *Neurobiology of Aging,* 9(1), 95–97.

1237. Gierz, Monika; Campbell, Scott S. & Gillin, J. Christian. (1987). **Sleep disturbances in various nonaffective psychiatric disorders.** *Psychiatric Clinics of North America,* 10(4), 565–581.

1238. Goodman, Catherine C. & Pynoos, Jon. (1988). **Telephone networks connect caregiving families of Alzheimer's victims.** *Gerontologist,* 28(5), 602–605.

1239. Gottlieb, Gary L.; McAllister, Thomas W. & Gur, Ruben C. (1988). **Depot neuroleptics in the treatment of behavioral disorders in patients with Alzheimer's disease.** 140th Meeting of the American Psychiatric Association (1987, Chicago, Illinois). *Journal of the American Geriatrics Society,* 36(7), 619–621.

1240. Grady, Cheryl L.; Haxby, J. V.; Horwitz, B.; Sundaram, M. et al. (1988). **Longitudinal study of the early neuropsychological and cerebral metabolic changes in dementia of the Alzheimer type.** *Journal of Clinical & Experimental Neuropsychology,* 10(5), 576–596.

1241. Granholm, Eric & Butters, Nelson. (1988). **Associative encoding and retrieval in Alzheimer's and Huntington's disease.** *Brain & Cognition,* 7(3), 335–347.

1242. Hart, Robert P.; Kwentus, Joseph A.; Harkins, Stephen W. & Taylor, John R. (1988). **Rate of forgetting in mild Alzheimer's-type dementia.** *Brain & Cognition,* 7(1), 31–38.

1243. Hart, Robert P.; Kwentus, Joseph A.; Wade, James B. & Taylor, John R. (1988). **Modified Wisconsin Sorting Test in elderly normal, depressed and demented patients.** *Clinical Neuropsychologist,* 2(1), 49–56.

1244. Hart, Siobhan. (1988). **Language and dementia: A review.** *Psychological Medicine,* 18(1), 99–112.

1245. Heindel, William C.; Butters, Nelson & Salmon, David P. (1988). **Impaired learning of a motor skill in patients with Huntington's disease.** *Behavioral Neuroscience,* 102(1), 141–147.

1246. Holman, B. Leonard; Johnson, Keith A. & Hill, Thomas C. (1988). **SPECT imaging in Alzheimer's disease.** Special Issue: Neuroradiology: Applications in neurology and neurosurgery. *Journal of Mind & Behavior,* 9(3), 385–398.

1247. Horner, Jennifer; Heyman, Albert; Dawson, Deborah & Rogers, Helen. (1988). **The relationship of agraphia to the severity of dementia in Alzheimer's disease.** *Archives of Neurology,* 45(7), 760–763.

1248. Huff, F. Jacob; Auerbach, Jonathan; Chakravarti, Aravinda & Boller, François. (1988). **Risk of dementia in relatives of patients with Alzheimer's disease.** *Neurology,* 38(5), 786–790.

1249. Johnson, Keith A.; Holman, B. Leonard; Mueller, Stephen P.; Rosen, T. John et al. (1988). **Single photon emission computed tomography in Alzheimer's disease: Abnormal iofetamine I 123 uptake reflects dementia severity.** *Archives of Neurology,* 45(4), 392–396.

1250. Kaszniak, Alfred W. (1988). **Cognition in Alzheimer's disease: Theoretic models and clinical implications.** *Neurobiology of Aging,* 9(1), 92–94.

1251. Kaye, J. A.; May, C.; Daly, E.; Atack, J. R. et al. (1988). **Cerebrospinal fluid monoamine markers are decreased in dementia of the Alzheimer type with extrapyramidal features.** *Neurology,* 38(4), 554–557.

1252. Kesslak, J. P.; Cotman, C. W.; Chui, H. C.; Van der Noort, S. et al. (1988). **Olfactory tests as possible probes for detecting and monitoring Alzheimer's disease.** *Neurobiology of Aging,* 9(4), 399–403.

1253. Kornreich, Sharon. (1988). **An Alzheimer patient's use of art as a form of constancy.** *Pratt Institute Creative Arts Therapy Review,* 9, 29–39.

1254. Koss, Elisabeth; Weiffenbach, James M.; Haxby, James V. & Friedland, Robert P. (1988). **Olfactory detection and identification performance are dissociated in early Alzheimer's disease.** *Neurology,* 38(8), 1228–1232.

1255. Kramer, Joel H.; Delis, Dean C.; Blusewicz, Matthew J.; Brandt, Jason et al. (1988). **Verbal memory errors in Alzheimer's and Huntington's dementias.** *Developmental Neuropsychology,* 4(1), 1–15.

1256. Krenz, Claudia; Larson, Eric B.; Buchner, David M. & Canfield, Connie G. (1988). **Characterizing patient dysfunction in Alzheimer's-type dementia.** *Medical Care,* 26(5), 453–461.

1257. Kreutzberg, Georg W. & Gudden, Wolfgang. (1988). **Alois Alzheimer.** *Trends in Neurosciences,* 11(6[120]), 256–257.

1258. Kumar, Vinod & Giabobini, Ezio. (1988). **Cerebrospinal fluid choline, and acetylcholinesterase activity in familial vs. non-familial Alzheimer's disease patients.** *Archives of Gerontology & Geriatrics,* 7(2), 111–117.

1259. Kurlan, Roger & Como, Peter. (1988). **Drug-induced Alzheimerism.** *Archives of Neurology,* 45(3), 356–357.

1260. Lampe, Thomas H.; Plymate, Stephen R.; Risse, Steven C.; Kopeikin, Hal et al. (1988). **TSH responses to two TRH doses in men with Alzheimer's disease.** *Psychoneuroendocrinology,* 13(3), 245–254.

1261. Levy, Linda L. (1987). **Psychosocial intervention and dementia: II. The cognitive disability perspective.** *Occupational Therapy in Mental Health,* 7(4), 13–36.

1262. Loring, David W.; Meador, K. J.; Mahurin, Roderick K. & Largen, John W. (1986). **Neuropsychological performance in dementia of the Alzheimer type and multi-infarct dementia.** *Archives of Clinical Neuropsychology,* 1(4), 335–340.

1263. Maletta, Gabe J. (1987). **Drug management of the geriatric Alzheimer's patient: Considerations for achieving effective treatment of behavioral problems.** *Journal of Geriatric Drug Therapy,* 2(1), 3–20.

1264. Mann, David M. & Esiri, Margaret M. (1988). **The site of the earliest lesions of Alzheimer's disease.** *New England Journal of Medicine,* 318(12), 789–790.

1265. Martin, Ronald L.; Gerteis, Gretchen & Gabrielli, William F. (1988). **A family-genetic study of dementia of Alzheimer type.** 139th Annual Meeting of the American Psychiatric Association (1986, Washington, DC). *Archives of General Psychiatry,* 45(10), 894–900.

1266. Masters, Colin L. & Beyreuther, Konrad. (1988). **The blood-brain barrier in Alzheimer's disease and normal aging.** *Neurobiology of Aging,* 9(1), 43–44.

1267. McCaffrey, Robert J.; Steckler, Rosemarie A.; Gansler, David A.; Roman, Lillian O. et al. (1987). **An experimental evaluation of the efficacy of suloctidil in the treatment of primary degenerative dementia.** *Archives of Clinical Neuropsychology,* 2(2), 155–161.

1268. McGrowder-Lin, Rachel & Bhatt, Ashok. (1988). **A wanderer's lounge program for nursing home residents with Alzheimer's disease.** *Gerontologist,* 28(5), 607–609.

1269. Molchanova, E. K.; Sudareva, L. O.; Selezneva, N. D. & Voskresenskaya, N. I. (1988). **Some distinctive features of the initial symptoms of Alzheimer's disease.** *Soviet Neurology & Psychiatry,* 21(2), 19–26.

1270. Mooradian, Arshag D. (1988). **Effect of aging on the blood-brain barrier.** *Neurobiology of Aging,* 9(1), 31–39.

1271. Morris, John C. & Fulling, Keith. (1988). **Early Alzheimer's disease: Diagnostic considerations.** *Archives of Neurology,* 45(3), 345–349.

1272. Morris, Lorna W.; Morris, Robin G. & Britton, Peter G. (1988). **The relationship between marital intimacy, perceived strain and depression in spouse caregivers of dementia sufferers.** *British Journal of Medical Psychology,* 61(3), 231–236.

1273. Moss, Robert J.; Mastri, Angeline R. & Schut, Lawrence J. (1988). **The coexistence and differentiation of late onset Huntington's disease and Alzheimer's disease: A case report and review of the literature.** *Journal of the American Geriatrics Society,* 36(3), 237–241.

1274. Mouradian, M. Maral; Mohr, Erich; Williams, Jill A. & Chase, Thomas N. (1988). **No response to high-dose muscarinic agonist therapy in Alzheimer's disease.** *Neurology,* 38(4), 606–608.

1275. Nappi, G.; Facchinetti, F.; Martignoni, E.; Petraglia, F. et al. (1988). **N-terminal ACTH fragments increase the CSF β-EP content in Alzheimer type dementia.** *Acta Neurologica Scandinavica,* 78(2), 146–151.

1276. Nebes, Robert D. & Brady, Christopher B. (1988). **Integrity of semantic fields in Alzheimer's disease.** *Cortex,* 24(2), 291–299.

1277. Neils, Jean; Brennan, M. M.; Cole, Monroe; Boller, François et al. (1988). **The use of phonemic cueing with Alzheimer's disease patients.** *Neuropsychologia,* 26(2), 351–354.

1278. Newhouse, P. A.; Sunderland, T.; Tariot, P. N.; Blumhardt, C. L. et al. (1988). **Intravenous nicotine in Alzheimer's disease: A pilot study.** *Psychopharmacology,* 95(2), 171–175.

1279. Norbiato, Guido; Bevilacqua, Maurizio; Carella, Francesco; Chebat, Enrica et al. (1988). **Alterations in vasopressin regulation in Alzheimer's disease.** *Journal of Neurology, Neurosurgery & Psychiatry,* 51(7), 903–908.

1280. Nybäck, Henrik; Nyman, H. & Schalling, D. (1987). **Neuropsychological test performance and CSF levels of monoamine metabolites in healthy volunteers and patients with Alzheimer's dementia.** *Acta Psychiatrica Scandinavica,* 76(6), 648–656.

1281. Oakley, Frances. (1987). **Clinical application of the model of human occupation in dementia of the Alzheimer's type.** *Occupational Therapy in Mental Health,* 7(4), 37–50.

1282. Ober, Beth A. & Shenaut, Gregory K. (1988). **Lexical decision and priming in Alzheimer's disease.** *Neuropsychologia,* 26(2), 273–286.

1283. Pardridge, William M. (1988). **Does the brain's gatekeeper falter in aging?** *Neurobiology of Aging,* 9(1), 44–46.

1284. Passeri, Mario; Cucinotta, Domenico; de Mello, Manuel & Bizière, Kathleen. (1987). **Comparison of minaprine and placebo in the treatment of Alzheimer's disease and multiinfarct dementia.** *International Journal of Geriatric Psychiatry,* 2(2), 97–103.

1285. Penn, R. D.; Martin, E. M.; Wilson, R. S.; Fox, J. H. et al. (1988). **Intraventricular bethanechol infusion for Alzheimer's disease: Results of double-blind and escalating-dose trials.** *Neurology,* 38(2), 219–222.

1286. Philpot, Michael P. & Levy, Raymond. (1987). **A memory clinic for the elderly diagnosis of dementia.** *International Journal of Geriatric Psychiatry,* 2(3), 195–200.

1287. Pomara, Nunzio; Stanley, Michael; Rhiew, H. Benjamin; Bagne, Curtis A. et al. (1988). **Loss of the cortisol response to naltrexone in Alzheimer's disease.** *Biological Psychiatry,* 23(7), 726–733.

1288. Probst, Alphonse; Cotrés, Roser; Ulrich, Jürg & Palacios, José M. (1988). **Differential modification of muscarinic cholinergic receptors in the hippocampus of patients with Alzheimer's disease: An autoradiographic study.** *Brain Research,* 450(1–2), 190–201.

1289. Quayhagen, Mary P. & Quayhagen, Margaret. (1988). **Alzheimer's stress: Coping with the caregiving role.** *Gerontologist,* 28(3), 391–396.

1290. Rai, G. S. & Wright, G. (1987). **Diagnostic tests for Alzheimer's disease for use in research.** *International Journal of Geriatric Psychiatry,* 2(3), 141–143.

1291. Represa, A.; Duyckaerts, C.; Tremblay, E.; Hauw, J. J. et al. (1988). **Is senile dementia of the Alzheimer type associated with hippocampal plasticity?** *Brain Research,* 457(2), 355–359.

1292. Riege, Walter H. & Metter, E. J. (1988). **Cognitive and brain imaging measures of Alzheimer's disease.** *Neurobiology of Aging,* 9(1), 69–86.

1293. Roberts, Eugene. (1988). **Beyond measurement: The pattern is the thing.** *Neurobiology of Aging,* 9(1), 97–100.

1294. Rubin, Eugene H.; Zorumski, Charles F. & Burke, William J. (1988). **Overlapping symptoms of geriatric depression and Alzheimer-type dementia.** *Hospital & Community Psychiatry,* 39(10), 1074–1079.

1295. Sahu, R. N.; Pandey, R. S.; Subhash, M. N.; Arya, B. Y. et al. (1988). **CSF zinc in Alzheimer's type dementia.** *Biological Psychiatry,* 24(4), 480–482.

1296. Salim, M.; Rehman, S.; Sajdel-Sulkowska, Elizabeth M.; Chou, Wen-gang et al. (1988). **Preparation of a recombinant cDNA library from poly(A+) RNA of the Alzheimer brain: Identification and characterization of a cDNA copy encoding a glial-specific protein.** *Neurobiology of Aging,* 9(2), 163–171.

1297. Sanborn, Beverly. (1986). **San Diego's Alzheimer's Family Center.** *Pride Institute Journal of Long Term Home Health Care,* 5(3), 13–18.

1298. Sano, Mary. (1988). **Using computers to understand attention in the elderly.** *American Behavioral Scientist,* 31(5), 588–594.

1299. Scarone, Silvio; Pieri, E.; Cattaneo, R.; Gambini, O. et al. (1988). **Neurofunctional assessment of early phases of Alzheimer's disease: A preliminary note on hemispheric EEG characteristics during cognitive tasks.** *Human Neurobiology,* 6(4), 289–293.

1300. Scheibel, Arnold B. & Duong, Taihung. (1988). **On the possible relationship of cortical microvascular pathology to blood brain barrier changes in Alzheimer's disease.** *Neurobiology of Aging,* 9(1), 41–42.

1301. Schneider, Lon S.; Severson, James A.; Chui, Helena C.; Pollock, Vicki E. et al. (1988). **Platelet tritiated imipramine binding and MAO activity in Alzheimer's disease patients with agitation and delusions.** *Psychiatry Research,* 25(3), 311–322.

1302. Selnes, Ola A.; Carson, Kathryn; Rovner, Barry & Gordon, Barry. (1988). **Language dysfunction in early- and late-onset possible Alzheimer's disease.** *Neurology,* 38(7), 1053–1056.

1303. Seltzer, Benjamin; Rheaume, Yvette; Volicer, Ladislav; Fabiszewski, Kathy J. et al. (1988). **The short-term effects of in-hospital respite on the patient with Alzheimer's disease.** *Gerontologist,* 28(1), 121–124.

1304. Sheridan, P. H.; Sato, S.; Foster, N.; Bruno, G. et al. (1988). **Relation of EEG alpha background to parietal lobe function in Alzheimer's disease as measured by positron emission tomography and psychometry.** *Neurology,* 38(5), 747–750.

1305. Shifflett, Peggy A. & Blieszner, Rosemary. (1988). **Stigma and Alzheimer's disease: Behavioral consequences for support groups.** *Journal of Applied Gerontology,* 7(2), 147–160.

1306. Small, Gary W. & Greenberg, David A. (1988). **Biologic markers, genetics, and Alzheimer's disease.** *Archives of General Psychiatry,* 45(10), 945–947.

1307. Smith, Gwenn. (1988). **Animal models of Alzheimer's disease: Experimental cholinergic denervation.** *Brain Research Reviews,* 13(2), 103–118.

1308. Smith, Robert C.; Kumar, Vinod; Khera, Gurbir; Elble, Rodger et al. (1988). **Brain morphological measures and CSF acetylcholine in Alzheimer dementia.** *Psychiatry Research,* 23(1), 111–114.

1309. Sokol'chik, E. I. (1988). **Affective disorders in Alzheimer's disease.** *Soviet Neurology & Psychiatry,* 21(2), 27–34.

132

1310. St Clair, David M.; Blackburn, Ivy M.; Blackwood, Douglas H. & Tyrer, Gillian M. (1988). **Measuring the course of Alzheimer's disease: A longitudinal study of neuropsychological function and changes in P3 event-related potential.** *British Journal of Psychiatry,* 152, 48–54.

1311. Stigsby, Bent. (1988). **Dementias (Alzheimer's and Pick's disease): Dysfunctional and structural changes.** *American Journal of EEG Technology,* 28(2), 83–97.

1312. Sulkava, Raimo; Viinikka, Lasse; Erkinjuntti, Timo & Roine, Risto. (1988). **Cerebrospinal fluid neuron-specific enolase is decreased in multi-infarct dementia, but unchanged in Alzheimer's disease.** *Journal of Neurology, Neurosurgery & Psychiatry,* 51(4), 549–551.

1313. Sunderland, Trey; Alterman, Ina S.; Yount, Donna; Hill, James L. et al. (1988). **A new scale for the assessment of depressed mood in demented patients.** *American Journal of Psychiatry,* 145(8), 955–959.

1314. Swearer, Joan M.; Drachman, David A.; O'Donnell, Brian F. & Mitchell, Ann L. (1988). **Troublesome and disruptive behaviors in dementia: Relationships to diagnosis and disease severity.** *Journal of the American Geriatrics Society,* 36(9), 784–790.

1315. Tariot, Pierre N.; Cohen, Robert M.; Welkowitz, Julie A.; Sunderland, Trey et al. (1988). **Multiple-dose arecoline infusions in Alzheimer's disease.** *Archives of General Psychiatry,* 45(10), 901–905.

1316. Tariot, Pierre N.; Gross, Michael; Sunderland, Trey; Cohen, Martin R. et al. (1988). **High-dose naloxone in older normal subjects: Implications for Alzheimer's disease.** *Journal of the American Geriatrics Society,* 36(8), 681–686.

1317. Tariot, Pierre N.; Sunderland, Trey; Cohen, Robert M.; Newhouse, Paul A. et al. (1988). **Tranylcypromine compared with l-deprenyl in Alzheimer's disease.** *Journal of Clinical Psychopharmacology,* 8(1), 23–27.

1318. Thal, Leon J. (1988). **Dementia update: Diagnosis and neuropsychiatric aspects.** *Journal of Clinical Psychiatry,* 49(5, Suppl), 5–7.

1319. Tham, Anne; Sparring, K.; Bowen, D.; Wetterberg, L. et al. (1988). **Insulin-like growth factors and somatomedin B in the cerebrospinal fluid of patients with dementia of the Alzheimer type.** *Acta Psychiatrica Scandinavica,* 77(6), 719–723.

1320. Thompson, I. M. (1987). **Language in dementia: I. A review.** *International Journal of Geriatric Psychiatry,* 2(3), 145–161.

1321. Tierney, Mary C.; Fisher, Rory H.; Lewis, Anthony J.; Zorzitto, Maria L. et al. (1988). **The NINCDS-ADRDA Work Group criteria for the clinical diagnosis of probable Alzheimer's disease: A clinicopathologic study of 57 cases.** *Neurology,* 38(3), 359–364.

1322. Urakami, Katsuya; Adachi, Yoshiki & Takahashi, Kazuro. (1988). **A community-based study of parental age in Alzheimer-type dementia in western Japan.** *Archives of Neurology,* 45(4), 375.

1323. Vinařová, E. & Vinař, O. (1987). **Lecithin in a psychiatric out-patient clinic.** 29th Annual Psychopharmacology Meeting (1987, Jeseník, Czechoslovakia). *Activitas Nervosa Superior,* 29(3), 219–221.

1324. Wasow, Mona & Coons, Dorothy H. (1987). **Widows and widowers of Alzheimer's victims: Their survival after spouses' death.** *Journal of Independent Social Work,* 2(2), 21–32.

1325. Weizman, Ronit; Dick, Jacob; Mosek, Abraham; Tyano, Sam et al. (1988). **Unaltered platelet [^{3}H]-imipramine binding in dementia of the Alzheimer type.** *Neuropsychobiology,* 19(2), 69–72.

1326. Wilcock, G. K.; Esiri, M. M.; Bowen, D. M. & Hughes, A. O. (1988). **The differential involvement of subcortical nuclei in senile dementia of Alzheimer's type.** *Journal of Neurology, Neurosurgery & Psychiatry,* 51(6), 842–849.

1327. Williams, Dianne E.; Vitiello, Michael V.; Ries, Richard K.; Bokan, John et al. (1988). **Successful recruitment of elderly community-dwelling subjects for Alzheimer's disease research.** *Journals of Gerontology,* 43(3), M69–M74.

1328. Wolf-Klein, Gisele P.; Silverstone, Felix A.; Brod, Meryl S.; Levy, Arnold et al. (1988). **Are Alzheimer patients healthier?** 39th Annual Scientific Meeting of the Gerontological Society of America (1986, Chicago, Illinois). *Journal of the American Geriatrics Society,* 36(3), 219–224.

1329. Wragg, Robin E. & Jeste, Dilip V. (1988). **Neuroleptics and alternative treatments: Management of behavioral symptoms and psychosis in Alzheimer's disease and related conditions.** *Psychiatric Clinics of North America,* 11(1), 195–213.

1330. Yatham, L. N.; McHale, Patrick A. & Kinsella, A. (1988). **Down's syndrome and its association with Alzheimer's disease.** *Acta Psychiatrica Scandinavica,* 77(1), 38–41.

1331. Zappoli, R.; Arnetoli, G.; Paganini, M.; Versari, A. et al. (1987). **Contingent negative variation and reaction time in patients with presenile idiopathic cognitive decline and presenile Alzheimer-type dementia: Preliminary report on long-term nicergoline treatment.** *Neuropsychobiology,* 18(3), 149–154.

1332. Zubenko, George S.; Brenner, Richard P. & Teply, Ivana. (1988). **Electroencephalographic correlates of increased platelet membrane fluidity in Alzheimer's disease.** *Archives of Neurology,* 45(9), 1009–1013.

1333. Zubenko, George S.; Cohen, Bruce M.; Reynolds, Charles F.; Boller, Francois et al. (1987). **Platelet membrane fluidity identifies a clinical subtype of Alzheimer's disease.** *Progress in Neuro-Psychopharmacology & Biological Psychiatry,* 11(6), 683–699.

1334. Zubenko, George S.; Reynolds, Charles F.; Perel, James M.; Decker, Cynthia et al. (1988). **Platelet membrane fluidity and treatment response in cognitively-impaired, depressed elderly: Initial results.** *Psychopharmacology,* 94(3), 347–349.

Section III. Subject Index

This is a subject index to entries in Section I. Subject Terms in this index are taken from the *Thesaurus of Psychological Index Terms,* (Fifth edition, 1988). The term used in the search to retrieve the references in this bibliography (*Alzheimers disease*) as well as the index term *Aged* are not included in this index. *See references* are used to refer to preferred forms of entry, or from conceptually broader terms to narrower ones. *See also* references alert the reader to more specific terms. Each document is indexed with the most specific terms that are appropriate for that document's content.

Accelerated Speech [See Speech Rate]
Accidents 679
Acetylcholine 26, 67, 95, 156, 208, 221, 225, 243, 281, 286, 303, 319, 352, 356, 361, 362, 364, 369, 604, 1008
Acetylcholinesterase 75, 80, 110, 111, 160, 218, 296, 349, 363, 400, 579, 824, 894
Acids [See Also Adenosine, Amino Acids, Deoxyribonucleic Acid, Gamma Aminobutyric Acid, Glutamic Acid, Glycine, Homovanillic Acid, Hydroxyindoleacetic Acid (5-), Nicotinic Acid, Phosphatides, Tryptophan, Tyrosine] 199
Acoustic Stimuli [See Auditory Stimulation]
Acquired Immune Deficiency Syndrome 204, 520, 532
ACTH (Hormone) [See Corticotropin]
Active Avoidance [See Avoidance Conditioning]
Activity Level 393, 553, 1055, 1060
Activity Therapy [See Recreation Therapy]
Adaptation [See Sensory Adaptation]
Adaptation (Sensory) [See Sensory Adaptation]
Addiction [See Alcoholism]
Adenosine 798
Adjudication 1142
Adjustment [See Also Related Terms] 456, 1132, 1171
Adrenal Cortex Hormones [See Hydrocortisone]
Adrenal Cortex Steroids [See Corticosteroids]
Adrenal Medulla Hormones [See Norepinephrine]
Adrenaline [See Epinephrine]
Adrenergic Blocking Drugs [See Hydroxydopamine (6-), Propranolol]
Adrenocorticotropin [See Corticotropin]
Adult Children [See Adult Offspring]
Adult Offspring 1171
Adults [See Adult Offspring, Middle Aged, Young Adults]
Advocacy 896
Aetiology [See Etiology]
Affective Disorders [See Affective Disturbances]
Affective Disturbances [See Also Major Depression, Manic Depression] 455, 726, 739, 1005
Afferent Pathways 303, 400
Age Differences 32, 82, 122, 153, 157, 293, 393, 514, 525, 574, 597, 599, 725, 796, 811, 857, 865, 901, 914, 1143

Aged (Attitudes Toward) 1126
Aging (Physiological) [See Physiological Aging]
Agitated Depression [See Major Depression]
Agrammatism [See Aphasia]
Agraphia 412
AIDS [See Acquired Immune Deficiency Syndrome]
Air Encephalography [See Pneumoencephalography]
Alcohol Abuse [See Alcoholism]
Alcoholic Hallucinosis [See Korsakoffs Psychosis]
Alcoholic Psychosis [See Also Korsakoffs Psychosis] 886
Alcoholism [See Also Korsakoffs Psychosis] 219
Alcohols [See Isoproterenol, Propranolol]
Alkaloids [See Also Atropine, Nicotine, Physostigmine, Pilocarpine, Scopolamine] 809, 946, 1008
Allergens [See Antigens]
Alpha Rhythm 811
Amantadine 981
Amatadine [See Amantadine]
Amentia [See Mental Retardation]
Amines [See Also Atropine, Catecholamines, Dopamine, Epinephrine, Imipramine, Meperidine, Methylphenidate, Norepinephrine, Physostigmine, Scopolamine, Serotonin] 948, 1051
Amino Acids [See Also Gamma Aminobutyric Acid, Glutamic Acid, Glycine, Tryptophan, Tyrosine] 12, 13, 26, 103, 279
Amnesia 383, 558, 631, 645, 665, 686
Amygdaloid Body 369
Anabolites [See Metabolites]
Analgesic Drugs [See Atropine, Meperidine, Procaine, Scopolamine]
Ancestors [See Grandparents, Parents]
Anesthetic Drugs [See Procaine]
Angiotensin 337
Angst [See Anxiety]
Anguish [See Distress]
Animal Biological Rhythms [See Animal Circadian Rhythms]
Animal Circadian Rhythms 393
Animal Drinking Behavior 393
Animal Ethology [See Animal Circadian Rhythms, Animal Drinking Behavior]
Animal Models 382
Anoxia 119

Anti Inflammatory Drugs [See Dexamethasone]
Antibiotics [See Amantadine]
Antibodies 7, 69, 200, 237, 275, 396, 844, 885
Anticholinergic Drugs [See Cholinergic Blocking Drugs]
Anticholinesterase Drugs [See Cholinesterase Inhibitors]
Anticoagulant Drugs 1104
Anticonvulsive Drugs 1059
Antidepressant Drugs [See Also Imipramine, Lithium Carbonate, Methylphenidate, Zimeldine] 980, 1055
Antiemetic Drugs [See Piracetam]
Antiepileptic Drugs [See Anticonvulsive Drugs]
Antigens 127, 331, 525, 803, 847
Antiparkinsonian Drugs [See Antitremor Drugs]
Antipsychotic Drugs [See Neuroleptic Drugs]
Antischizophrenic Drugs [See Neuroleptic Drugs]
Antispasmodic Drugs [See Atropine, Meperidine]
Antitremor Drugs [See Also Amantadine] 988
Anxiety 1162
Anxiousness [See Anxiety]
Apes [See Primates (Nonhuman)]
Aphasia [See Also Agraphia, Dysphasia] 447, 534, 545, 570, 606, 631, 633, 690, 699, 731, 734
Apnea 820, 848, 865
Apoplexy [See Cerebrovascular Accidents]
Apparatus [See Also Timers (Apparatus)] 804
Apprehension [See Anxiety]
Arecoline 951
Arecoline Hydrobromide [See Arecoline]
Arrhythmias (Heart) 974
Art Therapy 1102, 1103
Arterial Pulse 1005
Arteries (Anatomy) [See Carotid Arteries]
Arteriosclerosis [See Cerebral Arteriosclerosis]
Articulation (Speech) 680, 684, 740
Arts [See Music]
Asia [See Israel, Japan]
Asian Americans [See Asians]
Asians 469
Asphyxia [See Anoxia]
Assessment [See Measurement]
Assistance (Social Behavior) 1133, 1143, 1144, 1175

135

SUBJECT INDEX

Coronary Disorders [See Cardiovascular Disorders]
Corpus Striatum [See Basal Ganglia]
Correlation (Statistical) [See Statistical Correlation]
Cortex (Auditory) [See Auditory Cortex]
Cortex (Cerebral) [See Cerebral Cortex]
Cortical Evoked Potentials 384
Corticoids [See Corticosteroids]
Corticosteroids [See Also Hydrocortisone] 892
Corticotropin 72, 87, 143, 182, 316, 840, 892, 985, 1062, 1072
Cortisol [See Hydrocortisone]
Cost Effectiveness [See Costs and Cost Analysis]
Costs and Cost Analysis 1002
Counseling (Group) [See Group Counseling]
Counseling [See Also Related Terms] 1127
Counselor Role 1027
Courts [See Adjudication]
Cramps (Muscle) [See Muscular Disorders]
Cranial Nerves [See Optic Nerve]
Crises [See Family Crises]
Crisis (Reactions to) [See Stress Reactions]
Cues 576
Curriculum [See Health Education, Spelling]
Cyclic Adenosine Monophosphate 797, 799, 889

Daily Biological Rhythms (Animal) [See Animal Circadian Rhythms]
Day Care (Treatment) [See Partial Hospitalization]
Day Care Centers 960, 1013, 1024, 1036, 1117
Day Hospital [See Partial Hospitalization]
Death and Dying [See Euthanasia]
Death Rate [See Mortality Rate]
Decarboxylases 286
Deception [See Confabulation]
Decision Making 1156
Decoding [See Human Information Storage]
Delusions 582, 677, 1057
Dementia [See Also Presenile Dementia, Senile Dementia] 2, 27, 50, 73, 74, 86, 133, 141, 223, 244, 245, 274, 282, 288, 290, 332, 407, 411, 416, 425, 426, 432, 436, 438, 440, 448, 454, 458, 459, 462, 468, 469, 470, 471, 488, 489, 500, 504, 506, 509, 511, 512, 513, 519, 520, 521, 522, 524, 531, 537, 538, 551, 556, 561, 562, 565, 566, 568, 572, 577, 587, 588, 601, 602, 604, 605, 625, 626, 636, 655, 677, 704, 724, 726, 731, 742, 755, 785, 786, 787, 801, 803, 804, 808, 815, 816, 817, 824, 827, 832, 834, 835, 841, 850, 852, 871, 877, 884, 886, 898, 899, 954, 975, 983, 989, 993, 1020, 1024, 1025, 1037, 1049, 1053, 1059, 1061, 1103, 1105, 1107, 1111, 1130, 1135, 1141, 1146, 1150, 1152, 1170, 1188
Dementia (Presenile) [See Presenile Dementia]
Dementia (Senile) [See Senile Dementia]
Dementia Praecox [See Schizophrenia]
Dendrites 71, 89
Dentist Patient Interaction [See Therapeutic Processes]
Deoxyribonucleic Acid 284, 299, 819, 876
Depression (Emotion) 17, 28, 36, 61, 75, 224, 406, 476, 499, 527, 550, 616, 617, 618, 627, 641, 646, 750, 787, 815, 817, 823, 828, 848, 874, 884, 893, 964, 986, 1006, 1007, 1017, 1036, 1065, 1121, 1125, 1133, 1134, 1138, 1146, 1161, 1162, 1163
Deprivation [See Sleep Deprivation]
Design (Experimental) [See Experimental Design]
Detection (Signal) [See Signal Detection (Perception)]
Developmental Age Groups [See Also Middle Aged, Young Adults] 51
Developmental Differences [See Age Differences]
Devices (Experimental) [See Apparatus]
Dexamethasone 499, 792, 793, 815, 816, 823
Dexamethasone Suppression Test 487, 785, 786
Diagnosis [See Also Computer Assisted Diagnosis, Differential Diagnosis, Electroencephalography, Medical Diagnosis, Pneumoencephalography, Psychodiagnosis, Roentgenography] 18, 29, 38, 132, 416, 418, 445, 451, 461, 466, 490, 500, 506, 518, 549, 574, 656, 733, 744, 804, 810, 900, 909, 917, 919, 953, 1094
Dialysis [See Hemodialysis]
Diazepam 17
Diencephalon [See Also Hypothalamo Hypophyseal System, Hypothalamus, Thalamus] 187
Diets 521
Differential Diagnosis 425, 426, 428, 429, 432, 434, 436, 443, 474, 476, 477, 483, 484, 488, 489, 493, 494, 496, 503, 504, 506, 509, 511, 512, 516, 520, 524, 529, 531, 535, 551, 555, 561, 568, 585, 588, 605, 607, 617, 618, 628, 693, 714, 724, 755, 768, 785, 815, 822, 827, 832, 835, 874, 897, 926, 1107, 1183
Digestive System [See Gastrointestinal System, Liver]
Digit Span Testing 536, 611, 617
Discrimination (Cognitive) [See Cognitive Discrimination]
Discrimination Learning 602, 635, 681, 737
Discriminative Learning [See Discrimination Learning]
Diseases [See Disorders]
Disorders [See Also Related Terms] 475, 727, 797, 941
Disruptive Behavior [See Behavior Problems]
Dissociative Patterns [See Amnesia]
Distraction 682, 747
Distress 1129, 1159
Diurnal Variations [See Human Biological Rhythms]
Divided Attention 536
Dizygotic Twins [See Heterozygotic Twins]
DNA (Deoxyribonucleic Acid) [See Deoxyribonucleic Acid]
Dogs 341
Dopamine 110, 117, 143, 210, 292, 345, 372, 375, 389
Dopamine Metabolites [See Also Homovanillic Acid] 894
Downs Syndrome 4, 7, 15, 22, 37, 62, 100, 110, 122, 134, 145, 146, 155, 211, 230, 250, 253, 254, 259, 263, 277, 287, 313, 314, 329, 330, 332, 436, 456, 482, 485, 514, 528, 574, 625, 660, 773, 801, 844, 878, 1095
Doxepin [See Antidepressant Drugs]
Drinking Behavior [See Animal Drinking Behavior]
Drinking Behavior (Animal) [See Animal Drinking Behavior]
Drug Adverse Reactions [See Side Effects (Drug)]
Drug Dosages 936, 966, 974, 1043, 1044, 1060, 1083, 1085
Drug Effects [See Drugs]
Drug Interactions 379, 961, 1008
Drug Potentiation [See Drug Interactions]
Drug Synergism [See Drug Interactions]
Drug Therapy 68, 264, 297, 840, 872, 932, 934, 936, 938, 944, 945, 946, 947, 948, 950, 951, 956, 957, 958, 959, 961, 964, 965, 966, 967, 969, 971, 972, 973, 974, 976, 978, 979, 980, 981, 982, 983, 986, 987, 988, 990, 991, 992, 998, 999, 1000, 1004, 1005, 1006, 1007, 1008, 1011, 1012, 1014, 1015, 1016, 1019, 1022, 1025, 1029, 1030, 1032, 1034, 1037, 1038, 1039, 1040, 1042, 1043, 1044, 1045, 1046, 1051, 1052, 1053, 1055, 1056, 1057, 1058, 1059, 1060, 1062, 1063, 1065, 1066, 1069, 1070, 1071, 1072, 1073, 1074, 1075, 1077, 1078, 1079, 1080, 1081, 1085, 1086, 1087, 1088, 1089, 1090, 1092, 1104, 1106, 1112, 1115, 1116
Drugs [See Also Related Terms] 297, 365, 957, 1115
Dyskinesia 75
Dysphasia 735
Dysphoria [See Major Depression]
Dystonia [See Muscular Disorders]

Eating [See Also Diets] 915
Eating Patterns [See Eating] 794
Educational Background 908

SUBJECT INDEX

Glucose 48, 95, 138, 157, 383, 421, 610, 749, 861, 1096
Glutamic Acid 119, 172, 186, 286
Glycine 1045
Gonadotropic Hormones [See Prolactin]
Government Policy Making [See Also Laws, Legislative Processes] 928
Graduate Education [See Medical Education]
Grammar [See Semantics, Syntax]
Grandparents 1126
Gross Motor Skill Learning 1001
Group Counseling 1111, 1136, 1138, 1145, 1146, 1158, 1176, 1180, 1184
Group Psychotherapy [See Also Therapeutic Community] 949, 1174
Group Therapy [See Group Psychotherapy]
Grown Children [See Adult Offspring]
Growth Hormone [See Somatotropin]
Guardianship 898
Gymnastic Therapy [See Recreation Therapy]
Gyrus Cinguli 49, 256

Hair 860
Hallucinations 1058
Hallucinosis [See Korsakoffs Psychosis]
Haloperidol 1075
Halstead Reitan Test Battery [See Neuropsychological Assessment]
Handedness 205, 796, 857
Handicapped [See Brain Damaged, Health Impaired, Institutionalized Mentally Retarded, Partially Hearing Impaired, Visually Handicapped]
Happiness 1165
Head Injuries 201, 204, 657, 726, 970
Health [See Also Mental Health] 1135, 1167
Health Care Delivery [See Home Care]
Health Care Professionals [See Medical Personnel]
Health Care Services [See Also Community Mental Health Services, Mental Health Services] 952, 1050, 1118
Health Education 931
Health Impaired 1013, 1036
Hearing Impaired (Partially) [See Partially Hearing Impaired]
Heart Disorders [See Arrhythmias (Heart)]
Heart Rate Affecting Drugs [See Epinephrine]
Helping Behavior [See Assistance (Social Behavior)]
Hemispheric Specialization [See Cerebral Dominance]
Hemodialysis 883
Heredity [See Genetics]
Herpes Simplex 16, 248, 299, 876
Heterozygotic Twins 207
High Risk Populations [See At Risk Populations]
Higher Education [See Medical Education]

Hippocampus 7, 16, 35, 50, 71, 83, 89, 103, 118, 169, 187, 208, 222, 224, 231, 256, 338, 345, 360, 361, 377
Hiring [See Personnel Selection]
Histology 69, 322
Home Care 537, 1002, 1023, 1113, 1122, 1123, 1124, 1127, 1134, 1135, 1138, 1151, 1156, 1157, 1159, 1164, 1168, 1169, 1176, 1179, 1185
Homovanillic Acid 105, 110, 117, 143, 264, 577, 579, 824, 873, 894
Hormones [See Also Corticotropin, Epinephrine, Estradiol, Hydrocortisone, Norepinephrine, Oxytocin, Pituitary Hormones, Prolactin, Sex Hormones, Somatotropin, Thyroid Hormones, Thyrotropin, Thyroxine, Triiodothyronine, Vasopressi 24, 27, 111, 239, 290, 749
Hospital Environment 1067
Hospital Programs [See Also Therapeutic Community] 727, 994
Hospital Staff [See Medical Personnel]
Hospitalized Patients 581, 994
Human Biological Rhythms 293, 450
Human Females [See Mothers, Wives]
Human Information Processes [See Cognitive Processes]
Human Information Storage 546, 558, 623, 626, 658, 676, 702, 703, 770
Human Males [See Also Brothers] 1128
Human Sex Differences 293, 525, 865, 1152
Huntingtons Chorea 36, 81, 119, 162, 198, 222, 299, 455, 474, 500, 501, 539, 554, 559, 560, 563, 611, 612, 678, 688, 730, 745, 759, 766, 891, 935, 970
Hydrocephaly 2, 245, 503, 822
Hydrocortisone 67, 786, 792, 793, 815, 816, 842, 1043
Hydroxydopamine (6-) 351
Hydroxyindoleacetic Acid (5-) 105, 110, 264, 306, 577, 579, 873
Hydroxytryptamine (5-) [See Serotonin]
Hygiene [See Health]
Hyoscine [See Scopolamine]
Hyoscyamine (dl-) [See Atropine]
Hypersensitivity (Immunologic) [See Immunologic Disorders]
Hypertension 869, 884, 947
Hypothalamo Hypophyseal System 88
Hypothalamus [See Also Hypothalamo Hypophyseal System] 88, 238, 256, 293, 392
Hypoxia [See Anoxia]

Identical Twins [See Monozygotic Twins]
Illness (Physical) [See Disorders]
Illness Behavior 952
Illusions (Perception) [See Spatial Distortion]
Imipramine 224, 874
Immunogens [See Antigens]
Immunoglobulins 825

Immunologic Disorders [See Also Acquired Immune Deficiency Syndrome] 56, 134, 501
Immunology 11, 17, 24, 25, 27, 72, 81, 94, 111, 203, 237, 239, 275, 316, 519, 824, 862, 863, 1147
Immunopathology [See Immunology]
Individual Problem Solving [See Problem Solving]
Industrial Safety [See Occupational Safety]
Infections [See Infectious Disorders]
Infectious Disorders [See Also Acquired Immune Deficiency Syndrome, Herpes Simplex, Viral Disorders] 56, 348, 519
Influence (Interpersonal) [See Interpersonal Influences]
Information Exchange 1140
Information Processes (Human) [See Cognitive Processes]
Information Storage (Human) [See Human Information Storage]
Information [See Also Related Terms] 1172
Informed Consent 924
Injections [See Intravenous Injections]
Injuries [See Also Head Injuries] 553, 679
Insanity [See Mental Disorders, Psychosis]
Institutionalization 497, 537, 1111, 1124, 1155, 1156, 1171
Institutionalized Mentally Retarded 528
Institutions (Residential Care) [See Residential Care Institutions]
Insurance 501
Intellectual Development [See Language Development]
Intellectual Functioning [See Cognitive Ability]
Intelligence 543, 550, 704, 707
Intelligence Measures [See Wechsler Adult Intelligence Scale]
Intelligence Quotient 622
Interaction (Interpersonal) [See Interpersonal Interaction]
Interaction (Social) [See Social Interaction]
Interdisciplinary Treatment Approach 484, 995, 1131
Interference (Learning) 556
Internal Consistency [See Test Reliability]
Internal External Locus of Control 1151, 1162, 1187
Interpersonal Communication [See Conversation, Interviews]
Interpersonal Influences 1133
Interpersonal Interaction [See Also Assistance (Social Behavior), Conversation, Interpersonal Influences, Interviews, Participation] 968, 1163
Interpersonal Perception [See Social Perception]
Interviews 1173
Intoxication [See Toxic Disorders]
Intravenous Injections 951
Inventories 569

140

SUBJECT INDEX

Appendix

Strategy Used to Retrieve References for the Bibliography

James Whitfield, Carolyn Gosling, Sarah Mulholland

The following is the search strategy executed on the PsycINFO database (through BRS) to retrieve journal and dissertation records on Alzheimer's disease. Search statements are followed by explanatory comments. Statements for updating this strategy and for searching for more recent research in the PsycALERT database are also provided.

1__: alzheimer$.ti,id,de. (Searches for variations of the concept in the title, identifier and descriptor fields of the record. Using truncation allows for retrieval of variations such as Alzheimer or Alzheimers or Alzheimer's.)

RESULT   1218 DOCUMENTS

Strategies to Update the Search

PsycINFO: To retrieve records on Alzheimer's disease added to the PsycINFO database after the update for the present search (December 1988) use the following strategy:

1__: alzheimer$.ti,id,de.

2__: ..L/ 1 up gt 8812 (Limits previous set to updates added after December 1988).

PsycALERT: To retrieve citations of recently published journal articles from the PsycALERT database, use the following strategy:

1__: alzheimer$ (Searches for variations of the concept in all fields of the record)